CHROMIUM:
AN ESSENTIAL ELEMENT

If used properly, chromium can dramatically help build muscle and reduce fat. It can also significantly contribute to the reduction of cholesterol and to the control of blood sugar metabolism. Before you even measure the difference on a scale or with a blood test, you will feel it. With this fast and unique diet and exercise program, you will quickly discover how as you increase your chromium intake, you will look more fit, feel healthier and better able to cope with daily problems. In no time at all, you will wonder why you hadn't heard about chromium before.

THE CHROMIUM PROGRAM

BY JEFFREY A. FISHER, M.D.

Foreword by Isadore Rosenfeld, M.D.
Introduction by George Sheehan, M.D.
Preface by Gary W. Evans, Ph.D.

HarperPaperbacks
A Division of HarperCollins*Publishers*

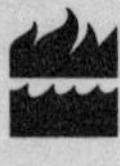

HarperPaperbacks *A Division of* HarperCollins*Publishers*
10 East 53rd Street, New York, N.Y. 10022

A hardcover edition of this book was published in 1990 by Harper & Row, Publishers.

First HarperPaperbacks printing: October 1995

Printed in the United States of America

HarperPaperbacks and colophon are trademarks of HarperCollins*Publishers*

10 9 8 7 6 5 4 3 2 1

For Liz

CONTENTS

ACKNOWLEDGMENTS

My thanks goes to those who shared the results of their research and scientific insight with me: Dr. Gary Evans, Dr. Richard Anderson, Dr. Edward Masoro, Dr. John Holloszy, Dr. Gilbert Kaats, Herb Boynton and Mark McCarty of Nutrition 21, and Steve Blechman of Twin Laboratories.

Several family members and friends also helped by listening to or reading the manuscript and offering their suggestions. Specifically, Howard Edsall and Linn Whitehouse frequently indulged me by allowing me to read entire chapters to them over the telephone.

I also thank Gary Guerriero, R.P.T., of the Eastside Sportsmedicine Center in New York for his assistance in formulating the exercise plan and Dr. Audrey Burkhart of Rutgers University Department of Food Science for her help with the nutritional analyses of the menus and recipes. My special thanks to Janet Whitehouse for so capably providing the illustrations of the exercises, working under difficult circumstances.

The enthusiasm for the project and the informed responses of my editor, Larry Ashmead, have been instrumental in the successful completion of this book. In addition, the contributions made by my assistant editor, Eamon Dolan, and my copyeditors, Judy Kahn and Pamela Montgomery, were invaluable.

In a separate category are those without whose contribution this book would not exist. My agents Herb and Nancy Katz have done far more than represent me. They have been involved in every aspect of *The Chromium Program* from conception to completion, and I am truly fortunate to be associated with them.

Finally, to my wife Liz, who not only worked tirelessly and creatively to develop all the menus and recipes, but allowed this book to become the dominant member of our family for several months, my undying love and gratitude.

FOREWORD

I am always excited about new concepts that have the potential for improving the quality of life. In his *The Chromium Program,* Dr. Jeffrey A. Fisher presents some interesting evidence suggesting that correcting a chromium-deficient diet may do just that. He also makes several other cogent recommendations that in my view are both sound and conservative.

According to recent research findings, most of the harmful consequences of obesity (including diabetes, cancer, and cardiovascular disease) are primarily due to too much fat in the wrong places, rather than to overweight in itself. Instead of perpetuating our preoccupation with what the scale tells us every morning, Dr. Fisher focuses on the problem of body composition and indicates how to reduce fat content and increase lean muscle tissue.

There is no guarantee that The Chromium Program will work for everyone who complains of fatigue or energy loss. But it's worth a try because it's safe and sensible.

Elevated levels of serum cholesterol are associated with an increased risk of coronary artery disease. Dr. Fisher reviews several recent studies which conclude that "enough" chromium in the diet can reduce the total cholesterol level and the level of its most harmful component, LDL. There is other intriguing evidence to suggest that chromium can also lower elevated blood sugar and insulin requirements in some diabetics.

The Chromium Program shows how to combine natural healthful foods into interesting and easily prepared menus. The simple exercise programs he recommends to accompany his diet are well within the capability of most people.

Dr. Fisher, whom I've known for several years both professionally and personally, is a scholar of great personal integrity. He has a broad knowledge of the field of disease prevention through life-style modification, of which this program is a worthwhile example. While there is still a great deal more to be learned about chromium, I am enthusiastic about this book because of its potential for helping so many at risk for serious disease.

Isadore Rosenfeld, M.D.
Clinical Professor of Medicine
Division of Cardiology
New York Hospital–Cornell Medical Center
New York, New York

INTRODUCTION

Decades ago in the early days of my practice I had as a patient a top executive of a steel company. One day he made a prediction of a future trend in medicine. "Trace metals," he said, "are going to be recognized as tremendously important." When I asked him how he had come to that opinion, he said it had occurred to him while thinking of the manufacture of steel. "If you can take an enormous quantity of iron and change its properties drastically with a handful of another metal, trace metals must be able to do the same thing to the human body."

My patient's prediction has come true. This book is evidence he was correct in his analogy. Trace metals are now of acknowledged importance. We still need research to catalogue their benefits and to determine their precise roles in the maintenance of the body. We cannot yet estimate the doses with precision and the outcomes with accuracy, but the pieces are gradually falling into place.

We know much more about some trace metals, and chromium is one of those, than about others. The documentation of the effects of chromium on health and fitness has reached a stage at which this book, devoted to the subject, could be written. In it Dr. Jeffrey Fisher examines what we know and what we conjecture about this vital trace metal.

In outlining this knowledge, he reminds us of the holistic approach to the care of our bodies. The use of any drug, diet, or nutrient cannot stand alone. We must pursue what the ancient Greeks prescribed for their athletes—a *regimen,* or a systematic plan to maintain health and improve performance. And of all the trace metals, chromium seems to be one that can help us achieve maximum body performance, not only in athletics but also in everyday activity.

George Sheehan, M.D.

PREFACE

Until the first part of this century millions of people throughout the world suffered from a disease that could have been eradicated. The disease was endemic goiter and its cause is a deficiency of iodine in the diet. As early as 1820 a French physician was using iodine to treat human goiter. Twenty years later a French botanist, Chatin, began studying the distribution of iodine in the environment and his results showed that goiter occurred in areas where the iodine content was low. He even went so far as to suggest that iodine be added to water in areas where goiter was prevalent. However, because there were some anomalies in his observations, Chatin's conclusions were discredited and iodine therapy was discarded for nearly fifty years.

In 1919 iodine was found to be a constituent of the hormone thyroxine, and medical professionals began to recognize the importance of iodine in the diet. Because thyroxine affects so many functions of the body, iodine deficiency leads to a broad spectrum of problems ranging from growth retardation to mental retardation. When iodine supplementation is initiated, impaired thyroxine function and its related health problems are virtually eliminated.

Iodine and chromium have much in common. Both are needed by vital hormones in the body, both must be taken into the body from the diet, and both are often deficient in the food we eat. Also, despite thirty years of research on this essential element, many health professionals do not recognize the important role chromium plays in the body.

Chromium is to this part of the twentieth century what iodine was to the first part. Once again people are faced with a preventable deficiency disease. This time the disease is impaired insulin action and its cause in many cases is a deficiency of the element chromium. Impaired insulin action causes glucose intolerance, elevated glucose levels in the blood, diabetes, elevated cholesterol levels, heart disease, obesity, and a host of other problems that have not yet been fully documented. I would be the first to admit that lack of chromium is not always the cause for impaired insulin action, but my research shows that many people with the condition respond to an increase in their chromium intake. In trials utilizing supplementation with chromium picolinate, cholesterol was lowered significantly in people with high blood cholesterol, and both glucose and cholesterol were lowered in adult onset diabetics. Another exciting discovery was that body fat could be decreased and lean body mass increased in athletes who were exercising and taking a chromium picolinate supplement. These scientific observations show that optimal body performance can be achieved without resorting to drugs, such as steroids, when specific nutrients, in this case chromium, are present in the diet in adequate quantities.

In this much needed book Dr. Fisher has taken chromium out of the formidable realm of technical scientific reports and brought it to the attention of the general public. In a skillful and understandable way Dr. Fisher reveals the importance of this element which so often is lacking in diets or is present in a form that the body can't use. Avoiding technical jargon and complex scientific analysis, he explains how chromium is linked to the action of the hormone insulin. Most important, he shows how careful selection and preparation of foods can eliminate a deficit in biologically useful chromium. Through his research in assessing diet composition, Dr. Fisher has been able to compile recipes and menus that provide a chromium-rich diet.

After reading this book, both the general public and

health professionals should realize that through adequate chromium intake many athletes will be able to increase their peak performance without resorting to illegal drugs and many people will be able to reduce health problems caused by impaired insulin function.

Gary W. Evans, Ph.D.
Professor of Chemistry
Bemidji State University
Bemidji, Minnesota

THE CHROMIUM PROGRAM

ONE

INTRODUCING CHROMIUM

This book will introduce you to a diet and exercise program that can make you look trimmer, be stronger, have more energy, and feel more self-confident. The program is based on my clinical experience and research, as well as that of others, with the remarkable nutrient chromium. *If used properly, chromium can dramatically help build muscle and reduce fat. It can also significantly contribute to the reduction of cholesterol and to the control of blood sugar metabolism.* If you increase your chromium intake to eliminate any deficit, you will look more fit, feel better able to cope with daily problems, and wonder, as I once did, why you hadn't heard about chromium before.

In the following chapters you are going to learn how chromium works. You'll read about some of the clinical evidence that documents these effects and about the experiences of some of my patients, friends, and relatives whose lives have been changed by chromium. But most importantly, you are going to learn how to take advantage of this information to enhance your own life—to tone and shape your body, to lower your cholesterol, and to help control your blood sugar.

The Chromium Program has two complementary components—diet and exercise. We'll discuss the best food sources of chromium and talk a bit about supplements. You'll be given an innovative, delicious, high-chromium meal plan, complete with many easy to prepare recipes, that adheres to high-fiber, low-fat dietary principles. The safe, weight-bearing exercises can be done by anyone at any age and can easily be incorporated into your life. As you apply what you learn in this book, the synergistic interaction between the high-chromium diet and the exercise program will become evident in the way you look and feel.

AS WITH ANY OTHER DIET OR EXERCISE PROGRAM, IT IS IMPORTANT FOR YOU TO CONSULT WITH YOUR PHYSICIAN BEFORE BEGINNING.

WHERE I BEGAN

I am often asked by patients if I practice what I preach, if I follow the recommendations I make to them. I usually answer, "No, I preach what I practice." I have never made a life-style suggestion to a patient, friend, or relative, regardless of the scientific documentation supporting it, unless I was convinced it worked. That invariably meant trying it on the ultimate guinea pig—myself.

Nine years ago, when I began counseling patients about optimal performance and energy level in daily activities and sports, I was aware of some of the early research that had been done on chromium. I felt that it might benefit some of my patients, so in the "king's taster" tradition, I wanted to try it myself. Over a period of a few months I increased the amount of chromium in my diet.

On the basis of the literature, I had decided to recommend increasing chromium intake to many of my patients, so I was really trying it to make sure there were no unexpected untoward effects. I didn't expect to see anything positive happen with me, since I was in good health before increasing my chromium intake. However, I did notice a definite increase in energy level. I realized that anecdotes, especially subjective ones such as my own experience, carry little if any scientific validity, but since there was some indication in the scientific literature as to why this might occur, I didn't totally discount it as a placebo effect.

THE WIFE OF A PROMINENT PHYSICIAN

The more I recommended chromium to my patients, the more it seemed to me that this phenomenon of increased energy was not a placebo effect—it was being reported too often.

I mentioned these observations at dinner one evening to Dr. X, one of the country's prominent physicians. We began talking about his wife's condition. She was a diabetic and was having difficulty controlling her blood sugar, despite being under the care of a highly respected endocrinologist. Among her main symptoms were fatigue and lack of energy. We both knew that most physicians, even good ones, are not particularly knowledgeable about nutrition and that nutrition can play an important role in the management of diabetes. So he suggested that his wife come to see me and my dietitian, for a dietary treatment program for her to follow in addition to her insulin treatment. I told him that one of the things I intended to do was to increase her intake of chromium. He admitted to knowing little about it and, after asking a few questions, said he would totally defer to my knowledge here.

After making some other adjustments in Mrs. X's diet, I told her about increasing her intake of chromium and why I thought she should do it. She agreed to give it a try. Two weeks later she called and reported, "I don't know what that chromium does, but I feel better than I've felt in the past few years." She said that she had mentioned her improved energy level to a friend, who wasn't a diabetic but who also often suffered from fatigue. Understandably, her friend was eager to try chromium, which she did without even seeing me or any other physician. Mrs. X's friend's results were identical to hers. (Although Mrs. X's friend experienced positive results, it's not a good idea to begin any program or take nutritional supplements without professional advice.)

This, of course, is not meant to imply that anyone with fatigue will instantly and miraculously improve after increasing chromium intake. Fatigue is a symptom of many conditions, which may need any of several different types of treatment. But I was seeing some wonderful results.

The majority of my patients who were experiencing these results from increasing their dietary intake of chromium seemed to have some abnormality in blood sugar. Their blood sugar level tended to be either too high, as with Mrs. X, or too low. (How chromium helps both ends of the blood sugar level spectrum will be discussed later.) Based on what I knew about chromium, this made sense, but several people, including myself and Mrs. X's friend, who apparently had normal blood glucose metabolism, were also experiencing energy increases. Either the standard methods of measuring blood sugar weren't sensitive enough to pick up subtle abnormalities in these patients, or some other mechanism was at work.

THE STORY OF EMMANUELLE GIRARD

Emmanuelle Girard was a 37-year-old art dealer, originally from Lausanne, Switzerland. Her primary residence was now in New York. Emmanuelle's life was fast-paced and tension-filled. She traveled extensively, often dealt with large sums of her clients' money, and had to make split-second decisions at art auctions.

Emmanuelle came to see me complaining of huge swings in her energy level which were definitely affecting her career performance. She would often have difficulty paying attention at dinner meetings with clients and consequently had lost some substantial commissions. After ruling out any obvious organic disease and determining that she was getting enough sleep to make up for jet lag resulting from frequent flights to Paris, Florence, and London, we analyzed her diet. Though it was better than most, even with all the air travel, the computer program confirmed my suspicion that she wasn't getting enough chromium. I explained how this might contribute to her lack of energy and asked her to talk with my dietitian about the best ways to add chromium to her diet.

Six weeks later Emmanuelle came back to see me. She told me that the difference in her energy level was truly remarkable. "I don't know if it's all in my head or not, but I don't care. I feel so good, I'm going to keep it up." She was now sharp and alert well into the evening and had just completed a large sale for one of her biggest clients.

THE STORY OF MY WIFE'S GRANDFATHER

My wife's grandfather, Howard Edsall, is a remarkable man. At age 85 he was more active mentally and physically than most people I know of any age. A former journalist and advertising executive, presently a fine arts publicist, he still regularly submitted articles to magazines. He read voraciously and discussed lucidly scholarly works on a variety of subjects, from philosophy to health. As intelligent and informed (and informative) as he was, I found his physical prowess even more impressive. He had a grip strength of 120 pounds, could chin twenty times with one hand, and could do pushups between two chairs on his fingertips! (If you don't think these are extraordinary accomplishments for anyone, try them yourself.)

But Howard sustained an injury, followed by the flu, and was unable to engage in his training routine for more than two months. When he was finally able to resume his regular exercises, he discovered his power had significantly deteriorated. His grip strength was less than half of what it had been, he found it difficult to chin with both arms, and he could hardly do any conventional pushups at all. I could see Howard, a proud and self-motivated man, beginning to get depressed.

Howard knew about research effectively debunking the myth that older people can't build muscle and had experienced the research findings himself ten years earlier when he successfully rehabilitated himself after another injury shelved him for three months. But he was also aware that none of the studies, nor his own prior history, included an octogenarian. Could it be possible, he wondered, that he had finally reached the point of no return?

I encouraged him not to give up, but to ease back into his exercise regimen with the aid of chromium. The effects were even better than I expected. Within two months after tripling his daily chromium intake, Howard realized definite results. First he reported feeling a "tingling" in his muscles when he worked out, as if they were awakening after a long sleep. Then he began to notice that his strength was gradually returning. After eight weeks his grip strength was back to what it had been before his injury and illness, and he was once again making me feel weak and puny as I watched him chin with one arm and do pushups on his fingertips.

These are only a few of the many successes I've seen with chromium. I've witnessed increases in energy and strength and improved cholesterol and blood sugar values. I have even heard reports of changes I at first thought apocryphal—better eyesight, healthier gums—but upon further investigation I discovered that at least some of these may be true, too.

Before we begin our discussion of chromium, the mechanisms by which it works, and the many exciting benefits this program has to offer you, some background is necessary.

TWO

THE FITNESS MOVEMENT SHAPES UP

The pollster George Gallup said that the fitness movement was the most fundamental change in American life-styles and attitudes that he had seen in his entire career. This certainly seemed to be the case in the 1970s and early 1980s. Following the introduction of aerobics in 1968 by Dr. Kenneth H. Cooper and Frank Shorter's remarkable triumph in the 1972 Olympic marathon in Munich, the fitness boom in the United States was born.

People began jogging, and soon running clubs sprang up all over the country. Running a race on the weekend before brunch became commonplace, and even the marathon, which covers 26.2 miles, a distance most of us thought more reasonably traveled in our cars than on foot, became a sport for Everyman. The New York City Marathon, which began in 1971 as a four-loop jog around Central Park, soon attracted 20,000 entrants (with many times that number turned away), millions of spectators and became a major media event. Other forms of aerobics—swimming, aerobic dancing, rowing machines, stationary bicycles—attracted increasing numbers of people to health clubs, which became hubs of social as well as physical activity. Americans had become fitness freaks!

But was Gallup wrong? Was the exercise boom just another hula hoop? In early 1989 *The Wall Street Journal* reported that "exercise is out," that health club membership had drastically declined, and that yuppies, the prime movers in the fitness boom, were becoming bored with exercise.

The Wall Street Journal was only partially right. The exercise movement isn't declining; it is changing. The number of runners may have dropped (to the relief of some of us who once again were able to experience some of the loneliness of the long-distance runner), but participation in other activities has been increasing. Two things are happening. One trend is an emphasis on low-impact aerobics; high-impact aerobics is out. Exercise walking has become the fastest growing type of activity for fitness in America.

The other trend is the emphasis on *whole body conditioning*. During the peak years of the running boom, the "in" look was gaunt, almost emaciated. Running 80 miles a week and racing just about every weekend, I suppose that was the way I looked. My father suggested I shop in the boys' department for clothes. I had a hard time convincing my parents and other nonrunners that marathon runners were actually healthy.

Now, runners and other athletes are doing much more *cross-training*. The best preparation for any sport is still the sport itself—runners run, swimmers swim—but these competitors are spending a good deal of time working on the parts of the body they don't use as much in their primary training. The increasing prominence of multifaceted competitive events such as biathlons and triathlons attests to that.

The most popular component of cross-training has become *resistance training*, or *body conditioning*. This used to be more commonly referred to as weight lifting or body building, but those terms usually conjure up images of Mr. Universe competitors or offensive linemen pumping iron, not an activity for everyone. But it *is* for everyone—for women as well as for men and for people of all ages. I admit to having been brought kicking and screaming into the conditioning age, but now that I'm here, I love it. I still put in the miles every week, but only about half of what I used to do. My running is supplemented with resistance training three times a week, and I feel (and, I am told, look) better. And resistance training can do the same for you.

THE MANY BENEFITS OF RESISTANCE TRAINING

Resistance training offers physical, psychological, and physiological benefits.

When a muscle is contracted against resistance, the net result is that the muscle gets stronger. (It may get bigger, too, and we'll discuss the details later.) A stronger muscle enhances performance, whether it be in a sports event, such as running, swimming, or tennis, or just in everyday activity. I've had patients tell me how much easier it is to accomplish tasks ranging from negotiating the subway to raking leaves after they've engaged in a resistance program for a while. Being stronger makes older people less likely to fall. Muscular weakness is the predominant cause of this common problem associated with aging.

Not only will a strengthened muscle perform better, but it will also look better. A program of resistance training or body conditioning will reduce body fat, increase lean tissue, improve muscle tone, give muscles better definition, and sculpt the body. You may not end up looking like Mikhail Baryshnikov or Florence Griffith-Joyner, but the look of the relaxed, but ready athlete is a goal to shoot for. At the very least, your clothes will fit better and your posture and carriage will be better. All of these physical changes dramatically enhance appearance.

The psychological benefits of conditioning are in many ways a direct result of enhanced performance capability and appearance. This is especially true for women and the elderly.

Women have told me that good body conditioning and a look of strength in how they move make them feel less vulnerable, more in control. Because they look stronger, there is less chance that someone will try to take advantage of them physically. But it also works wonderfully in the board room or in closing a deal. People who feel stronger compete better and with less anxiety.

Most of my elderly patients have told me that the thing they fear most about growing old is not dying, but losing their ability to care for themselves. Being stronger can help boost an older person's self-confidence and ability to remain independent.

I'm almost ashamed to admit that before I began doing research on resistance training, I didn't know about the physiological benefits it can confer. I was under the impression, as perhaps you are, that weight lifting was not really good for people. Not only did I think that it does not afford the protection from cardiovascular disease that endurance activities such as running or walking do, but I also believed it could raise blood pressure. I didn't do it, and I didn't recommend it to any of my patients.

But, when I started reading the scientific literature on resistance training and talking to exercise physiologists around the country, I made what was to me an amazing discovery: *Resistance training, properly done, can reduce risk for heart disease.* (We'll discuss how it does that later on.)

The idea that resistance training raises blood pressure also turns out to be false. Some studies on patients with high blood pressure have shown that, although blood pressure goes up acutely during the exercise (it also does during endurance exercise such as running), in the long run resistance training can actually lower blood pressure. This has been demonstrated in both adolescents and adults. However, to achieve this result, the training needs to be carefully supervised and it works best as an adjunct to aerobic exercise. If you have high blood pressure, it's imperative you discuss with your physician whether you should do resistance training and what type of program is appropriate for you.

These misconceptions may have come from reading about power lifters, who may be strong, but aren't necessarily healthy. Also, it seems that most of the exercise physiologists in the United States are aerobically oriented (many of them are runners), so some of them may just not have looked beyond their own interest to acquire useful information and to correct misconceptions in other areas.

Besides conferring protection from cardiovascular disease and helping to reduce blood pressure, resistance training makes it easier to lose weight and sustain weight loss by increasing the percentage of lean muscle tissue and reducing that of body fat. We're going to emphasize in this book that percentage of body fat is much more important than actual weight—you'll be able to become unchained from your scale. Conditioning can also result in actual weight loss as well. One of the reasons is that muscle burns calories at a much higher rate than fat, so the more muscle tissue one has, the more calories one burns.

This doesn't mean that you should jettison your aerobic program. Aerobic exercise and resistance training are helpful in overlapping ways, and we'll talk later about how to integrate them.

Before we look at the safe way to get all these benefits with the Chromium Program, we have to look at a deadly way to achieve some of them as a frame of reference.

THE DANGEROUS ENHANCER: ANABOLIC STEROIDS

The widespread use of anabolic steroids is evidence that the enhanced appearance that can result from resistance training can be taken to narcissistic extremes. Unfortunately, this isn't limited to a few fanatics on muscle beach. Not only are most (up to 90 percent) competitive body builders using anabolic steroids, but so are athletes in a variety of other sports. The 1988 Olympics in Seoul will most likely be remembered as the "games of steroid abuse." Several Bulgarian weight lifters were disqualified and sprinter Ben Johnson of Canada lost his world record and gold medal when a test of his urine showed traces of stanazolol, an anabolic steroid.

A substance that promotes the building of tissue is called anabolic. Steroids are a group of compounds derived from other body substances. The steroids that are derivatives of the male sex hormone testosterone have an anabolic effect. Steroid use by healthy persons for nontherapeutic reasons is increasing dramatically, but it is not something new. Reportedly, Adolf Hitler's SS troops were given anabolic steroids to increase their aggressiveness. In 1954 John B. Ziegler, the physician for the United States weight lifting team, reported that Russian athletes were using them. In 1956 Ziegler, along with the pharmaceutical company Ciba, developed the oral anabolic agent methandrostenolone (Dianabol), and in the late 1950s American athletes began using anabolic steroids. At that time their potential deleterious effects were not known, and Dr. Ziegler later said that he wished that chapter could have been removed from his life.

Today a great deal is known about the dangerous side effects of anabolic steroids and much of this information has been made available to those most likely to use these drugs. Even so, many people continue to use them in a Faustian bargain, neglecting warnings about their health for the sake of being able to lift a few more pounds, to run a tenth of a second faster, or to achieve a little more muscle definition. Anabolic steroids are being used by body builders, football players, wrestlers, track and field athletes, and, surprisingly, even endurance performers, who apparently use them to hasten recovery between workouts. Although elite athletes are the most visible users, the feeling in the sports community is that users among recreational athletes form an even larger group. And many people may use them not to enhance athletic performance, but merely to try to make themselves more attractive to others.

Perhaps most disturbing is the prevalence of anabolic steroid abuse among teenagers. A survey in the *Journal of the American Medical Association* indicated that one in every fifteen high school seniors admitted to having used steroids (so the actual number is probably larger), and in most cases the abuse had begun a few years earlier, at a stage in their development when the potential negative effects can be even greater than in adults. Best estimates are that there are now more than a million users of anabolic steroids in the United States, with adolescents accounting for a quarter to a half of them.

The side effects of anabolic steroid use are myriad (see tables below). Effects that occur frequently and are not life-threatening are classified medically as minor effects, but that does not mean they do not have serious consequences in the life of the individual. Some of the minor effects can occur in both sexes. These include personality alterations (usually extreme aggression and mood swings), sleep disturbances, altered libido, acne, and baldness.

Some side effects are limited to specific groups. Women may experience masculinization, including male pattern baldness, deepening of the voice, increased

MINOR SIDE EFFECTS OF ANABOLIC STEROIDS			
	MEN	WOMEN	ADOLESCENTS (BOTH SEXES)
Personality changes	X	X	X
Sleep disturbance	X	X	X
Altered libido	X	X	X
Acne	X	X	X
Masculinization		X	X
Enlarged clitoris		X	
Increased body and facial hair		X	X
Breast development	X		X
Baldness	X	X	X
Growth retardation			X
Precocious puberty			X

MAJOR SIDE EFFECTS OF ANABOLIC STEROIDS (ALL AGES AND SEXES)
Cholesterol imbalance
Peliosis hepatis
Liver tumors (benign and malignant)
Hepatitis
Leukemia (rare)
Wilms's tumor

Source: Adapted from R. E. Windsor and D. Dumitru, Anabolic steroid use by atheletes, *Postgraduate Medicine, 84* (4):37–48, 1988.

body hair, and enlargement of the clitoris. All of these changes are considered irreversible! Men may experience gynecomastia (enlargement of the breasts) and a shrinking of the testes, effects brought about by the fact that anabolic steroids suppress the body's production of normal amounts of testosterone. Most males on anabolic steroids have severely depressed levels of the male sex hormone. In adolescent males anabolic steroids can cause enlargement of the penis, shrinking of the testes, increased facial and body hair, deepening of the voice and acne, some of the same effects seen in women. Also, preadolescents and adolescents are at risk for premature closure of the growth plates of the bones, leading to a decrease in ultimate height.

And these are just the minor effects! One of the most common major side effects is a cholesterol imbalance, especially a reduction of the protective HDL (high-density lipoprotein) cholesterol and an increase in the detrimental LDL (low-density lipoprotein) cholesterol. A profile of this kind is associated with increased risk for coronary artery disease.

Another common major side effect is hepatitis, which probably occurs because anabolic steroids are metabolized by the liver. Some major side effects occur relatively infrequently, but can be fatal when they do. Liver tumors, both benign and malignant, have been reported. Another life-threatening condition associated with steroids is peliosis hepatis, the formation in the liver of large blood-filled spaces.

Two other types of potentially fatal malignancies may be associated with anabolic steroid use. Wilms's tumor, a kidney malignancy usually seen in young children, has been reported in two otherwise healthy adult men who were taking anabolic steroids. Five cases of leukemia have been documented in users of anabolic steroids. These cases were in patients who were taking steroids for reasons other than their muscle-building effect, but the risk of developing leukemia may apply to all users.

There are two other important considerations. Although not commonly thought of as a risk factor for HIV (AIDS) transmission, many anabolic steroids are injected, and there is evidence that steroid users, particularly adolescents, engage in the dangerous habit of needle sharing. Not that this is an AIDS-prone group, but anytime needles are shared, the possibility of transmission exists. And, in fact, HIV infection has been documented in body builders who inject anabolic steroids.

Besides the side effects we've already discussed, there are many others that are difficult to chronicle because they result from the use of illegally obtained steroids (a large percentage of the drugs used), which can, and do, contain a variety of contaminants. Any of these contaminants can cause adverse reactions.

Yet, in spite of all these dangers, use continues. It's amazing that people we think of and who think of themselves as health-conscious would virtually risk their lives for a few fleeting moments of glory. But perhaps it isn't, when we consider that ours is a "win now at all costs" society. There are even reports that anabolic steroid use *increased* after the Ben Johnson incident. After all, didn't he run a world record while on the drugs? The lesson learned was only to be more careful to avoid detection. This is not to imply that anabolic steroid users aren't responsible for the consequences of their own actions—they most certainly are—but they are just as much a product of the pervasive "quick-fix" mentality.

A NATURAL ALTERNATIVE

Happily, most of us haven't fallen prey to the sort of extremes that lead to taking anabolic steroids. But, we all do want that better looking body, don't we? If there were a safe, natural alternative to anabolic steroids that could help tone and define muscle and reduce fat, wouldn't you want to use it?

For several years the health food industry has been proclaiming that there are some nutrients that have an anabolic effect. Because of all the negative publicity surrounding the use of anabolic steroids, the television news program "CBS This Morning" ran a segment about the so-called anabolic aids available over the counter. In it Dr. Victor Herbert of Mt. Sinai Hospital in New York discussed these products and dismissed them as completely ineffective. Dr. Herbert has had many confrontations with the nutrition industry. While in some cases he may have overlooked benefits that might be obtained from some nutrients (if not from the products he criticized), in this case he was right. None of the substances Dr. Herbert mentioned has ever been documented to have a genuine muscle-building effect.

There is, though, one nutrient that has been demonstrated to have an anabolic effect, that has been shown in controlled clinical studies to increase the development of muscle tissue while at the same time reducing body fat. That nutrient is the trace mineral chromium, which can enhance all the benefits of resistance training and do much more. How chromium works in the body and how you can make it work for you to improve your health and appearance are the subjects of the rest of this book.

THREE

THE PIONEERING WORK OF GARY EVANS

The ultimate duty of a physician, of course, is to his patients, and I was observing some exceptional results in those I put on a chromium program. Since I was so gratified with what was happening, I continued to recommend increased intake of chromium.

However, just practicing the art of medicine isn't enough. I was making some encouraging clinical observations, but they remained just that. In order for me to be absolutely certain that the effects I had been observing were indeed related to chromium intake, I needed some more input from the science of medicine. I was aware of some research that had been done several years earlier and wanted to investigate this further personally, but conducting clinical experiments in a private practice setting is generally impractical. Fortunately, these clinical trials had already been conducted by someone else. It wasn't until I learned of the work of Dr. Gary Evans that I fully understood the potential of chromium nutrition. Dr. Evans did not discover the physiological function of chromium nor had he done most of the early research on it, but his studies put it all in perspective for me.

Gary Evans is professor of chemistry in the Minnesota State University system at Bemidji, Minnesota, and an expert in trace mineral nutrition. Although Dr. Evans had done some earlier work on chromium, much of his research in the past had concentrated on another mineral, zinc. While working as a scientist at the United States Department of Agriculture laboratory in Grand Forks, North Dakota, he discovered the most bioavailable, or best absorbed, form of zinc.

Dr. Evans and his colleagues were working with a devastating skin disease of infants, known as acrodermatitis enteropathica, or AE. The severe skin pathology in AE is the result of a failure to absorb zinc. After much experimentation, Dr. Evans found that a particular form of zinc, called zinc picolinate (zinc plus picolinic acid), was highly successful in alleviating AE. Further studies by him and other scientists determined that zinc picolinate was the most bioavailable form for everyone, not just those with AE.

From this work Dr. Evans reasoned that if zinc picolinate worked so well, might picolinic acid enhance the availability of other minerals? Picolinic acid is a natural substance produced in the body from the essential dietary amino acid tryptophan and is an excellent "chelator," or binder of minerals. In their chelated form the minerals are much more readily absorbed and used by the body. Thus, the binding property of picolinic acid allows it to increase markedly the absorption of minerals with which it combines.

Dr. Evans had always been fascinated with the effects of chromium in the body and felt it hadn't been studied nearly enough. He had done some experiments with chromium at the USDA in the early 1970s, but had turned to other projects. Now he directed his attention to chromium picolinate.

He first tested it in laboratory animals to determine its absorption and toxicity. He found that not only was chromium picolinate absorbed well, but it was about as nontoxic as any natural substance we ingest. He was unable to feed enough chromium picolinate to the laboratory animals to cause any side effects at all, let alone any toxic effects. The next step was to conduct some clinical trials in human subjects.

Working with Dr. Ray Press and Dr. Jack Geller at Mercy Hospital in San Diego, California, Dr. Evans found that chromium picolinate lowered cholesterol in patients in whom it was elevated and reduced blood sugar in diabetics. Both of these results had been demonstrated in the past with other forms of chromium, although not as convincingly as with chromium picolinate. (Chromium's effects on cholesterol and blood sugar will be described in detail in the next chapter.)

These were stimulating results, but Dr. Evans didn't stop there. He began testing the muscle-building capability of chromium picolinate. Working with Dr. Muriel Gillman, he conducted two separate studies at his university. In the first study he recruited ten entering freshman who were in average condition and had enrolled in weight training classes. The students were divided into two groups. One group of students were given 200 micrograms of chromium picolinate each day for six weeks. The other group were given an inactive placebo. (For experimental purposes, so that dosages can be controlled, supplements are often used instead of food sources.) It was a double-blind study, that is, neither Dr. Evans nor the participants knew which group was getting the drug. Both groups followed a prescribed weight lifting protocol for three hours a week. Measurements were taken at the beginning and end of the study and included percent of body fat, lean body mass, and circumferences of the biceps and calf muscles.

In the group on the placebo the lean body mass increased only about 0.08 lbs (less than 2 ounces), which was not significant. In the group given chromium picolinate, the lean body mass increased (about 3.5 pounds)—*30 times more than those on the placebo!* The calf and biceps circumferences of the group on chromium also increased significantly (see Figure 1).

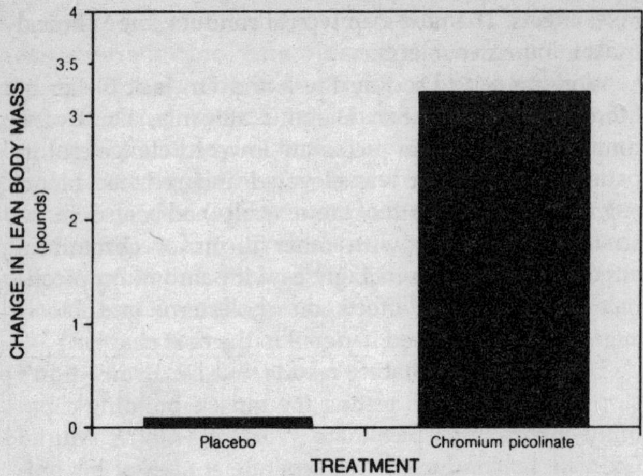

Figure 1. Effect of supplemental chromium on lean body mass in Evans's first study. Ten volunteers supplemented their usual diets with either 200 micrograms of chromium (chromium picolinate) or placebo daily for six weeks. During that time they followed a prescribed weight training program (see Appendix D). At the end of the six weeks, the lean body mass of those on chromium had increased by 3.5 lbs, whereas there was only a 0.08 lb change in lean body mass in those on the placebo. (From G. W. Evans and others, submitted for publication.)

Dr. Evans knew that as exciting as these results were, they had to be validated. He next selected a much larger group of thirty-one men, not just in average condition as in the first study, but trained football players. The athletes, divided into two groups, took either 200 micrograms of chromium from chromium picolinate or placebo for six weeks while following a weight training program. As with the other study, it was double-blind. Since this was near the end of the football season and the participants were in such good condition before the study began, Dr. Evans was not sure if the chromium would still prove to have a significant effect.

However, the results of this study confirmed the first

(see Figure 2). In the group on chromium, the lean body mass increased significantly after only fourteen days and continued to increase to 5.69 pounds at the end of the study. The magnitude of muscle gain in some of the participants in Dr. Evans's studies with safe and natural chromium paralleled that seen with dangerous anabolic steroids. Although the group on placebo also gained lean body mass (they were, after all, on a weight training program), they gained 42 percent less and it didn't show up significantly until the end of the six-week period.

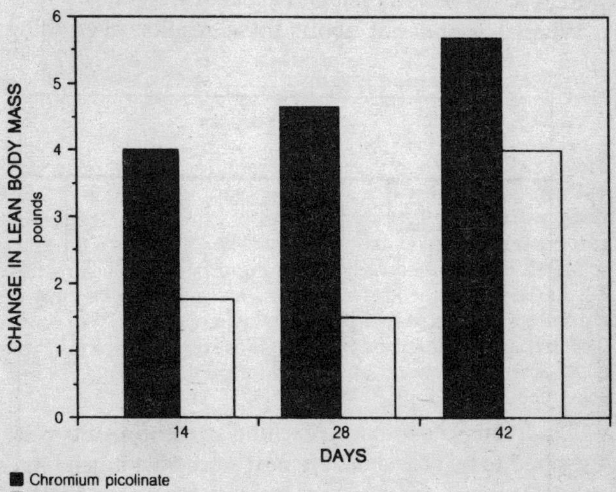

Figure 2. Effect of supplemental chromium on lean body mass in Evans's second study. Thirty-one football players took supplements of either 200 micrograms of chromium (chromium picolinate) or placebo for six weeks while participating in a supervised weight training program (see Appendix D). The group on chromium increased lean body mass by 4 pounds after two weeks and by 5.69 pounds by the end of the six weeks. In the group on placebo, there was less than a 2 lb increase after 14 days and only 4 lbs at the end of 6 weeks, 42% less than the group on chromium. (From G. W. Evans and others, submitted for publication.)

And that's not all. In the group on chromium, total body fat decreased by 22 percent, from 15.8 percent to 12.2 percent (Figure 3). This is remarkable, considering that their average starting body fat of 15.8 percent was already quite low. Just as remarkable, the group on chromium actually lost weight, 2.63 pounds during the six weeks. Since they gained 5.69 pounds of lean mass (muscle), and since muscle weighs more than fat, they lost more fat than they gained muscle. These are ideal results for anyone who wants to shape up—an increase in lean muscle, a loss of body fat, and a loss of weight!

When I found out about these results, everything

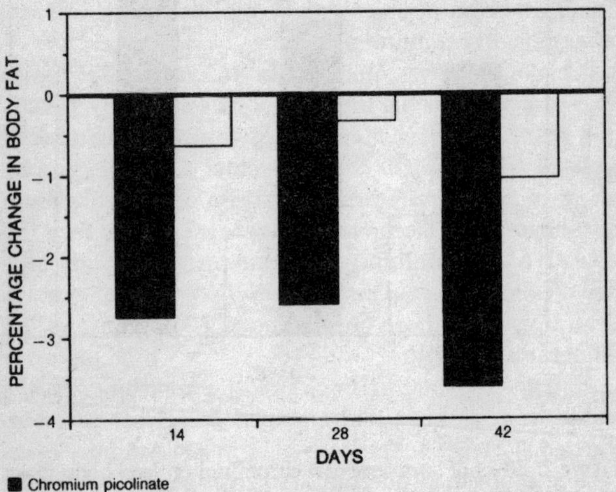

Figure 3. Effect of supplemental chromium on body fat. In the thirty-one football players who participated in Dr. Evans's second study, there was a significant loss of body fat in the group on chromium. At the completion of the six-week study, those on chromium had lost 7.5 lbs (3.6 percent) of body fat. This was a highly significant result, compared with the group on placebo, which lost only 2 lbs (1 percent) of body fat. (From G. W. Evans and others, submitted for publication.)

began to fall in place. The effect on muscle development, body fat, and weight tied in with other ways good chromium nutrition can be of benefit—cholesterol and blood sugar regulation. This is why my patients who were increasing their chromium intake were feeling more energetic and stronger, especially the ones who were sticking to an exercise regimen. The work of Dr. Evans helped me formulate a more specific diet and exercise program for my patients.

Since Dr. Evans conducted these trials, there have been several more studies on the effect of chromium on body composition, both validating and expanding upon the initial observations. As did Dr. Evans's work, all of them involved supplementing the diet with different strengths of chromium picolinate.

One of them was quite similar to Dr. Evans's studies except that it was the first to involve females. Dr. Deborah Hasten of Louisiana State University gave fifty-nine college students of both sexes either a dietary supplement of two hundred micrograms a day of chromium picolinate or a placebo for twelve weeks while they followed a weight lifting program. In this study, the females fared best. They gained almost twice as much lean muscle as those on placebo (2.7 kilograms vs. 1.5 kilograms).

But the most surprising, almost astonishing, results came from a study that I helped design. It was conducted at a large weight loss clinic in San Antonio, Texas where more than one hundred overweight volunteers were given either placebo, 200 micrograms or 400 micrograms a day of chromium picolinate for more than two months. Unlike previous studies, the subjects were not given any specific instructions regarding diet or exercise. It can, of course, be assumed that many of them were motivated to lose weight, but since the study followed all the correct scientific procedures (the subjects were randomly assigned to either the placebo or one of the two chromium groups, and the study was conducted double-blind so that neither investigators or subjects knew who was in which group) the most motivated would most likely be evenly distributed among the three groups. Body fat at the end of the study was measured by underwater immersion, generally recognized as the most accurate way to determine body composition.

The group on placebo showed no significant changes in body composition between pre- and post-test measurements, but the group on chromium picolinate showed highly significant changes—a decrease in body fat and an increase in lean muscle. On average, the chromium-treated group lost 4.2 pounds of fat accompanied by a 1.4 pound increase in fat-free mass. Although the changes tended to be greatest in the group on 400 micrograms of chromium picolinate, the results were not, according to statistical principles, significantly different from the group on 200 micrograms.

When I and my colleagues published these results, and I subsequently appeared on television to discuss them, I was naturally excited to report these findings, but I was also concerned that they were going to be blown out of proportion. Analyzing this study, one could be tempted to conclude that chromium picolinate is a true "magic bullet" for weight loss and muscle gain, since there was no controlled exercise program. Is that really possible? The only correct answer at this time is we don't know. It is biochemically plausible, but a great deal more clinical trials of this sort are needed. Indeed, they are already underway.

Besides these, and some other human studies, there have also been several studies on body composition in animals, primarily in pigs, at Louisiana State University, Virginia Polytechnic Institute and the University of Kentucky. These studies invariably demonstrated that chromium picolinate increased lean muscle mass and decreased fat. While data from animals cannot universally be extrapolated to humans, pig physiology is in many ways remarkably similar to our own. At the very least, chromium picolinate will probably lead to our eating leaner pork chops.

I can't promise that you'll achieve the same degree of lean tissue increase or fat loss as the athletes in Dr. Evans's studies. (You probably won't unless you are advanced enough in weight training and condition to follow his ambitious program, described in Appendix D.) But if you adhere to the chromium diet and the simple exercise program described in detail later on, you will notice some significant changes in the contour of your body—much more and sooner than you would have achieved with exercise alone. And you will experience the other rewards that adequate chromium intake brings.

FOUR

WHAT CHROMIUM IS AND HOW IT WORKS

Up to now I've described some clinical observations of the benefits increased chromium intake has brought and some experimental demonstrations of chromium's ability to accelerate the development of muscle and loss of fat. But I haven't really told you anything about what chromium is and how it works.

If you're like most people, you've never thought of chromium as a nutrient. Most people know something about different vitamins, and many have heard of some less commonly mentioned nutrients, such as selenium, but few are familiar with chromium. The word itself isn't new to most people, but at an informal survey I conducted one evening at a party, everyone I questioned thought I meant the metallic alloy. When I explained I was talking about the nutritive properties of chromium, I had to listen to all the predictable jokes about gnawing on car bumpers.

But the metallic form has nothing to do with the nutritional form. Chromium exists in two chemical states or valences, a term that refers to its ability to combine with other substances in chemical reactions. The metallic alloys and other industrial applications utilize hexavalent chromium, or Cr^{+6}; the nutritional form is trivalent chromium, or Cr^{+3}. This is of more than academic importance. Hexavalent or industrial chromium can be toxic, whereas trivalent or nutritional chromium has extremely low toxicity, probably about that of water. From now on, all our discussion will refer to trivalent chromium.

Chromium is a trace mineral, required by our bodies in minute quantities; the intake recommended by the National Research Council is 50 to 200 micrograms per day (one microgram is one-thousandth of a milligram or one-millionth of a gram). But it is an essential mineral and performs a function without which we cannot live. *Chromium is a required cofactor for all of the actions of the hormone insulin and the actions of chromium directly parallel those of insulin.* A cofactor is a substance with which another substance must unite in order for that second substance to perform a specific function or bring about a specific effect.

The function of insulin that people are most familiar with is control of blood sugar. And, the original research on chromium involved the interaction between chromium and insulin in regulating blood sugar. But that's only a small part of what insulin does in the body. Its effect on blood sugar doesn't explain all the results I have seen in patients, nor does it explain the muscle-building effect of chromium discovered by Dr. Evans. However, these effects are all related to the interaction between chromium and insulin and this will soon become clear to you when we discuss all the ways insulin (and therefore chromium) works.

A BRIEF HISTORY OF CHROMIUM

If there were a United States of Essential Nutrients, chromium would be the Hawaii. Although fluoride is officially given credit for being the most recently designated essential mineral, if we consider human nutrition, that distinction more properly belongs to chromium.

In 1957 the late Klaus Schwarz and Walter Mertz were doing experiments with laboratory rats and noticed that their animals developed an impaired ability to metabolize sugar, so-called glucose intolerance, while being fed a standard commercial diet. When chromium-containing fractions of yeast or yeast concentrates were added to the rats' diets, their blood sugar became normal. Trivalent chromium was identified as the active component of a molecule the exact structure of which wasn't known but which was called glucose tolerance factor, or GTF.

To investigate this further, Mertz and Schwarz intentionally deprived rats of chromium. They discovered that, despite having adequate amounts of insulin, the animals' blood sugar control was impaired. This occurred after only three weeks on a chromium-deficient diet, but one intravenous dose of chromium restored their sugar metabolism to normal! These numbers don't apply to humans, but they illustrate the dramatic effect that chromium was discovered to have on glucose tolerance.

This same phenomenon was soon found to exist in other animals, including monkeys. The more severe the chromium deficiency, the more the symptoms resembled diabetes, including high blood sugar and sugar in the urine. But even in these situations, chromium was able to reverse the symptoms. *Dr. Mertz postulated that chromium, as GTF, acts as a cofactor to bind insulin to tissues and therefore improves the efficiency of insulin.*

Since the relationship between chromium deficiency and glucose intolerance had now been shown in monkeys as well as rats, the probability that it also existed in humans was increased, but it still needed to be demonstrated. As with many important scientific discoveries, this connection was arrived at serendipitously (as was the original observation in laboratory rats). In 1977 Dr. K. N. Jeejeehboy and his colleagues reported a patient who had undergone removal of most of her intestine and was relegated to total intravenous feeding for the rest of her life. After three and a half years the woman developed signs of diabetes—elevated blood sugar, weight loss, and loss of sensation—which did not improve with insulin. But, within two weeks of adding chromium to her daily intravenous fluids, her blood sugar, neurological function, and weight were back to normal. Other instances have been reported in which as a result of the inadequate amounts of or absence of chromium in intravenous feeding, glucose intolerance developed slowly as with this woman or as rapidly as within five months. The condition in these cases was corrected quickly with the addition of chromium.

Probably as a result of the demonstration in humans of the critical role chromium plays in blood sugar control (plus all the data that had accumulated in animals), in 1980 the National Research Council of the National Academy of Sciences—the institution that sets the recommended dietary allowances (RDAs) of nutrients—declared that chromium was an essential nutrient, and safe and adequate intake was set at 50 to 200 micrograms per day.

In 1994, as a result of all the studies conducted on chromium since 1980, the Food and Drug Administration proposed a Reference Daily Intake of 130 micrograms a day. This is probably too low, but it's a step in the right direction and further acknowledgment of just how important chromium is to so many aspects of our metabolism.

HOW CHROMIUM HELPS BUILD MUSCLE

We'll talk more about the effects of chromium on blood sugar later, but let's focus now on the central point of the Chromium Program: the ability of chromium to accelerate muscle development and fat loss.

I've told you that I witnessed this in several patients and that it was documented in studies by Dr. Gary Evans. But how does it work? The answer is that chromium helps build muscle in the same way it aids in

HOW INSULIN (AND CHROMIUM) HELP BUILD MUSCLE
Increased uptake of amino acids Increased assembly of amino acids into protein Decreased breakdown of muscle protein

blood sugar control, that is, as an essential *cofactor* to insulin.

The major actions of insulin are represented in simple terms in Figure 4. As you can see, besides affecting the disposition of blood sugar, insulin also is intimately involved in protein and fat metabolism. The actions of insulin are actually much more complex than this and the effects on carbohydrate, protein, and fat are interrelated, but for our discussion it's easier to think about them separately.

When you eat a meal containing sugar or other forms of carbohydrate, it triggers a release of insulin from the pancreas, the organ in your body that produces the insulin. In the presence of its necessary cofactor chromium, the insulin "escorts" the sugar across cell membranes where it can be utilized for energy production.

Although not as commonly known, almost exactly the same thing happens when protein is eaten. The breakdown of ingested protein into its amino acid building blocks stimulates a release of insulin. In the same fashion as with sugar, insulin directs the amino acids into cells, such as muscle cells, where they are assembled into proteins that constitute body tissues.

Insulin's participation in protein synthesis, or anabolism, is not limited to bringing the raw materials to the muscle cell. It promotes the assembly of amino acids into protein through its effect on the cell's genetic material, DNA and RNA. And, in addition, it slows the breakdown, or catabolism, of body protein. The net effect of all of this is increased protein available for building tissue.

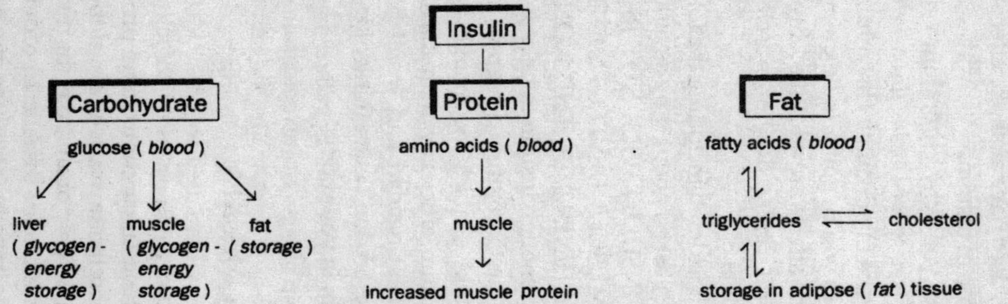

Figure 4. The major actions of insulin. Although insulin performs other functions in the body, its three main ones are to aid in the regulation of carbohydrate, protein, and fat metabolism.

Carbohydrates: Insulin promotes the entry of glucose (sugar) from the blood into liver and muscle cells, where it is stored as glycogen (the storage form of carbohydrate) and into fat cells, where it is also stored.

Protein: Insulin promotes the entry of amino acids (protein building blocks) into muscle cells, where they are assembled into muscle protein (see table p. 32 for further details about how insulin accomplishes this).

Fat: Insulin's effect on fat metabolism is complex and not completely understood. Essentially, it helps regulate the balance between the blood and storage forms of cholesterol and triglycerides. This is important in controlling both risk of heart disease and weight.

When combined with resistance exercise, this results in more muscle development and fat loss. Insulin is the body's primary anabolic hormone. Testosterone, the substance from which anabolic steroids are derived, does have anabolic effects, but they are secondary to those of insulin.

Now it should be clear to you why chromium can help build muscle. *Chromium is necessary for insulin to help build muscle.* When the presence of adequate chromium is combined with the exercises you're going to be doing in the Chromium Program, the effects are additive: chromium + resistance training = a double dose of muscle-building and fat-losing potential.

I would never even have considered including the following caution had I not been asked about it by several body builders. INJECTING INSULIN WILL NOT RESULT IN ACCELERATED MUSCLE DEVELOPMENT AND CAN BE LIFE-THREATENING IN THE NON-DIABETIC. You already have enough insulin to help develop muscle. The point of the Chromium Program is that adequate chromium intake enables the insulin in your body to work at maximum efficiency with maximum results. More insulin isn't needed and won't be better—it will be much worse! So don't even think of increasing the amount of insulin in your body.

INSULIN RESISTANCE: AN IMPORTANT UNIFYING CONCEPT

You now know that chromium, as an essential cofactor for insulin, is important in blood sugar control and protein metabolism that can accelerate muscle development. Chromium also plays a crucial role in fat metabolism and protection from heart disease. In order to explain this role to you, we have to introduce you to insulin resistance, a concept that ties all the functions of insulin together. As you read these next few pages, keep in mind that the story of insulin is in many ways the story of chromium.

When carbohydrate, fat, and protein reach the bloodstream, they stimulate a release of insulin from the pancreas. The insulin directs these food constituents to where they are most needed—generally to muscle, liver, or fat cells where they are used for energy (carbohydrate), used to build tissue (protein), or stored (fat) (see Figure 4). Insulin seems to do this by attaching to specific receptors on the surface of the cell which then send a "message" to the cell telling it to let the carbohydrate, fat, or protein enter. Under normal conditions tissues are responsive, or *sensitive,* to insulin, and only small amounts of it are required to dispose efficiently of the carbohydrates, fat, and protein.

In some cases, however, the body tissues are *insulin-resistant,* and the small amounts of insulin normally secreted can't do the job. Either there aren't enough receptors on the cell surface for insulin or they don't "recognize" the insulin (see Figure 5). As a result the nutrient constituents cannot be transported into the cell. When this occurs, the pancreas doesn't give up easily. It secretes more and more insulin to try and overcome the insulin resistance of the tissues. If a person on one side of a closed door hears well, you need knock only softly to gain admittance. If, however, the person is hard of hearing, you will have to knock very loudly to get them to open the door. Insulin-resistant tissues are like the hard-of-hearing person, and the compensatory increased insulin levels in the bloodstream are the loud knocks.

The classic example of insulin resistance is diabetes. In the most common type of diabetes, Type II or non-insulin dependent diabetes mellitus (NIDDM), there is not a deficiency of insulin; rather there are excess amounts secreted by the pancreas in an attempt to compensate for the insulin resistance of the cells. In these cases the high insulin levels may be fairly effective in

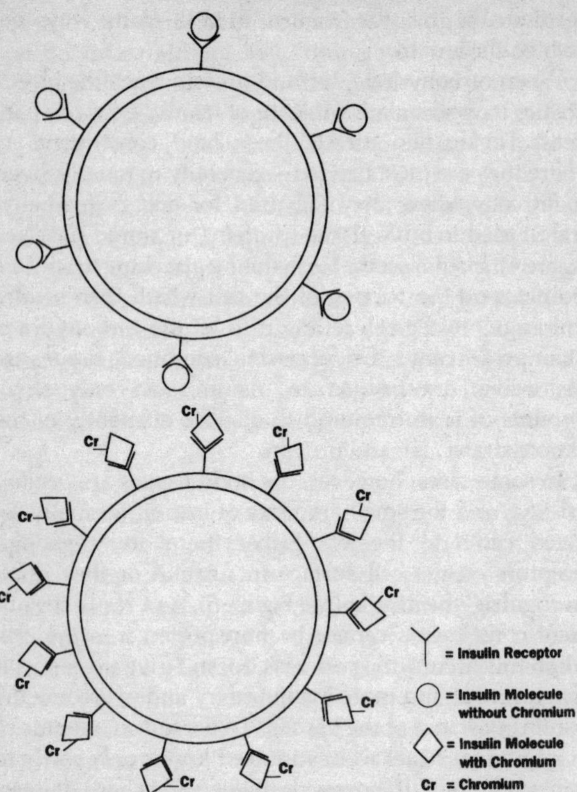

Figure 5. Possible mechanisms by which chromium enhances the effects of insulin. Insulin works by attaching to specific receptors on the surface of cells. In order to work best, the insulin molecules must either have enough receptors to attach to, physically conform (fit) to the receptors, or both. The upper diagram represents the situation in which there is less than an optimal amount of chromium available, and the lower figure represents the situation with adequate chromium. Although it is not known exactly how it occurs, chromium is thought to either increase the number of insulin receptors on the cell surface or help insulin fit better into the receptors, or possibly a combination of the two mechanisms. Whichever mechanism or combination of mechanisms exists, chromium is essential for insulin to function optimally.

directing enough sugar from the blood into the cells, so that blood sugar levels don't rise too high. Obviously, they are not completely effective since, by definition, diabetics have elevated blood sugar. The high amount of insulin also handles protein metabolism pretty well.

But those with NIDDM do pay a price for having continually elevated levels of insulin, even if their blood sugar is reasonably well controlled. This toll is exacted primarily in the area of fat metabolism. Under normal circumstances insulin promotes formation in fat cells of small amounts of triglycerides, a storage form of fat. If the tissues are properly sensitive to insulin, only enough fat is deposited to insulate our organs and provide energy reserves and normal blood levels of triglycerides and cholesterol are maintained.

However, when tissues are insulin-resistant and there is a resultant increased production of insulin, as in NIDDM, the high levels of insulin promote excess fat storage (leading to obesity), cause an increase in the blood of triglycerides and cholesterol, and cause a decrease in high-density lipoproteins (HDL), or "good" cholesterol. All of this increases risk for coronary artery disease. It is highly probable that the high frequency of this condition in diabetics is linked to insulin resistance and high insulin levels. Besides this, high insulin levels contribute to hypertension, another risk factor for heart disease. Although not definitely known, the elevation in blood pressure probably occurs, at least in part, because the elevated insulin causes an increase in sodium retention.

But not only diabetics have insulin resistance. One of the world's leading diabetes researchers, Dr. Gerald Reaven of Stanford University, found that 25 percent of all nondiabetics he tested were insulin-resistant. These people had normal blood sugar and appeared healthy in every way—normal weight, normal cholesterol, normal blood pressure. However, in order to keep their blood sugar at a normal level, they had to secrete high levels of insulin and therefore were prone to the same consequences of high insulin levels as diabetics.

Dr. Reaven has suggested that there is a constellation of related symptoms, all associated with insulin resistance and high blood levels of insulin, that increase risk for coronary artery disease. He probably should have called it Reaven's syndrome, but modestly has named it syndrome X. Anyone with insulin resistance—about 1 in 4 healthy-appearing individuals according to Dr. Reaven—is prone to develop syndrome X and therefore to be at risk for the number one killer in industrialized countries, coronary artery disease.

So, here are the three possible general situations (there may be variations; for example, not all diabetics have elevated blood pressure):

	NORMAL	DIABETIC	NONDIABETIC BUT INSULIN-RESISTANT
Blood sugar	Normal	Elevated	Normal
Blood insulin	Normal	Elevated	Elevated
Blood lipids	Normal	Elevated	Normal or elevated
Blood pressure	Normal	Elevated	Normal or elevated

How do you know if you have insulin resistance, and, if you do, what can you do about it? As with many conditions, it appears that insulin resistance is part genetic, part environmental. If you have a parent who is diabetic, who has coronary artery disease, or has any of the components of syndrome X, it might not be a bad idea to discuss being checked for insulin resistance with your physician. The best test for this condition is quite sophisticated and is still a research tool. But a glucose tolerance test that measures insulin levels at the same time blood sugar levels are measured is a good substitute. This can

CHARACTERISTICS OF SYNDROME X
Insulin resistance
High blood levels of insulin
Elevated triglyceride levels
Decreased HDL cholesterol
Hypertension

FACTORS THAT ENHANCE INSULIN SENSITIVITY
Ideal body weight
Exercise (aerobic and resistance)
High soluble fiber intake
Adequate chromium nutrition

determine whether elevated insulin levels are present, and hence whether insulin resistance exists.

Whether or not you decide to get tested, you can do quite a bit to reduce the environmental factors that contribute to insulin resistance. The goal is to keep your tissues as sensitive as possible to insulin, so that insulin levels stay as low as possible and the risk of syndrome X will also be low. Insulin resistance tends to increase with age, but this can be at least partially counteracted by factors in our control.

Obesity is often an effect of insulin resistance, but it can be a cause as well. Keeping weight within an ideal range increases insulin sensitivity. Physical exercise, both aerobic and resistance, heightens tissue insulin sensitivity. So does eating a diet high in soluble fiber—the kind found in oat bran, beans, fruits, and vegetables. And, most relevant to the point of our program, *appropriate chromium nutrition can increase insulin sensitivity.* Since we've already learned that chromium is an essential cofactor for insulin, this should not be surprising. Chromium makes insulin more efficient, so less is needed.

CHROMIUM AND INSULIN RESISTANCE

Look again at the characteristics of syndrome X, with all the features of insulin resistance. Now look at the list of signs and symptoms of chromium deficiency (see the table below) as determined by Dr. Richard Anderson of the United States Department of Agriculture Human Nutrition Research Center and one of the country's most prominent chromium scientists. *The consequences of chromium deficiency and insulin resistance seem nearly identical*—completely logical from what we've learned about the interaction of chromium and insulin.

Several clinical studies have put the chromium deficiency–insulin resistance theory to the test. In epidemiological investigations populations with a low incidence of diabetes have relatively high tissue levels of chromium. When chromium has been administered to diabetics with insulin resistance (and high insulin levels), blood sugar has improved, cholesterol and triglycerides have dropped to normal levels, and insulin levels have dropped. The elevated blood sugar and blood fats were the result of insulin resistance, which was improved by the essential cofactor chromium (Figures 6 and 7). Chromium seems to help insulin attach to the cell receptors by making it easier for the receptors to recognize it. In

SIGNS AND SYMPTOMS OF CHROMIUM DEFICIENCY
Impaired glucose tolerance
Elevated blood levels of insulin
Glycosuria (sugar in the urine)
Elevated blood sugar
Elevated serum cholesterol and triglycerides

Source: Adapted from R. A. Anderson, Chromium metabolism and its role in disease processes in man, *Clinical Physiology and Biochemistry,* 4:31–41, 1986.

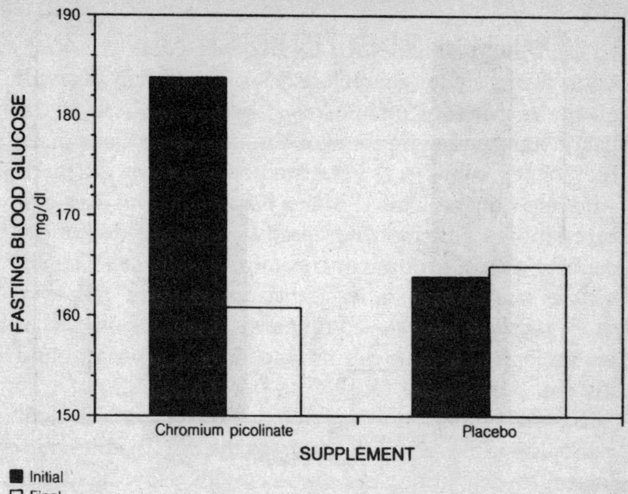

Figure 6. Effect of supplemental chromium on fasting blood sugar. The diets of eleven diabetic patients were supplemented with 200 micrograms daily of chromium (chromium picolinate) or placebo for six weeks. At the end of that period, fasting blood glucose had decreased approximately 12 percent in the patients on chromium, whereas it remained unchanged in those on placebo. (From R. I. Press, J. Geller, and G. W. Evans, The effect of chromium picolinate on serum glucose, glycosylated hemoglobin and cholesterol of adult onset diabetics, FASEB Journal, 1989; 3:A761.)

our analogy of the hard-of-hearing person, chromium is like a "hearing aid" for the cell.

Chromium supplementation has also worked at the opposite end of the blood sugar spectrum in hypoglycemia. You may find it puzzling that the same substance can both lower and raise blood sugar. But chromium does not act on the blood sugar itself, but helps improve insulin sensitivity to create a more even and appropriate pattern of insulin activity. In this way, chromium can help prevent excessive rises or excessive falls in blood sugar levels (Figure 8).

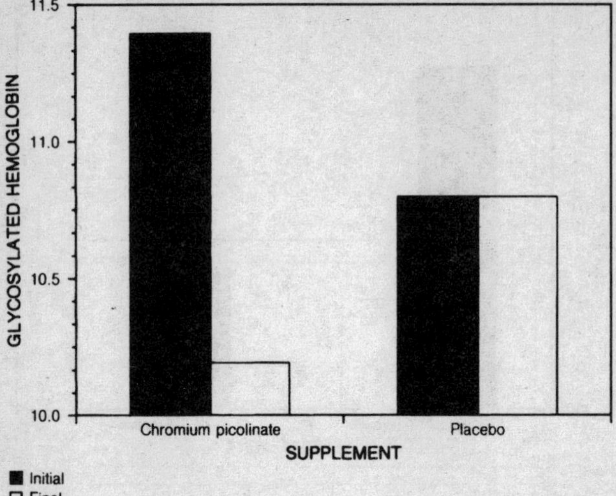

Figure 7. Effect of supplemental chromium on glycosylated hemoglobin. The diets of eleven diabetic patients (the same patients in the blood glucose study) were supplemented with either 200 micrograms daily of chromium (chromium picolinate) or placebo for six weeks. At the end of that time, the level of glycosylated hemoglobin (a marker of control of diabetes) had decreased more than 10 percent in the patients on chromium, but remained the same in those on placebo. (From R. I. Press, J. Geller, and G. W. Evans, The effect of chromium picolinate on serum glucose, glycosylated hemoglobin and cholesterol of adult onset diabetics, FASEB Journal 1989; 3: A761.)

These effects of chromium in normalizing both high and low blood sugar explain the improvements I have witnessed over the years in both diabetic and hypoglycemic patients. And it also clears up the mystery of why I noticed improvement in blood fats and blood pressure in those who had normal blood sugar. Although early on I didn't know enough about chromium to test for insulin resistance (I routinely do now), these patients most likely were insulin-resistant, which was improved by increasing chromium intake.

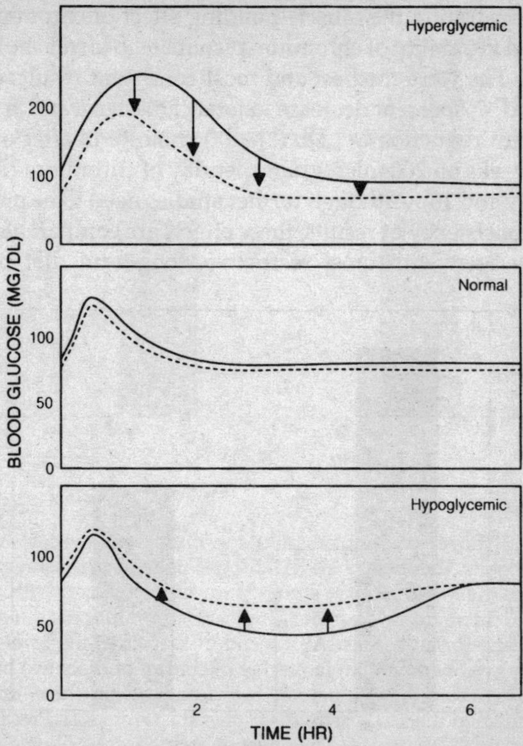

Figure 8. Effects of supplemental chromium on hyperglycemic, normal, and hypoglycemic individuals. Solid line depicts blood glucose values before supplementation, and dashed line after chromium supplementation. (From R. Anderson, in *Trace minerals in foods,* ed. Kenneth T. Smith. New York and Basel: Marcel Dekker, 1988.)

There have been several tests in which elevated cholesterol, elevated triglycerides, and reduced HDL ("good") cholesterol in nondiabetics have improved following chromium supplementation. Subjects who had the highest insulin levels (insulin resistance) tended to improve the most. Dr. Evans and his colleagues, before demonstrating the muscle-building effect of chromium, tested the ability of chromium picolinate to lower cholesterol. His were the best and most consistent results obtained: a 7 percent decrease in total cholesterol and an 11 percent reduction in LDL ("bad") cholesterol after only six weeks on 200 micrograms per day of chromium (Figures 9 and 10). Although further studies need to be made for consistency of results, these effects are comparable to those seen with most restrictive, long-term diet pro-

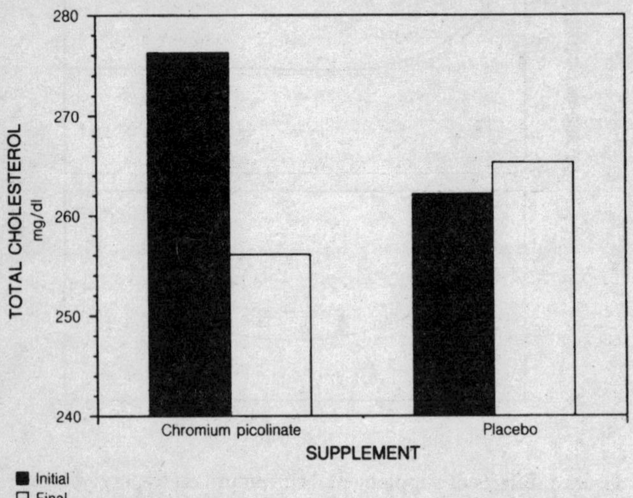

Figure 9. Effect of supplemental chromium on serum cholesterol. Twenty-eight patients with elevated serum cholesterol levels were given either 200 micrograms daily of chromium (chromium picolinate) or placebo for six weeks. At the end of that period, the total cholesterol of those on chromium was reduced by 7 percent, whereas the levels of those on placebo were essentially unchanged. Other studies have shown similar results. (From R. I. Press, J. Geller, and G. W. Evans, The effect of chromium picolinate on serum cholesterol and apolipoprotein fractions in human subjects, *Western Journal of Medicine,* Vol 152 (1): 41–45, 1990.)

grams (no dietary changes were made with Dr. Evans's subjects). Dr. Evans didn't check for insulin resistance, but it's reasonable to assume that it existed in those who improved.

If chromium supplementation can improve cholesterol levels, and high cholesterol is associated with coronary artery disease, it follows that chromium deficiency could be associated with coronary artery disease. In 1980 Dr. Abraham Abraham at Hebrew University in Jerusalem induced atherosclerosis in rabbits and corrected it with chromium supplementation. In 1984 Dr. Monique Simonoff and her colleagues in France found that the chromium concentration in the blood of patients with coronary artery disease, demonstrated by angiograms, was much lower than the concentration in patients without coronary artery disease. This study was conducted on 150 patients and confirmed an earlier, smaller one.

Ten years before Dr. Reaven proposed syndrome X as a group of symptoms associated with insulin resistance, researchers from the Miami Heart Institute had postulated that chromium deficiency was the cause of insulin resistance, which in turn caused blood sugar abnormalities, high serum cholesterol, high triglycerides, and atherosclerosis (Figure 11). Their hypothesis was remarkably similar to Dr. Reaven's except that they backed up a step and proposed chromium deficiency as the cause.

So, this leaves us with the following: Insulin resistance is related to many serious conditions—diabetes, coronary artery disease (including elevated cholesterol, elevated triglycerides, and reduced HDL cholesterol), obesity, hypertension, and muscle wasting. *Chromium is intimately associated with the way insulin works, and chromium deficiency is probably a major contributor to insulin resistance and hence all the above conditions.*

Understanding this allows us to link the muscle-

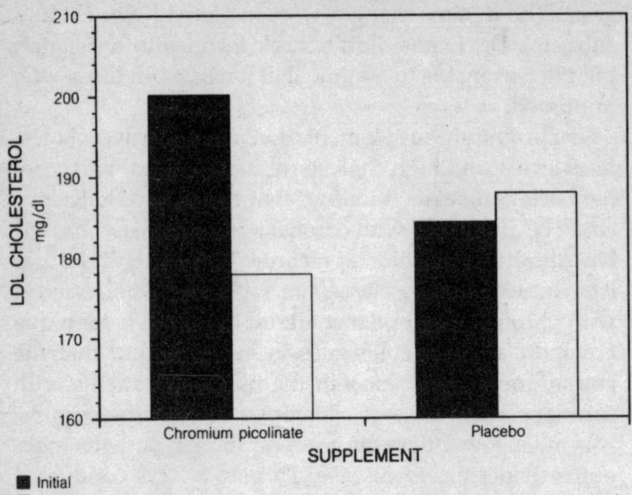

Figure 10. Effect of supplemental chromium on LDL cholesterol. Twenty-eight patients with elevated serum cholesterol levels were given either 200 micrograms daily of chromium (chromium picolinate) or placebo for six weeks. At the end of that period, the LDL cholesterol of those on chromium was reduced by 11 percent, whereas the levels of those on placebo were essentially unchanged. (From R. I. Press, J. Geller, and G. W. Evans, The effect of chromium picolinate on serum cholesterol and apolipoprotein fractions in human subjects, *Western Journal of Medicine,* Vol 152 (1): 41–45, 1990.)

building effects of chromium with reducing the chance of developing insulin resistance or improving it if it already exists. *The more lean body tissue and the less fat we have, the more sensitive our tissues are to insulin.* Even if you don't look fat, as you get older, the amount of lean tissue in your muscles decreases and the amount of fat increases. By following the Chromium Program of diet and exercise, you can increase your lean body mass and reduce insulin resistance and all the risks associated with it. Therefore, although the main focus of the chromium diet and exercise program is to help you build

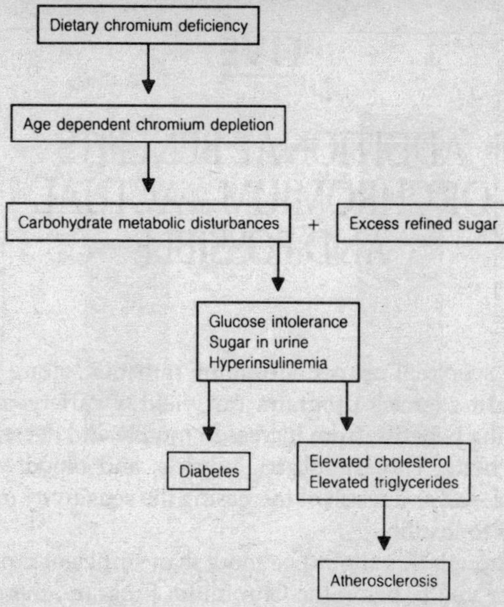

Figure 11. Postulated sequence of events as to how chromium deficiency leads to diabetes and atherosclerosis. (Adapted from E. Boyle, B. Mondschein, and H. Dash, Chromium depletion in the pathogenesis of diabetes and atherosclerosis, *Southern Medical Journal, 70*(12):1449–1453, 1977.)

muscle and lose fat, with all the attendant benefits, from everything we've covered in this chapter it should now be obvious to you that the Chromium Program can do much, much more.

FIVE

ADDITIONAL BENEFITS OF CHROMIUM—ACTUAL AND POSSIBLE

We've seen that proper chromium nutrition, along with the right exercise program, can yield a variety of astounding benefits, from increased muscle and decreased fat to better cholesterol, triglyceride, and blood sugar control—all as a result of increasing the sensitivity of our tissues to insulin.

Although this should be more than sufficient motivation for you to begin the Chromium Program, there are still other rewards you may experience. The results we've discussed so far are well documented. The benefits I'm about to present to you are less so. Some of them have been demonstrated in clinical studies or at least alluded to. Others might be expected on the basis of theory and are known from anecdotal reports. Still others are theory only. But all are interesting and worth describing. As we go through them, I'll let you know how solid the evidence is for each.

No matter how startling the results and how many stories I heard, I always remain skeptical until I find documentation in the scientific literature. But an anecdote plus a plausible mechanism heightens interest and belief.

By no means am I trying to present chromium as a panacea for everything from hangnails to cancer, but, since it is an essential cofactor for insulin—a hormone that has many actions in addition to those we have already discussed—a wide range of potential applications does exist.

WEIGHT LOSS

The evidence for chromium's effect on weight loss is part clinical, part theoretical, and part anecdotal. Besides the trial I helped design that was described earlier, there are two studies that have demonstrated weight loss with increased chromium intake. In the larger of the two trials of chromium picolinate with weight-training athletes, Dr. Gary Evans and his colleagues found a 2.63 pound weight loss in the group on chromium, concomitant with a 5.69 pound increase in muscle. Earlier, in 1981, Dr. Rebecca Riales and Dr. Margaret Albrink at the University of West Virginia had found a 1.5 pound weight loss over a three-month period in a group on chromium. This amount was small but statistically significant. (The reasons for this smaller decrease in weight may be related to the type of chromium used in the study, which we will discuss when we talk about the bioavailability of chromium.)

In addition to these studies, anecdotal reports seem to support a relation between increased chromium and weight loss. I have heard from numerous patients, friends, and relatives of all ages that they lost weight when they increased their chromium intake. For example, my mother-in-law, Linn Whitehouse, is a well-trained marathon runner, who was sidelined for almost two years with a chronic injury. As a substitute, she began swimming. However, while swimming is an excellent activity for promoting fitness, it generally doesn't lead to the same weight loss as running. Consequently, Linn gained 9 pounds in less than a year, which remained until she began increasing her chromium intake. After three months on chromium, she lost almost all 9 pounds—without changing her diet or increasing her exercise at all!

How can chromium promote weight loss? One possible mechanism is insulin resistance. Recall that high blood levels of insulin, which occur as a consequence of tissues' resistance to insulin, promote excessive deposition of fat. Chromium reduces insulin resistance, which in turn decreases the storage of adipose (fatty) tissue and increases its metabolism.

Another way could be by decreasing hunger. By helping to stabilize blood sugar levels, chromium diminishes the desire to eat. In addition, insulin stimulates the synthesis in the brain of serotonin, a member of a family of chemicals called neurotransmitters, which facilitate communication between brain cells. Increased amounts of serotonin in the brain can help promote a feeling of satiety. Consistent with what we've been saying about chromium's role as an essential "partner" to insulin, increasing chromium intake should help insulin perform this job better as well.

Also, carbohydrate ingestion elevates metabolic rate, an effect known as carbohydrate-mediated thermogenesis. Here again insulin seems to be involved; this type of thermogenesis has not been seen in animals that are diabetic or insulin-resistant. Insulin activates an energy-burning enzyme known as the "sodium pump," which may account for the carbohydrate-mediated thermogenesis. Chromium could enhance this action.

LONGEVITY

In the 1930s, Dr. Clive McKay at Cornell University discovered that systematically restricting calories of laboratory mice by about 30% throughout their entire life significantly increased their maximum lifespan. In the 1970s and 1980s, Dr. Roy Walford, a renowned pathologist and gerontologist at UCLA School of Medicine not only repeated these experiments, but he showed that restricting calories of mice beginning in middle age rather than at birth had the same effect.

Dr. Edward Masoro of the University of Texas discovered a possible mechanism by which caloric restriction increases lifespan. As we age, sugar molecules in our bloodstream tend to attach to proteins throughout the body. This happens slowly but relentlessly and has the cumulative effect of diminishing cell function and eventually causing cell death and physiologic aging. This is essentially what happens in diabetes, only at a much accelerated pace.

When Dr. Gary Evans heard of Dr. Masoro's work he reasoned that, since chromium has been demonstrated to reduce the attachment of sugars to proteins in diabetes (this is what is measured in the "glycosylated hemoglobin" blood test that diabetics frequently have to take to check the progress of their condition), perhaps it might also extend the lifespan of laboratory mice in the same way that caloric restriction does. And he was right! He divided a group of newborn rats into 3 categories and supplemented their diets with either chromium picolinate or two other types of chromium which studies have shown to be less effective—chromic chloride or chromium nicotinate. At various ages, blood was drawn to check glycosylated hemoglobin. What he found were 2 things: (1) the rats on chromium picolinate lived much longer than the rats on the other forms of chromium—at 41 months, all of the animals on chromic chloride or chromium nicotinate had died while *80% of the rats fed chromium picolinate were still alive*; (2) The changes in the blood levels of glycosylated hemoglobin exactly paralleled the increase in lifespan.

These results demonstrate that chromium, specifically in the form of chromium picolinate, increases longevity in laboratory animals, probably by retarding hyperglycemia and attachment of sugar to protein. *This is the first reported instance of any nutrient having lifespan-extending properties.* It is difficult at this time to determine what this means for humans, and of course, because we live so long, it is difficult to perform life extension experiments in humans. In order to do these type of studies on humans, scientists look for biomarkers of aging that can act as surrogates for measuring actual lifespan. Glycosylated hemoglobin or other proteins are one such biomarker. A study needs to be done looking at this biomarker in non-diabetics and until it, or some similar study is done, this is merely an extremely interesting and provocative laboratory result.

OSTEOPOROSIS

The mineral most commonly presumed to be deficient in osteoporosis is calcium, but, following some elegant reasoning, Dr. Evans and his colleagues investigated whether chromium might also play a role. Most scientists believe that calcium loss is the result of decreased production of estrogen, primarily the form in the body known as estradiol. Without enough estradiol, calcium gets filtered through the kidneys and is excreted. One of the important biochemical building blocks in women's bodies for estradiol is a hormone produced by the adrenal glands called DHEA. But, as women age, less DHEA is produced and therefore less estradiol. It has been discovered that one of the reasons that DHEA production decreases with age is that insulin resistance increases, leading to elevated levels of insulin in the blood which block DHEA synthesis. Therefore, Dr. Evans reasoned, if insulin resistance could be controlled, insulin levels would decrease, more DHEA and then more estradiol would be produced and calcium loss from bone would be decreased. What better, he thought, to reduce insulin resistance than tried and true chromium picolinate. And that's exactly what he found. For a period of sixty days, twenty-seven post-menopausal women took either placebo or 200 micrograms of chromium picolinate per day. In the women on chromium picolinate, plasma insulin levels decreased 37.6% and plasma DHEA increased 24%. Concomitantly, urinary calcium excretion decreased by almost 20%. These results suggest that chromium, through its effect on insulin, might be effective in preventing osteoporosis. This work needs to be expanded and include sophisticated measurements of bone density before we can be certain about chromium's role as an osteoporosis preventive, but it certainly looks encouraging.

IMPROVED VISION

The discovery of chromium's effect on vision began with an anecdote told me by a friend, who is not a professional but is intelligent and well informed in scientific and medical matters. The only time he ever read the tabloids was in the barber shop while he was waiting his turn. He would often take the paper with him to the barber's chair in case there might be some additional wait, but his reading would be interrupted when he took his glasses off. After increasing his chromium intake, he noticed that he could continue to read even without his glasses.

As astute as I know my friend to be, I still thought his story apocryphal and told him so. But he had already anticipated that and had searched the scientific literature. To my surprise, he sent me three articles by Ben Lane, an optometrist who had associated low tissue levels of chromium with myopia (nearsightedness). Although Dr. Lane had originally used hair analysis as his means of measuring chromium level (not a very reliable method), when I called him he told me that he had since confirmed his findings using more precise methodology.

Dr. Lane told me it is well established that the ciliary

muscle, the tiny muscle that controls the shape of the lens in the eye (and hence the ability of the eye to focus), is quite dependent on glucose metabolism for energy. Therefore, anything that could improve tissue utilization of glucose would improve the function of the ciliary muscle. I'm sure you've guessed that chromium and insulin fit the job description.

My discussion with Dr. Lane also explained why my friend, who did not have myopia but presbyopia (a form of farsightedness), responded to chromium, even though the papers I had read referred only to myopia. According to Dr. Lane, any improvement in the ability of the lens to change shape can improve vision.

HEALTHIER GUMS: THE HAYNES-THOMAS EFFECT

About two months after increasing his chromium intake, my friend Dr. Charles Thomas, a former professor of biochemistry at Harvard Medical School and now president of the Helicon Foundation in San Diego, told me he had just returned from his dentist who said that his gums were in better condition than they had been in for years. Dr. Thomas avoids talking about himself as much as possible, so I knew he felt this was something significant. Shortly afterward, I heard similar reports from Robin Haynes, Dr. Thomas's administrative assistant, and also from my wife.

After checking with several periodontists and dentists for additional observations and searching the scientific literature for a possible explanation, I found that periodontal disease, one of the most widespread maladies in western society, was more common in diabetics and that it was one of the early signs of impaired glucose tolerance. Increasing chromium intake to improve insulin function could positively affect the health of the gums.

This still doesn't establish a correlation between chromium and gum health in the cases of Dr. Thomas, Ms. Haynes, and my wife, none of whom are diabetic or even insulin-resistant. But I cannot ignore the fact that three people had such similar experiences. My theory is that they all had either borderline chromium nutrition or a slightly increased need for chromium which, when met, manifested itself in better gums.

ACNE

A possible connection between chromium and acne is not based on my personal observations, but primarily on a hypothesis by M. McCarty that appeared in the journal *Medical Hypotheses* in 1984. McCarty reports a communication to him by a physician who had observed rapid improvement of acne in a child treated with high-chromium yeast. Since acne tends to wax and wane on its own, uncontrolled clinical observations such as this need to be treated with skepticism, so McCarty undertook a search of the scientific literature.

McCarty found a number of publications dating as far back as the 1930s indicating that measures that enhance insulin activity may have value in the treatment of acne. In some studies insulin was injected directly into the acne lesions. When tolbutamide, the first oral drug for diabetes was introduced, there were reports that it was effective in treating acne. In another study, although patients with acne didn't have abnormal glucose tolerance tests, their "skin glucose tolerance" was found to be significantly impaired. These studies were inconclusive and this approach to treatment has fallen into disfavor. However, according to Dr. Arthur Balin, a noted dermatologist and biochemist, the data remain interesting because there is a possibility that insulin might improve acne by increasing production of essential fatty acids in the skin. Although we as yet have no clinical trial that documents its effectiveness, we can still develop a mechanism whereby chromium might aid acne as an unexpected and welcome side benefit.

INSOMNIA AND ADDICTION

The topics in this chapter have progressed from most to least documented, and this is the final one.

When we were discussing the ways chromium could enhance weight loss, I mentioned the neurotransmitter chemical serotonin, which can promote a feeling of satiety. Other actions of serotonin include improved sleep and reduced cravings. Insulin (and therefore possibly chromium) aids in the production of serotonin and so might enhance these actions.

You may have heard that the dietary amino acid tryptophan has proven successful in several studies in relieving insomnia. Here's how it works: Tryptophan is a precursor to serotonin, which is the compound that actually induces sleep. For tryptophan to be converted to serotonin, however, it must first enter the brain, a process facilitated by insulin, and therefore potentially enhanced by chromium. (Because there have been several reports recently that tryptophan supplements may cause blood abnormalities and severe muscle aches, until the cause of this is discovered, the Food and Drug Administration has recommended against the use of tryptophan supplements.)

In addition to relieving insomnia, increased serotonin concentrations in the brain have also been associated with reduced craving for nicotine, alcohol, and narcotics. We're leaping a giant theoretical chasm when we suppose that chromium, as a cofactor to insulin which can increase serotonin synthesis, could be effective in the treatment of smoking addiction, alcohol addiction, and drug addiction, but I think it's worthy of some study.

Meanwhile, we'll be happy to settle for building stronger, trimmer bodies, controlling cholesterol, and controlling our blood sugar.

SIX

ADDING CHROMIUM TO YOUR DIET

DIETARY DEFICIENCY OF CHROMIUM

In 1985 Dr. Richard Anderson of the Department of Agriculture Human Nutrition Research Center in Beltsville, Maryland, studied the chromium intake of 32 people on self-selected diets, that is, eating what they normally ate. The participants were selected at random and included 10 males and 22 females from 25 to 65 years old, a representative cross-section of the population. He found that *90 percent of the participants in his study took in less than 50 micrograms of chromium per day, the minimum amount recommended by the National Research Council* (Figure 12). The average dietary intake was about 25 micrograms, only half the recommended minimum; there were almost as many people who consumed less than 10 micrograms per day (a severe deficiency) as there were who consumed 50 micrograms or more.

Dr. Anderson's study is generally considered the most accurate one to date, but other investigations have confirmed the low level of chromium consumption in the United States today. *Therefore, it is highly likely that your diet is deficient in chromium.*

Why does the diet of most Americans contain so little chromium? There are three reasons, the first two of which are related and under our control.

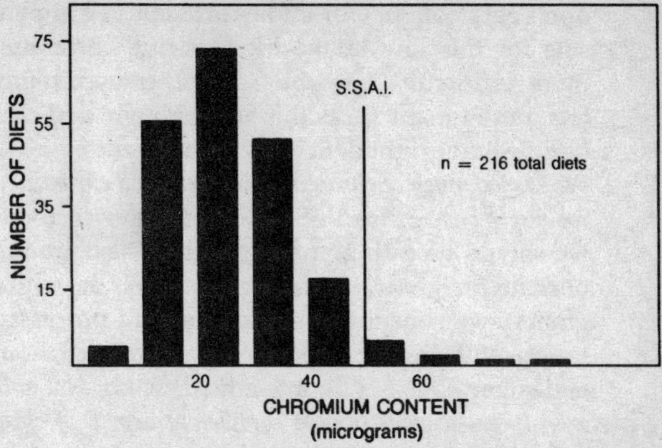

Figure 12. Frequency distribution of dietary chromium intake. Diets from 32 people (10 males, 22 females) were collected for 7 consecutive days (total of 216 diets) and analyzed for chromium. The average daily chromium intake was 33 micrograms for the men and 25 micrograms for the women. Ninety percent of the diets were below 50 micrograms in chromium content, the minimum amount recommended by the National Research Council.

SSAI = suggested safe and adequate intake.

(From R. A. Anderson and A. S. Kozlovsky, Chromium intake, absorption & excretion of subjects consuming self-selected diets, *American Journal of Clinical Nutrition 41:* 1177–1183, 1985.)

1. *We don't eat enough of the foods that are richest in chromium.* The best source of chromium is brewer's yeast, obviously not a staple of the American diet except perhaps as beer (which we will discuss shortly). Other foods high in chromium are organ meats such as liver and kidney, which are too high in cholesterol to be eaten regularly, no matter how much chromium they contain. Whole grains—whole wheat and buckwheat, for example—also contain moderate amounts and, while the consumption of these has been increasing, we still

don't eat enough. Our bodies attempt to compensate for this low intake by digesting chromium more efficiently, absorbing more and excreting less, but in many cases this isn't enough, and borderline or outright deficiency is the result.

2. *We eat too much of chromium-deficient and chromium-robbing foods.* Instead of the chromium-rich foods we should be eating, many of which also are important for general good health (such as whole grains), we consume large amounts of processed foods, with high concentrations of refined flour and sugar. This is a double-edged sword. *Not only are processed foods almost completely devoid of chromium, but they deplete the body's precious chromium supply.*

   The large amount of sugar in processed foods stimulates the release of insulin to help metabolize the sugar. Of course, insulin's essential cofactor, chromium, is also mobilized. This chromium, once summoned, cannot be reused and is excreted in the urine. In the average American diet up to 25 percent of calories come from simple sugars, so this depletion cycle is quite important. *It has been demonstrated that diets high in simple sugars (35% of the total calories) stimulate urinary chromium losses up to 300* percent, as compared with a more sensible diet consisting of only 10% simple sugars.

3. *We may eat foods grown on low-chromium soil.* Many of the vitamins and minerals we need to sustain life are also required by plants to grow. Therefore, when we eat the plants directly or consume the animals that foraged on the plants, we consume the plants' supply of these nutrients.

But there are some nutrients essential for humans that aren't required by plants. The plants will grow well whether the nutrients are present in the soil or not. If the nutrients happen to be present, the plants will accumulate them as they grow. If the nutrients are not in the soil, they will not be present in the plant tissue.

Three minerals fall in this category—iodine, selenium, and chromium. Iodine has been studied for more than a hundred years, and the iodine-rich and iodine-poor soils of the world have been mapped out. It was discovered that several areas in the United States had iodine-poor soil and to compensate table salt was fortified with iodine. The incidence of goiter (a result of iodine deficiency) declined markedly in these areas, but goiter remains common in other parts of the world, such as India, where iodine deficiency still exists.

Selenium has been studied less, but we know that the soil content throughout the world is variable. Just as with iodine, health problems have been associated with the selenium content of the soil. In China, for example, a rare form of heart disease called Keshan's disease has been attributed almost entirely to selenium deficiency in the soil of just a few provinces.

Chromium, the new kid on the block of essential nutrients, has hardly been studied at all in this manner. While it is known that there are differences in soil content from region to region, the high-chromium and low-chromium areas haven't been well identified yet. Of course, the important thing to know is where your food was grown, not whether your house sits on chromium-rich soil. With modern technology and transportation, the food you buy in the supermarket could have originated almost anywhere.

In contrast with the first two reasons most of our diets are deficient in chromium—what we don't eat enough of and what we eat too much of—the chromium content of the soil in which our food is grown is not really under our control. But it is another cause of the widespread dietary deficiency of chromium.

CHROMIUM DEPLETION: THE ATHLETE'S DILEMMA

As common as dietary deficiency of chromium is, there is another factor we must contend with to assure ourselves of good chromium nutrition—*chromium depletion.* We've already mentioned that eating highly processed foods is one way our bodies can lose chromium, and there are others as well.

John, a patient of mine, is a man after my own heart—a dedicated runner. He is a successful newspaper executive but still finds time to run 70 miles a week and compete in races two or three times a month. John is also committed to good nutrition and when I first saw him, he had been eating an almost exemplary diet. His complaint was that he frequently felt tired. Although 70 miles of running a week sounds like enough to make anyone tired, John was fit and was not overtraining. He shouldn't have been fatigued.

Diet analysis showed that John was obtaining about 110 micrograms of chromium from his daily food intake, more than double the minimum recommended amount. Under ordinary circumstances, this should have been enough chromium, but I still suggested that John add a chromium supplement to his diet. Several studies have shown that strenuous physical activity, such as running, can deplete the body of chromium. When we exercise, our muscles use carbohydrate for fuel, which requires insulin and chromium for proper metabolism. Urinary excretion of chromium is increased nearly fivefold 2 hours after a strenuous 6-mile run, the excretion rate is about six times greater, and the 24-hour urinary chromium losses are almost twice as high on a run day as on a nonrun day (see table below). Trained athletes tend to lose less chromium after exercising than untrained ones, probably a way our body has of conserving its chromium supply, but chromium depletion still occurs.

EFFECT ON URINARY CHROMIUM EXCRETION OF RUNNING 6 MILES			
	PRERUN	2 HOURS POSTRUN	POSTRUN : PRERUN
Urinary chromium concentration (parts per billion)	0.15	0.72	4.7
Urinary excretion (nanogram/hour)	6.3	31.3	6.3

Adapted from W. W. Campbell and R, A. Anderson, Effects of aerobic exercise and training on the trace minerals chromium, zinc and copper, *Sports Medicine*, 4:9–18, 1987.

Within one month after beginning a chromium supplement, John reported to me that he no longer felt fatigued. His race performance had also significantly improved. I can't be certain whether this was due to a physiological effect of the chromium on carbohydrate utilization during competition, the psychological effect of improved mind set because John simply felt better, or a combination of the two. Dr. Richard Anderson and his colleagues at the United States Department of Agriculture Research Center recently found that chromium is important for the deposition of glycogen (the storage form of carbohydrate) in muscle, so a plausible biochemical mechanism exists. Even though this hasn't yet been demonstrated in humans, Dr. Anderson has stated that he believes that less than optimal chromium nutrition could impair an endurance athlete's performance.

John's increased chromium requirement could have been met by redesigning his diet according to the high-chromium menu plan in this book. But he was already eating quite healthfully and was comfortable with his diet, so in his case a supplement made more sense. Many of the other athlete patients I've seen were eating the typical American high-fat, high-sugar diet. Unlike John, their diets needed total revamping. For them, the Chromium Program menu plan not only provided enough chromium to take care of their athletic needs, but corrected their other dietary deficiencies—and excesses—as well. Each case must be considered individually.

Chromium depletion does not apply only to running, but to all strenuous athletics—bicycling, swimming, aerobic dancing, perhaps even brisk walking. And weight lifting, because more chromium is needed to help build muscle, increases chromium demands as well.

Of course, if you don't exercise, you won't have this "problem," but that's obviously not the solution. We're all aware of the many benefits of regular aerobic and conditioning exercise. Just as you must increase caloric intake when you exercise vigorously in order to keep up with your body's greater metabolic demands, so should you increase chromium intake to match the increased requirement of exercise.

OTHER CAUSES OF CHROMIUM DEPLETION: AGE, STRESS, AND PREGNANCY

Walter is typical of many of my older patients. He was 76, had elevated triglycerides, had mild hypertension, and, although not diabetic, had an abnormal glucose tolerance test and elevated blood insulin levels. In short, he showed the signs of insulin resistance we discussed in Chapter 4. Reducing dietary fat, increasing fiber, restricting salt, and starting a walking program all helped, but Walter's blood test values and blood pressure were still not in the desirable range. It wasn't until I increased his chromium intake, which in his case included a high-chromium diet and a chromium supplement, that all his tests became normal.

Tissue chromium levels are highest in people in their teens and twenties and decline progressively with each succeeding decade. In fact chromium is the only nutritional "heavy metal" (a description of its atomic weight) that shows a continuing decrease in tissues with age.

Although everywhere in the world older people tend to have lower levels of chromium stores than younger ones, there are variations that suggest that the decline might be at least partly avoidable. The tissue chromium levels of people in the Near East, Far East, Africa, and parts of Europe average 2½ to 13 times higher than the levels of people in the United States, at any age. The diets in these regions are higher in chromium and lower in processed foods that deplete chromium, so that even though it appears that depletion does increase with age, a dietary deficiency can be avoided by high chromium intake.

Walter, my patient, had been eating a typical chromium-deficient American diet for most of his life. And now, living alone, he had lost interest in food preparation and was probably eating a diet even more processed and refined (and chromium-deficient) than ever. Since chromium depletion is intimately associated with insulin resistance, it's not surprising Walter had elevated blood pressure and abnormal lab values. Nor was it surprising that replenishing his depleted chromium stores corrected his problems.

Another chromium depleter is stress. Any form of stress increases carbohydrate and protein utilization. Since chromium, as a partner of insulin, is an essential cofactor for these processes, stress can deplete chromium. Although we don't usually characterize it as such, exercise is a form of stress. There are both "good" and "bad" forms of stress, and exercise, unless carried to extremes, is, of course, a "good" form. Other stresses, both good and bad, that increase chromium requirements and can deplete chromium stores include pregnancy, physical trauma (including surgery), severe emotional trauma, and cold.

SUMMARY OF FACTORS CONTRIBUTING TO CHROMIUM DEFICIENCY

- Chromium Deficient Diet
  - Low consumption of foods rich in chromium
  - High consumption of chromium-deficient and chromium-robbing foods (simple sugars and highly processed foods)
  - Consumption of foods grown on low-chromium soil
- Chromium Depletion
  - Increased consumption of refined foods
  - Exercise
  - Aging
  - Stress
  - Pregnancy

So, because of chromium-deficient diets, chromium depletion, or, most likely, a combination of the two, most of us are living with our chromium nutrition in precarious balance. In most cases, if a daily net loss occurs, it will be so small as not to be noticed. But if the loss continues, the long-term consequences could have a decidedly negative effect on health and performance.

HIGH-CHROMIUM FOODS

In spite of some of the barriers to achieving optimal chromium nutrition and maintaining adequate chromium stores, we can achieve these goals with a little thought and careful planning. Being aware of the reasons most diets are chromium-deficient and knowing the factors that deplete chromium are the first steps in that direction. In the next chapter you will be given a complete high-chromium menu plan. But first, let's talk about some of the high-chromium foods. Not only will this help you understand the selections upon which the menu plan is based, but it will help you design your own high-chromium meals.

The table below lists the foods that have the highest concentration of chromium. The foods are listed in descending order according to their chromium content, although amounts differ slightly from analysis to analysis (possibly reflecting the variability of soil chromium). The list is fairly short, although not complete. (You will be introduced to other chromium-containing foods in the menu plan, and you can find the amount of chromium in many foods in Appendix B.) In order to achieve a high-chromium diet, you need to combine the chromium-rich ingredients listed here into an interesting variety of palatable preparations. And that is exactly what the menu and recipe section of this book will do for you.

Brewer's yeast is by far the richest source of chromium. Baker's yeast and brewer's yeast are different forms of the same yeast organism. Baker's yeast is used as a leavening agent; brewer's is used in preparing beers and ales and, in a dried form, as a nutritional supplement. The two are not interchangeable. Some people are concerned about sensitivity or allergy to both brewer's and baker's yeast and try to eliminate both from their

FOODS HIGHEST IN CHROMIUM

- Brewer's yeast
- Dried liver and kidney
- Cracked wheat
- Wheat bran
- Whole wheat
- Wheat germ
- Cornmeal
- Buckwheat
- Molasses
- Apples (skin)
- Beer
- Prunes
- Cheese
- Clams
- Melon
- Mushrooms
- Lobster
- Shrimp
- Spices and herbs (pepper, thyme)

diet. I share the opinion of many physicians that yeast sensitivity does exist, but that it is not common. It seems to be a currently popular "*wastebasket*" diagnosis for vague symptoms for which no other explanation is immediately apparent.

It's unlikely you consume much brewer's yeast. If you haven't tried it, you will be pleasantly surprised by its nutty taste and the many ways it can be combined with other foods (especially as recommended in the Chromium Program). You might want to consider consuming some of it as beer. The brewer's yeast used in the brewing process makes beer and ale a good source of chromium. There are differences in the amount of chromium from brand to brand, probably as a result of slight differences in the brewing process. The most comprehensive study found that Carling's Black Label, a brand available mostly in the northeast, is highest in chromium. Some other regional and nationally available beers that contain relatively high amounts of chromium are National Bohemia, Moosehead, Schaefer, Miller, Miller Light, and Pabst.

What about nonalcoholic beers? Although I know of no study documenting this, I suspect they don't contain the high amounts of chromium found in alcoholic beer, since brewer's yeast, used in the fermentation process to make alcohol, isn't employed in making them.

Although liver and kidney have relatively high concentrations of chromium, their high cholesterol content precludes their being included in the Chromium Program. The other foods listed in the table—most whole grains, apples with skin, shellfish, mushrooms, prunes, and cheese—have been incorporated into the Chromium Program menu. Lobster and shrimp are high in cholesterol, but contain almost no saturated fat, so they can be eaten occasionally as part of a healthful diet. Cheeses require more caution, because they contain large amounts of cholesterol and saturated fat.

THE PARADOX OF BIOLOGICALLY ACTIVE CHROMIUM

Over and over you've heard the expression "You are what you eat." Of course, our nutrition is not the only determinant of our condition, but within the context of how nutrition does affect our condition, the expression should more correctly be "You are what you eat, digest, absorb, and deliver to your tissues."

In order for nutrients to affect how the body functions, they must get to the cells in a usable form. This is called *biological activity* and is especially important for minerals, such as chromium, which are never biologically active by themselves. They must be part of a larger molecule.

When it was originally discovered that chromium was necessary for blood sugar control, Mertz and Schwarz knew that chromium was not acting alone to make insulin more efficient, but was part of a larger compound. Although they didn't know the structure of this compound, they called it glucose tolerance factor, or GTF. Since it is now known that chromium also enhances other functions of insulin—control of cholesterol and triglycerides and building of muscle—most scientists have dropped the term GTF in favor of the broader, more descriptive term *biologically active chromium,* or *BAC.* The exact structure of BAC has still to be determined.

Even though the structure of this compound remains elusive, there are ways to test whether any chromium compound or a food that contains chromium possesses biological activity. Most chromium-containing foods have been tested in this way, and it has been found that, for the most part, *there is little relationship between the total amount of chromium a food contains and how much of it is biologically active.* The foods highest in biologically active chromium are listed in the table below.

FOODS HIGHEST IN BIOLOGICALLY ACTIVE CHROMIUM
Brewer's yeast
Beer
Liver
Lobster tail
Shrimp
Whole grains
Mushrooms
Black pepper

If you compare this list with the list of foods highest in chromium (page 44), which indicates whether a food contains significant amounts of chromium regardless of its state of activity, you'll see several foods make both lists. Brewer's yeast not only contains the highest amount of chromium, it is the best source of biologically active chromium. And beer, because its chromium comes from brewer's yeast, also contains appreciable amounts of the biologically active form. But some foods high in total chromium concentration are low in biologically active chromium. Eggs, cheese, and most fruits and vegetables fall in this category.

Of course, while the foods highest in biologically active chromium are emphasized in the Chromium Program menus, this does not mean that these are the only acceptable foods. It would be impossible to design a healthful diet from just this short list, and no amount of chromium could make up for an otherwise unbalanced and nutrient-deficient diet.

CONVERTING CHROMIUM INTO BIOLOGICALLY ACTIVE CHROMIUM

Fortunately, most of us have the ability to convert chromium in foods from a biologically inactive form to the active form. Since the exact structure of biologically active chromium isn't known, we don't know the exact process by which the conversion occurs. But we aren't completely in the dark. Scientists do have some ideas about the structure of this important compound, which might help us construct a diet to enhance the conversion of inactive to active chromium.

About twenty years ago Dr. Mertz postulated that the biologically active chromium molecule was a complex of chromium, niacin, and three amino acids—glycine, cysteine, and glutamic acid. But after several years of unsuccessfully attempting to determine the exact structure of this compound, Dr. Mertz abandoned the effort. Since compounds with roughly this composition have been demonstrated to have biological activity, many scientists still assume that this combination of chromium, niacin, and the three amino acids is the biologically active chromium.

Although I think the evidence is stronger in favor of a structure other than the complex suggested by Dr. Mertz, the menus of the Chromium Program contain adequate amounts of tryptophan (the amino acid dietary precursor of niacin), glycine, cysteine, and glutamic acid. All these amino acids can be obtained from complete protein. Since vitamin B_6 is necessary for the conversion of tryptophan to niacin, care has been taken to ensure the menus contain sufficient amounts of it as well (most dietary surveys have indicated that most American diets are deficient in vitamin B_6).

Dr. Gary Evans believes that chromium picolinate is the biologically active chromium molecule, not the complex suggested by Dr. Mertz. The following points support his suggestion. Chromium picolinate has been isolated from brewer's yeast, the richest source of biologically active chromium. He has demonstrated biological activity for chromium picolinate in humans for all major areas of insulin action; it has lowered cholesterol, reduced blood sugar in diabetics, and enhanced and accelerated muscle development. Dr. Evans has determined the exact structure of chromium picolinate.

It's easy to see why it might be difficult to determine which of the two compounds is the active form (or if, indeed, only one of them is). Picolinic acid, the substance that combines with chromium to form chromium picolinate, is structurally almost identical to niacin and both have the same nutritional building blocks (tryptophan and vitamin B_6). So even though I believe that chromium picolinate is the biologically active chromium, the menus provide for both possibilities.

This discussion of biologically active chromium gives us another item to add to our list of factors affecting chromium nutrition. We now know that it is affected not only by what we eat and how it is depleted, but also by the form in which it is present in the body.

THE ROLE OF CHROMIUM SUPPLEMENTS

If your diet contains adequate amounts of the foods richest in biologically active chromium and foods with inactive chromium and the raw materials necessary to convert it to the active form, in most cases your body will have an adequate supply. But some people in some circumstances might want to take a chromium supplement as well.

I often recommend supplements to people who are at risk for chromium depletion or who have increased demands for chromium. John, my runner patient, was one example. Despite being on a diet high in biologically active and potentially biologically active chromium, he was fatigued, a symptom I thought might be related to chromium depletion. A supplement seemed warranted because of his high level of athletic activity.

Supplements seem appropriate also for older patients. Aging depletes chromium, and it's more difficult for older people to get adequate amounts of chromium in any form. I would certainly recommend that supplements be considered by anyone subject to stress. For example, pregnant women might discuss with their obstetrician a supplement to compensate for the chromium depletion that occurs with pregnancy.

Another group who should consider a supplement are diabetics and hypoglycemics. For reasons as yet unknown patients with sugar metabolism problems seem to have difficulty converting inactive into active chromium, even if the necessary raw materials are present. This makes it more difficult to design high-chromium diets for them that are also nutritionally balanced, so I frequently recommend supplements.

Then there are those who seem unable or unwilling to change old eating habits enough to follow the menu plan in the Chromium Program. Tom is just such a patient. A professional photographer, he leads a hectic life, working irregular hours, traveling frequently, and more often than not eating on the run. Both my dietitian and I have shown him how he can fit the high-chromium diet into his pattern of activity, and Tom always promises, but never changes. Although I may not approve of this behavior, it's my job to help patients. My only choices are to let him continue his chromium-deficient diet or to suggest a supplement.

Finally, we must take individual differences into account. The late Dr. Roger Williams of the Clayton Institute of Biochemistry at the University of Texas pioneered the concept of biochemical individuality, which is, simply put, that no two people have the identical biochemistry. Although the recommended dietary amounts of most vitamins and minerals are calculated to take a range of individual requirements into account, they are not necessarily the optimal amounts for any one individual. Also, even if someone is not diabetic, his or her individual biochemistry might be inefficient in converting inactive to active chromium. Such a person might well benefit from a chromium supplement.

The menu plan of the Chromium Program should work well for most people. However, if one or more of the special circumstances we've just discussed apply to you, you might want to discuss with your physician the possibility of adding a chromium supplement.

CHOOSING A SUPPLEMENT

There are many different types of chromium supplements. Which is best?

The most commonly available, and the cheapest, are the inorganic chromium supplements, usually sold as chromium chloride. Products labeled "natural trivalent chromium" may sound special, but they are usually just chromium chloride.

Chromium chloride is not biologically active, so it must be converted into the active form in the body. Just as with chromium in food, some people can do this, some can't. In addition, inorganic chromium is poorly absorbed, only about 0.5 to 1.0 percent of the amount ingested.

Several clinical studies have demonstrated that inorganic chromium can lower cholesterol and help control blood sugar, but other studies have failed to show such results. This disparity may reflect the inability of some people in these studies to absorb chromium or to convert it into the active form. Because of this possibility, the Food and Drug Administration has stated that there is no rationale for using inorganic chromium in supplements.

You may also see supplements in which chromium is chelated to amino acids. While some feel that this type of compound may be more absorbable than inorganic chromium, the evidence is scanty. The chromium–amino acid complexes are definitely not biologically active, so they, like inorganic chromium, must be converted in the body. They are usually more expensive than inorganic chromium without offering much of an advantage.

High-chromium brewer's yeast tablets are also available. Although biologically active and much more absorbable than other forms of chromium *(about 10 to 25 percent of the amount ingested),* the concentration is comparatively low (despite the label high-chromium), so several large tablets must be taken. And, there is the question of yeast sensitivity for some people.

The newest form of supplement, and the one I think is best, is chromium picolinate. We've already mentioned that chromium picolinate is a good candidate for the true biologically active chromium. It is relatively well absorbed, and it is quite cheap. I've recommended it to many patients and have seen excellent results. I've also heard several reports of its effectiveness from other sources.

Anthony Escobar, a trainer from Salt Lake City, Utah, works with many professional athletes, including several in the National Football League and the National Basketball Association. He feels that chromium picolinate definitely has increased strength and endurance in many of his clients. Although his observations are no substitute for hard scientific data, Tony's years of work with professional athletes make his observations hard to discount. Besides all these reasons, every clinical and laboratory study conducted in the past 5 years on the metabolic effectiveness of chromium—whether on cholesterol, triglycerides, blood sugar, body composition, longevity or osteoporosis—has employed chromium picolinate. And in some studies, chromium picolinate has been pitted head to head with chromium chloride, chromium nicotinate, or both, and has always been demonstrated to be superior.

Lastly, there is chromium polynicotinate. This supplement is loosely based on Dr. Mertz's concept of a

CHROMIUM SUPPLEMENTS		
SUPPLEMENT	DOSE YIELDING 200 MICROGRAMS	BIOLOGICAL ACTIVITY
Inorganic chromium	1 small capsule	–
Chromium-amino acid complex	1 small capsule	–
High-chromium yeast	3–4 large tablets	+
Chromium picolinate	1 small capsule	+
Chromium polynicotinate	1 small capsule	?

chromium-niacin complex as the biologically active form. But, the structure of chromium polynicotinate has never been identified, so you really don't know what you're getting. And, to my knowledge, chromium polynicotinate has never been tested in humans, so we don't know if it has biological activity.

Whichever supplement you choose, don't take more than 200 micrograms. Even though all studies have shown that nutritional chromium is remarkably non-toxic, at this point there is no research indicating that more is necessarily better.

Finally, remember that a supplement should be just that—something taken in addition to the primary source of food intake. Even if you decide to include a supplement in your program, you should still adhere to the high-chromium menu plan. Not only are you about to find out how delicious these meals are, but a supplement can never replace a well-balanced, complete nutritional program.

SEVEN

THE CHROMIUM PROGRAM DIET: EATING YOUR WAY TO A FIRM, LEAN BODY

The Chromium Program has two components, both necessary to achieve the maximum benefits from the mineral. They complement one another and are meant to be used together. The high-chromium diet supplies the requisite amount of chromium, and the exercise plan allows for optimal utilization of the chromium in building muscle, increasing strength and energy, reducing body fat and weight, and lowering cholesterol.

In the next chapter you'll be presented with a six-week menu plan that will provide approximately 200 micrograms of chromium a day from natural sources. There is also an extensive collection of recipes that will allow you to create your own high-chromium meals.

Besides being chromium-rich, the diet plan has been carefully constructed in other ways to help you develop a firm, lean body. It provides the correct percentage of calories from carbohydrates, fats, and protein and supplies the key micronutrients to help you best use these calories in conjunction with the exercise plan.

In addition, the menus and recipes are in accordance with the most up-to-date dietary recommendations for the promotion of health in general.

1. The menus and recipes are low in total and saturated fat content and cholesterol. Healthful monounsaturated fats (from olive oil and canola oil) and

selected polyunsaturated fats (from vegetable oils and fish) are emphasized wherever fat is used; the meals and recipes contain almost no saturated fat at all. Although there is some cholesterol (primarily from shellfish, which is a good source of chromium), the total amount is still far below the American Heart Association's (AHA) recommendation of less than 300 milligrams per day. Besides, it is well recognized that saturated fat can elevate blood cholesterol levels much more than dietary cholesterol itself.

3. Also in accordance with AHA recommendations, the diet plan is low in total sodium content, much less than 3 grams per day.
4. The menus and recipes are high in complex carbohydrates and fiber, both soluble (from legumes and fruit, to help control cholesterol and blood sugar) and insoluble (from whole grains and vegetables, to add bulk to the intestinal contents). The chromium content and the proper amounts and types of fat and fiber work together to aid in the reduction of serum cholesterol and moderation of blood sugar levels.
5. The menus and recipes include many fruits and vegetables that are rich in beta carotene (for example, carrots, melon, spinach, romaine lettuce, and vegetables in the cabbage family such as broccoli). Beta carotene is believed to help protect against a variety of cancers.
6. Although designed to ensure adequate intake of a few specific nutrients, the menus provide the recommended dietary allowances (RDA) for all vitamins and minerals. The Chromium Program diet is a diet for complete good health.

This diet plan has several features that will make it easier for you to increase muscle and lose fat and that will make it easier for you to incorporate the menus into your eating habits. So, before beginning to prepare and savor these meals, take some time to familiarize yourself with the highlights of the plan.

GROUPS BASED ON PHYSICAL ACTIVITY

While everyone on the Chromium Program has as goals the loss of body fat and increased strength, different people engage in different amounts and types of physical activity. Menus are designed for three different groups of people to take these differences into account. So, to begin, place yourself in the appropriate group.

Group I includes most of us—active people who are interested in being fit and in increasing strength and endurance for everyday activity and occasional athletics. You belong in this group if you engage in athletic activity, such as walking, low-impact aerobics, or tennis, up to three times a week. Even though your life-style is far from sedentary, athletics are not as much a part of your life as they are for those in groups II and III. (If you feel that your present level of activity doesn't even justify inclusion in this group, consider yourself part of it anyway. Adhering to the exercise component of the Chromium Program will qualify you for membership in group I.)

Group II members are the endurance athletes: runners, swimmers, cyclists, cross-country skiers, scullers, triathletes, and anyone who performs aerobics just about every day. Although group II is defined to include competitive athletes, such as runners who race at least once a month, participation in competitive events is not an absolute criterion for inclusion. For instance, my wife Liz and I are both in this group even though we don't compete much any more. I run an average of 5 to 6 miles a day six times a week, run 10 to 12 miles on Saturday (my "positive" addiction), and weight train three or four times a week. Liz runs, swims, or takes an aerobic class every day and supplements with weights three times weekly. So, if aerobic exercise is part of your daily life and you take it seriously, put yourself in this group even if you don't compete regularly.

Group III are the body builders and anyone trying to "bulk up," such as some football players, boxers, and wrestlers. Members of this group work out with heavy weights almost every day, compete in body building contests, or compete in college or professional sports. There should be no question as to whether you belong in group III; to paraphrase J. P. Morgan, if you have to ask, you're not in this group.

BODY FAT VERSUS BODY WEIGHT

Since our primary goal is loss of fat and increase of lean muscle, the caloric requirements have been developed from the basic premise that *all members of each group have a specific desirable level of body fat—not weight.* The only variable for body fat within each group is sex (men inherently have more muscle and less fat than women, so their target body fat percentage will be lower).

Our central purpose is toning and firming rather than shedding pounds, but if losing weight is one of your goals you will almost certainly accomplish that as well on the Chromium Program. Even though muscle weighs more than fat, recall that the athletes on a weight-training program in Dr. Gary Evans's study lost weight at the same time they increased muscle and decreased fat (see Chapter 3). The reasons for this aren't perfectly clear—it may be that chromium increases metabolism in adipose tissue even more than in muscle tissue—but whatever the reason, it happened for Gary's subjects and probably will for you, too.

DETERMINING BODY FAT PERCENTAGE

As we're more concerned with loss of fat and inches than pounds, our aim is a specific body fat percentage, not a specific weight. A person might be within an "ideal" weight range, yet have too much body fat, and, conversely, someone who is well-muscled might be "overweight."

Before going any further, you should estimate your body fat percentage. There are many methods of determining body fat, but for our purposes the following method will more than suffice. (If you are interested in more sophisticated techniques, see Appendix C.)

Dr. Jack Wilmore, an exercise physiologist at the University of Texas, has devised a procedure that requires only a tape measure, scale, and special chart. Men and women follow the same procedure but use different charts and measurements. Men tend to deposit fat around the abdomen (so-called abdominal fat distribution) and women around the hips (gluteofemoral fat distribution). This accounts for the difference in determining body fat.

For men, weigh yourself first thing in the morning. Then measure your waist at the exact level of the belly button. Using a straight edge, draw a line on the chart (Figure 13) between your waist measurement and your weight. The point where this line intersects the percent fat scale is a reasonably close approximation of your body fat.

For women, measure your hips at their widest point. Using a straight edge, draw a line on the chart (Figure 14) between your hip measurement and your height (not your weight). The point where the line crosses the percent fat scale is your body fat.

Men should have between 10 and 18 percent body fat and women between 17 and 25 percent. The "average" man has more than 20 percent fat and the "average"

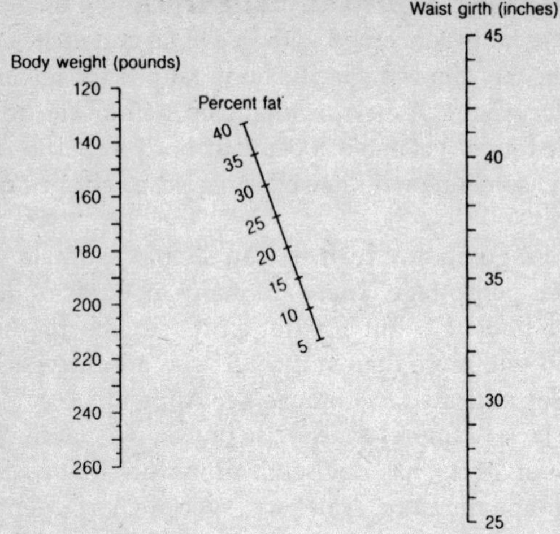

Figure 13. Estimation of relative fat in men from body weight and waist circumference.

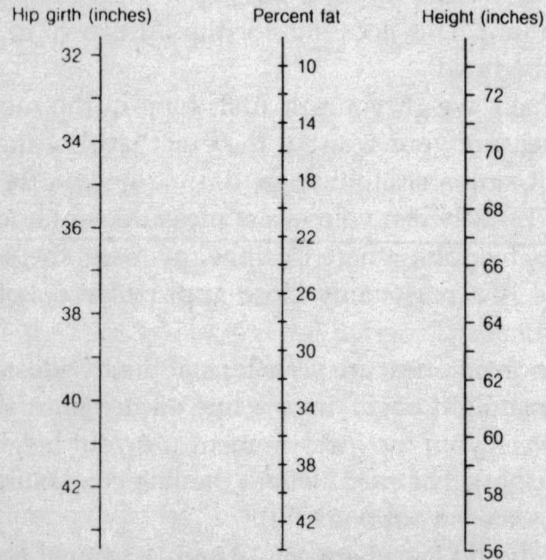

Figure 14. Estimation of relative fat in women from height and hip circumference.

woman more than 30 percent (see the table on pages 84–86).

PROTOTYPES FOR EACH GROUP

Within the context of body fat percentage, prototypes for each of the three groups have been developed. Don't be concerned if your present body fat doesn't match the prototypes, because we're going to discuss how to tailor your diet so that you will reach that goal.

For group I, the ideal prototype male has 17 percent body fat, well below the average percentage but by no means an unrealistic number. The Chromium Program diet and exercise plans will make that percentage easy to attain.

If your body fat already measures 17 percent, the diet and exercise plans will make it simple for you to maintain that level. However, even if your body fat exceeds 17 percent, *you will eat as though you've reached your goal and follow the same diet as those already at 17 percent body fat.* This concept, called *"life at goal weight,"* was developed and used successfully by Dr. Gilbert Kaats, a weight control and fitness expert in San Antonio, Texas.

Although we've assigned a weight of 160 pounds to our group I male with 17 percent body fat, you don't have to try to reach that goal. For every group weight is dependent on other factors, such as height and bone structure, and is not our main focus. *The primary aim of* The Chromium Program *is to help you become healthier and look better, and as long as you reach (and maintain) 17 percent body fat, your weight will automatically be within an acceptable range.*

The prototype group I female has 22 percent body fat. (Remember, women have higher body fat content than men, so the higher percentage doesn't mean women in this group are less fit than men.) As with the men, whatever your actual body fat was determined to be on the

PERCENT BODY FAT FOR DIFFERENT REFERENCE GROUPS

MALES	BODY FAT PERCENTS	FEMALES
Lowest male measured	3	
Gymnasts, wrestlers	4	
Medically unsafe for most males	5	
Swimmers, body builders (finalists)	6	Lowest female measured
Basketball centers	7	
Cross-country skiers	8	
Racquetball players	9	
Basketball forwards, soccer players	10	Average for female anorexic patients
Distance runners, defensive backs	11	
Basketball guards, linebackers	12	
Offensive backs	13	
Basketball players, quarterbacks	14	Gymnasts
"Ideal" fit male, maximum for professional athletes	15	Racquetball players
Average 25-year-old in an exercise program	16	
Power lifters, shot putters, discus throwers	17	Aerobic dance/ jazzercise instructors

PERCENT BODY FAT *(Continued)*

MALES	BODY FAT PERCENTS	FEMALES
Average 35-year-old in an exercise program	18	Cross-country skiers
Maximum percent before coronary risk factors begin	19	Swimmers, average 25-year-old in an exercise program
Military's "desired" percent for males (all ages)	20	Tennis players, Alpine skiers
Average 45-year-old in an exercise program	21	Hurdlers, basketball players, volleyball players
Military's maximum allowable percent for 21- to 27-year-olds	22	"Ideal" fit female, maximum for professional athletes
Average 55-year-old (or older) in an exercise program	23	Average 35-year-old in an exercise program
Military's maximum allowable percent for 28- to 39-year-olds	24	Maximum percent before coronary risk factors begin
Average or typical American male at age 35	25	Average 45-year-old in an exercise program
Military's maximum allowable percent for 40 years and up	26	Military's desired percent for females (all ages)
Classified as morbidly obese	27	

PERCENT BODY FAT *(Continued)*

MALES	BODY FAT PERCENTS	FEMALES
	28	Military's maximum allowable percent for 17- to 20-year-olds
	29	Average 55-year-old in an exercise program
	30	Military's maximum allowable percent for 21- to 27-year-olds
	31	Average 65-year-old in an exercise program
	32	Military's maximum allowable percent for 28- to 39-year-olds
	33	Average for typical American female at age 35
(Athletic groups are world class or professional levels)	34	Classified as morbidly obese
	35	Military's maximum allowable percent for 40 years and up

Source: Dr. Gilbert R. Kaats.

chart, follow the "life at goal weight" concept and use the menus as if you already were at 22 percent—because you soon will be. We have assigned a weight of 125 pounds to our ideal prototype woman in this group, but this need not be your ideal weight, as long as you reach and maintain 22 percent body fat.

Group II, composed of endurance athletes, will be lighter and leaner than group I, but the same principles apply. The prototype group II male has much lower body fat than the group I prototype—only 11 percent. If you were correct in placing yourself in this group, your estimation according to the chart probably came close to that number. It's all right to be a little higher than the target percentage, but if you're higher than about 15 to 16 percent, perhaps group II is not the correct classification for you; group I may be more appropriate, at least until your fitness level improves. Remember, even if they don't compete regularly in endurance events, members of group II are serious athletes, which is why most men in this group are probably already quite close to 11 percent body fat.

We've assigned a weight of 150 pounds to our ideal prototype group II male, but, in keeping with our principle that body fat is what's important, it is the 11 percent body fat, not a particular weight, that should be your goal.

The prototype group II female has 17 percent body fat. We've assigned 120 pounds to the ideal prototype. As we've said before, concentrate on reaching and maintaining the ideal body fat percentage and the weight will take care of itself. If you belong in this group, your body fat is probably already close to 17 percent. If you're more than a few percent above 17 percent, perhaps you belong in group I for a while.

Better than any other, members of group III illustrate the concept we've been emphasizing—that body composition is what's important, not weight. If you're in this group, you almost certainly are heavier than groups I and II, but probably are leaner than either of them as well. This does not imply that group III is the ideal body type—that's an individual decision—but this group does demonstrate that a person can be much heavier than the standard height-weight charts and still have a low percentage of body fat.

Our prototype group III man has 9 percent body fat, a low amount but fairly typical of serious body builders and some football players and wrestlers. The weight of the prototype group III man is more than the other groups, about 180 pounds, but, as with the weights for groups I and II, this can vary according to height and frame and shouldn't be a main consideration.

The prototype group III woman is also leanest and heaviest of all the groups. She has 14 percent body fat and we've chosen 135 pounds as the average ideal weight.

The following table summarizes the target body composition (percent fat) for males and females in the three groups. Remember, although weight loss is likely on the Chromium Program, *the goal is fat loss and muscle gain.* The number of calories in the menus and their specific breakdown into carbohydrates, protein and fat—in conjunction with the exercise plan—have been formulated to help you achieve your ideal body composition.

MEN		WOMEN	
GROUP	BODY FAT	GROUP	BODY FAT
I	17%	I	22%
II	11%	II	17%
III	9%	III	14%

EXERCISE PLAN FOR GROUPS

The different body fat goals for the three groups are a reflection of the type and amount of exercise members of the groups perform. Specific exercises—what to perform and how to perform them—will be covered in detail in Chapter 9.

Group I will follow the weight training regimen three or four times a week and also perform some form of aerobic exercise three or four times per week. Each exercise session will be about 30 to 40 minutes.

Group II will exercise every day or at least six days a week. Since members of this group are endurance athletes, they will run (or its equivalent) 35 miles or more per week. In addition they will follow the weight training regimen for 20 to 30 minutes six times a week.

Group III already weight trains six or seven days a week, for at least 1 hour each day. They will continue this regimen and add 30 minutes of aerobic exercise three or four times a week.

DETERMINING CALORIC REQUIREMENTS

In determining the caloric requirements for each of the groups, we used a formula developed by Dr. Oliver Owen of Temple University Medical Center in Philadelphia. He studied many men and women of different body compositions and devised a formula that takes body fat into account in evaluating caloric needs. Actually, it is the lean body mass, not the fat, that is the most important factor in determining caloric needs, because, as we mentioned earlier, the more lean tissue a person has, the more calories the person burns. However, one measurement is dependent upon the other, since lean body mass is everything in the body except fat; in other words, lean mass equals total body weight minus body fat. We used some of Dr. Owen's findings in deciding the caloric needs for our three groups and added an exercise factor to his formula.

Most menu plans or diets simply assume that the average person burns 14 to 15 calories per pound, without taking into account body fat percentage and level of activity. The Chromium Program is designed to provide the optimal intake for firming and toning the body, so not only have all the elements that could affect this been addressed, they have been individualized as well. Even though determination of caloric requirements and caloric expenditure is still somewhat inexact, this program is more precise and up-to-date in that area than any you'll encounter. Based on the target body fat percentage and the exercise factor, the daily caloric requirements for the prototypes in the groups are as follows:

	GROUP I	GROUP II	GROUP III
Females	1,550–1,600	1,800–1,850	2,050–2,100
Males	2,050–2,100	2,300–2,400	2,700–2,800

After a while, as you become more and more comfortable with the Chromium Program and more in harmony with how your body works, you will become (as my friend Dr. George Sheehan says) the "good animal," that is, you'll almost intuitively know how many calories you require for your target body fat and your daily activity. For now, though, use the following guidelines as an aid.

Within a group, not everyone will need the same number of calories every day. All members of the group will have the same range of body fat percentage as their goal, and all will do about the same amount of exercise, but they will differ in weight (mostly because of height and frame size) and in daily nonexercise activity (because of life-style).

This means that not everyone within a group will eat

the same portion sizes. As it would make the menus too crowded to list all these possible variations, *the portion sizes are given for the prototype male and female.* The portions for males are listed first; any difference for females follows the item and is designated "F." Since caloric intake is higher for males, most of the changes for females are omissions. (Remember, group I prototype males weigh 160 pounds, females 125; group II males weigh 150 pounds, females 120; group III males weigh 180 pounds, females 135). If you feel your ideal weight is more or less than the prototypes (and can still reach and maintain the target body fat for your group), increase or decrease your portion sizes accordingly.

To allow for adjustments for individual differences, the calories were set for prototypes who are relatively inactive except when doing the exercises on the Chromium Program. If you are otherwise active throughout the day (for example, if you're a mother with small children, a salesperson, or anyone else who does not sit at a desk most of the day), you may want to increase your portion sizes to satisfy your increased caloric requirements.

In all cases, if you deviate from the portions recommended for the prototypes, let your body fat—estimated by the chart in this chapter or by some of the other methods described in the next chapter—be your guide. If it reaches and stays at the target for your group, you know you've estimated your caloric requirements correctly.

CARBOHYDRATES, FATS, AND PROTEIN

The breakdown of calories into the right proportions of macronutrients—carbohydrates, fats, and protein—is as important as the number of calories we consume. Not only does this affect our exercise performance and the ability to lose fat and build muscle, but our overall health as well.

It is now well accepted by almost all health authorities that the consumption of complex carbohydrates from grains, fruits, and vegetables is important for good health. Besides being the primary fuel for exercise (which gives us a special interest in them), carbohydrates are the best source of fiber. You've undoubtedly heard of the benefits of both soluble fiber (control of cholesterol and blood sugar) and insoluble fiber (increased bulk of intestinal contents with reduced risk of digestive diseases).

The U.S. Senate Select Committee on Nutrition has advised that Americans consume approximately 55 percent of daily calories from carbohydrates and that at least 45 percent of these calories be complex, with the remainder from simple sugars. But, these recommendations don't take into account the amount needed for exercise, so all groups in the Chromium Program will derive more of their daily calories from carbohydrates than recommended by the government.

Group I will get about 60 percent of their calories from carbohydrates. Groups II and III, who will be exercising more, not only need more calories than Group I, but need a little more of them as carbohydrates. Each of these groups will derive about 65 percent of their daily calories from complex carbohydrates. With all three groups, almost all the carbohydrates will be the more healthful complex carbohydrates.

The U.S. Senate Select Committee on Nutrition and the American Heart Association recommend that we get no more than 30 percent of our daily calories from fat and that this should be divided equally among saturated, monounsaturated, and polyunsaturated fats. As you know, saturated fat is associated with increased serum cholesterol (and hence increased risk of cardiovascular disease) and some forms of cancer as well; monounsaturated and polyunsaturated fats are considered much more healthful. The Chromium Program uses almost no saturated fat; almost all fat is monounsaturated (olive oil, canola oil) or polyunsaturated (the oil in fish). And, even though the fat is the "good" kind, the total amounts are below the government and American Heart Association maximum recommendations.

Those in group I will derive about 25 percent of their daily calories from fat. Since groups II and III are consuming a higher percentage of carbohydrates, the percentage of calories from fat is reduced; it is only 20 percent of daily caloric intake.

PROTEIN

The U.S. Senate Select Committee on Nutrition recommends that we get 12 to 15 percent of daily calories from protein. It is rare to find someone who doesn't exercise intensely who is deficient in protein, but some athletes may need more than was previously thought.

Recent research, primarily by Dr. Peter Lemon at Kent State University, has determined that both strength training and endurance training may increase protein requirements by 50 percent. Although carbohydrate is the main fuel, up to 15 percent of energy for exercise can come from amino acids, the building blocks of protein. If they are not replaced, not only won't we be able to increase lean body mass, we may actually lose some muscle.

Most weight lifters have gone overboard on protein, however, consuming as much as 25 to 30 percent of daily calories from protein. This does them no good and most likely can do harm. Several studies have shown an association between excessive protein intake and risk of osteoporosis, cancer, heart disease, and kidney disease.

Anyone attempting to increase muscle mass needs

protein to build tissue. The key is to consume enough to support both endurance exercise and muscle development, but not so much as to increase risk for any ill effects. Although both groups II and III need more protein than group I, this should not be an increased *percentage* of calories as protein. The National Research Council's recommended dietary allowance (RDA) of protein is 0.8 to 1.0 grams per kilogram of body weight. Since groups II and III will be consuming more calories than group I, the absolute amount of protein intake will increase sufficiently to meet their needs without any increase in the percentage of calories as protein.

Some research indicates that protein needs for groups II and III may even be a little higher. However, since much of the protein in the Chromium Program diet is high-quality protein (a better balance of amino acids and utilized by the body more efficiently) less is needed to achieve the same important protein balance.

Chief among these high-quality proteins is whey (found in the products Diet Fuel and Twinfast), the portion of milk that remains after another protein, casein, is precipitated, as in the manufacture of cheese. Whey is made of proteins called lactalbumin, which have the highest biological value of any protein and recently have even been shown to have an immune-stimulating effect. As heavy exercise may slightly suppress the immune system, this could potentially be helpful to groups II and III.

Albumin, from egg whites, is also used frequently as a protein source in the Chromium Program and is close behind whey protein in biological quality. Fish, legumes, and lean meat provide high-quality protein as well.

CONVENIENCE IN THE MENU PLAN

The menus and recipes in the Chromium Program have been devised for superior nutrition and to help you achieve the results you want, but with equal emphasis on the esthetics of eating. For most of us dining is and should be a pleasurable experience. With that in mind, the Chromium Program menu plan, unlike the spartan meals in most diets, has been designed to fuel your soul as well as your workouts.

The menus and recipes in the Chromium Program are original and delicious, but you're not going to have to spend hours in the kitchen to prepare them. We certainly don't want to dissuade you if you love to dice, grind, and chop. Cooking for some people is a creative activity, and you'll have an opportunity here to exercise your artistic muscles. But most people don't like to or aren't able to spend a good part of every day in the kitchen. Liz, who created these menus, truly enjoys developing her culinary talents, but can spare the time only a few days a week and the same assumption has been made for you.

You're going to be spending some time every day exercising and putting chromium to work to help shape your body, lower your cholesterol, and control your blood sugar. And, of course, you also have the rest of your life to live. While the diet and exercises of the Chromium Program are going to take commitment, the real point of the program is to enhance your life, not intrude upon it.

To that end, the diet plan incorporates two important features: the use of leftovers and the use of ready-made products. Liberal use is made of leftovers, but not at the expense of taste. Many of the recipes are calculated to yield more servings than you need for a meal, and you will be instructed to save the extra portions for another lunch or dinner later. In almost all cases the leftovers aren't used as the same meal reheated, but are transformed in creative ways.

Several superior-tasting, ready-made products that are rich in chromium and other nutrients are recommended. If you haven't explored this option before, you're going to be surprised at how easy it is to make healthful and delicious meals using these products. The specific brand names mentioned in the menus and recipes have been chosen for their taste, quality of ingredients, and ease of use. Every one of them has been tested and compared with similar products and has come out on top in its category. Most are available nationwide in either supermarkets or health food stores or can be ordered by you or your store from the manufacturer or distributor. The brand-name products and a few general items with which you may not be familiar are listed in Appendix A, The Chromium Program Food Resource List. The resource list tells where the products can be obtained and gives acceptable alternatives, in case it is too difficult to get the suggested product or you simply prefer another brand.

A FEW WORDS ABOUT BEVERAGES

In order to streamline the menus, specific beverages aren't recommended with each meal. The only ones that are mentioned are orange juice, root beer, optional beer or wine, and wheatgrass juice (all good sources of chromium). (Twinfast shakes and Diet-Fuel are meal substitutes and supplements rather than beverages.) What's best to drink routinely?

There is no question that water is the best liquid to drink and it should be consumed in large quantities. This is especially true in the Chromium Program since you're going to be physically active and will need plenty of water to replenish fluid lost during exercise. Also, the high fiber content of the menus further increases water requirement. Drink tap water, bottled water, or filtered water, according to your taste, but whichever you choose, drink a minimum of six to eight glasses a day.

Coffee and tea are acceptable in moderation. Some research studies have associated increased coffee consumption with elevated cholesterol, although no consensus has been reached on this point. My recommendation is to limit coffee to two cups a day, whether it's regular or decaffeinated (the cholesterol elevation, if it exists, does not seem to be related to the caffeine content but to the kind of bean used). If you like to drink coffee (a morning cup is one of the pleasures of my day), occasionally try Creole coffee—coffee with a little blackstrap molasses. The molasses adds some chromium and the combination has an unusually good taste.

As for soft drinks, avoid the sugar-containing chromium depleters. Unless you're among the small number of people who apparently have a sensitivity to aspartame (Nutrasweet), an occasional sugar-free soda is all right. Best in this category is sugar-free root beer, a reasonably good source of chromium, and we've included it a few times in the menus.

In general, stay away from fruit juices unless they are diluted (with water, seltzer, sparkling mineral water, or salt-free club soda), except for the orange juice as specified in the menus. Undiluted or in larger quantities than we have recommended, they're just too concentrated a source of sugar (even if it's "natural") to drink regularly.

We don't generally think of milk as a beverage, but some people do. It can be a good source of calcium and there's no real objection to it (unless you're lactose intolerant). If you choose to drink milk, make it skim, low fat, or buttermilk, since milk adds not only to the nutrients consumed but also to the calories, fat, and cholesterol.

CHOREOGRAPHING YOUR DAYS AND WEEKS

Just as no one portion size can be right for everyone, neither can one menu plan. The menus are meant as guidelines and suggestions to enable you to incorporate delicious, high-chromium, nutrient-rich meals into your diet. They needn't be followed to the letter as long as you learn to stay close to the nutritional values they are designed to provide.

Alter the meals according to your schedule—workouts, business activities, family routine. For example, snacks in the morning and afternoon are recommended for group III. If this doesn't coincide with your schedule, you can omit one of the snacks and try to make up the calories and nutrients at another time, either by having more at the remaining snack or adding to one of your meals.

The lunches were generally designed to be convenient whether you eat home most days or are away from home. Suggestions are given for eating lunch out and for take-out food. Obviously, you can alter this to fit your own schedule.

Almost certainly there will be some recipes and meals that you prefer to others. If so, substitute whenever you feel like it. For breakfast especially, many people (myself included) enjoy eating the same thing practically every day. With the exception of eggs, do this as you desire. And, of course, you can switch the recipes around, creating your own menus.

We find it easier, and you may too, to order or prepare certain essential ingredients in quantity and in advance. For example, you're going to be introduced to fromage blanc, a delicious nonfat, spreadable cheese. Since you'll most likely use this product quite often, order as much as your freezer will accommodate. Some greens and herbs are good sources of chromium, especially when fresh. Fresh spinach, basil, parsley, and others can be stored in the freezer, so you'll have them when you want them, even if they are out of season. Finally, you can make foods such as muffins (either the high-chromium and quick chromium), spreads (such as the high-chromium spread and half-the-fat hummus), and treats (such as high-chromium gingers) in large quantities to last for several meals or several days. It's always a good idea to read through the menus a week or two in advance so you can arrange your time and effort in the most convenient and enjoyable way for the best results.

EIGHT

THE CHROMIUM PROGRAM DIET: MENUS AND RECIPES

Information about specific brand names and unfamiliar products is given in the Resource List in Appendix A.

MENUS

GROUP I

WEEK 1

Sunday

BREAKFAST (BRUNCH)

2 buckwheat pancakes ✪ with 4 ounces fromage blanc and 1 tablespoon blackstrap molasses (sulfured or unsulfured—see Resource List)

1 Alvarado Street Bakery sprouted wheat bagel with 1 slice of smoked salmon, 1 slice sweet onion, and 1 tablespoon Fromage Blanc (F: ½ bagel, ½ slice lox, 1 teaspoon Fromage Blanc)

½ melon (F: ¼ melon)

½ cup berries

F: portions for women; ✪: recipe included

SNACK

1 high-chromium muffin ✪ with 1 tablespoon Sorrell Ridge conserve *or* 2 high-chromium gingers ✪
1 apple with 1 tablespoon high-chromium spread ✪ and 5 dates (F: omit spread and dates)

DINNER

1 serving corn meal pizza crust ✪ or Grain Dance whole wheat pizza shell with 3 ounces tomato zucchini sauce ✪ (Save leftovers for Monday lunch.)
1 serving corn meal scallops ✪
3 ounces instant Casbah tabouly—follow directions on package but substitute 2 tablespoons olive oil for the amount suggested and add 2 teaspoons balsamic vinegar (F: use 1½ tablespoons olive oil)

Nutritional Information (PER DAY)

	MALE	FEMALE
Calories	2,020	1,570
Carbohydrate g (%)	317 (60)	243 (60)
Fat g (%)	55 (24)	43 (24)
Protein g (%)	83 (16)	68 (17)
Cholesterol mg	210	204
Sodium mg	2,337	1,883
Chromium mcg	219	172

Monday

BREAKFAST

1 high-chromium muffin ✪ with 1 tablespoon de-oiled peanut butter and 1 tablespoon Sorrell Ridge conserve (F: omit peanut butter and conserve)
1 banana
6 ounces skim or 1%-fat milk

LUNCH

1 cup Golden Couscous tomato minestrone soup (F: omit)

1 serving shrimp salad ✪ with wheat sprouts in 1 whole wheat mini pita bread (may use any available sprouts but wheat sprouts preferable) *or* 1 slice leftover corn meal pizza (see Sunday) and Golden Couscous tomato minestrone soup (F: omit soup)

SNACK

1 sliced apple with lemon

4 cups air-popped popcorn with 1 tablespoon grated parmesan cheese and Vegit (F: add 1 tablespoon brewer's yeast)

DINNER

2 ounces whole wheat elbow pasta and ½ cup Kashi pilaf with 1 serving primavera sauce ✪ or 2 tablespoons de-oiled ready-made pesto mixed with 2 ounces fromage blanc (Save leftovers for Tuesday dinner.)

salad of mixed greens, green pepper, mushrooms, and tomatoes with ¼ cup vinaigrette dressing ✪ (F: 1 tablespoon dressing)

3½ ounces mandarin oranges *or* 1 fresh orange

Nutritional Information (PER DAY)

	MALE	FEMALE
Calories	2,169	1,571
Carbohydrate g (%)	340 (60)	256 (62)
Fat g (%)	66 (26)	39 (22)
Protein g (%)	78 (14)	66 (16)
Cholesterol mg	171	171
Sodium mg	1,907	1,290
Chromium mcg	222	245

Tuesday

BREAKFAST

1 cup Shredded Wheat 'N Bran, ¼ cup Fiber One, and ¼ cup Mueslix with 6 ounces skim milk, ½ banana, and 1 teaspoon molasses

LUNCH

1 fresh tomato sandwich ✪

3 cups salad of romaine lettuce, mushrooms, green pepper, cucumber, onion, celery, water chestnuts, and ½ avocado with 2 tablespoons vinaigrette dressing ✪ (F: omit avocado)

1 large sour dill pickle

SNACK

2 high-chromium gingers ✪

1 pear

DINNER

1 serving minestrone alla Burrini ✪ (Save leftovers for Wednesday dinner.)

2 ounces roast chicken stuffed with 1 cup leftover pasta-Kashi mixture (see Monday) roasted in red wine and sage

1 beer (optional) (F: omit)

1 serving frozen shake ✪ *or* 1 slice apple spice cake ✪

Nutritional Information (PER DAY)

	MALE	FEMALE
Calories	2,112	1,690
Carbohydrate g (%)	333 (60)	280 (62)
Fat g (%)	65 (25)	42 (21)
Protein g (%)	87 (15)	80 (17)
Cholesterol mg	82	82

Sodium mg	2,013	1,934
Chromium mcg	213	202

Wednesday

BREAKFAST

1 poached egg
1 slice whole grain, sprouted bread
½ melon *or* 1 orange

LUNCH

1 serving curried chicken and rice salad ✪ with sprouts in 1 whole wheat pita bread
or 1 serving Jaclyn's split pea soup
1 high-chromium muffin ✪

SNACK

4 dates with 1 tablespoon de-oiled peanut butter (F: 1 tablespoon high-chromium spread)
2 whole wheat pretzels

DINNER

2 servings ribollita made with leftover minestrone alla Burrini (see Tuesday) ✪ (F: 1 serving)
salad of dark greens with 2 tablespoons vinaigrette dressing ✪
2 servings acorn squash souffle ✪ (F: 1 serving)

Nutritional Information (PER DAY)

	MALE	FEMALE
Calories	2,052	1,502
Carbohydrate g (%)	309 (57)	228 (57)
Fat g (%)	72 (29)	50 (28)
Protein g (%)	75 (14)	56 (15)
Cholesterol mg	426	362

Sodium mg	1,150	913
Chromium mcg	220	198

Thursday

BREAKFAST

1 Casbah breakfast cup

LUNCH

1 serving Casbah tabouly (follow directions on package but substitute 2 teaspoons olive oil for amount suggested and add 2 teaspoons balsamic vinegar) stuffed in a whole wheat pita with ¼ avocado, diced fresh tomato, and sprouts (F: omit avocado)

SNACK

1 high-chromium muffin ✪
2 cups air-popped popcorn with 1 tablespoon grated Parmesan cheese and Vegit (for F only)
1 apple

DINNER

2 servings whole wheat noodles with peanut sauce ✪ (F: 1 serving)
salad of romaine lettuce with 2 ounces Fromage Blanc–Vegit salad dressing variation ✪
2 ounces seafood (lobster) salad with 2 tablespoons vinaigrette dressing ✪
1 slice apple spice cake *or* 1 serving nonfat yogurt dessert ✪

Nutritional Information (PER DAY)

	MALE	FEMALE
Calories	2,083	1,635
Carbohydrate g (%)	341 (63)	261 (61)
Fat g (%)	54 (22)	43 (23)

Protein g (%)	82 (15)	70 (16)
Cholesterol mg	92	97
Sodium mg	1,640	1,555
Chromium mcg	207	190

Friday

BREAKFAST

4 ounces fresh orange juice
1 cup Shredded Wheat 'N Bran and 1½ tablespoons wheat germ with 6 ounces skim milk and 1 banana (F: ½ banana)
1 slice Food for Life seven-grain sprouted cinnamon raisin toast with 1 tablespoon de-oiled peanut butter and 1 tablespoon sugar-free apple butter (F: omit)

LUNCH (OUT)

1 bowl vegetable or tomato-based soup
3 ounces salmon or fish fillet, poached, broiled, or grilled with lemon, wine, and herbs (F: 2 ounces)
salad of mixed greens and ¼ avocado with 1 tablespoon house dressing

SNACK

4 cups air-popped popcorn with Vegit
1 whole wheat pretzel
1 stick Panda licorice *or* 1 high-chromium ginger ✪ (F: omit)

DINNER

1 baked potato stuffed with 1 serving Fantastic Foods Shells 'n Curry prepared in water instead of oil *or* 1 serving half-the-fat hummus ✪
2 servings Jaclyn's mushrooms and
1 serving grilled broccoli ✪

1 slice apple spice cake ✪ *or* 1 serving frozen shake ✪

Nutritional Information (PER DAY)

	MALE	FEMALE
Calories	2,051	1,633
Carbohydrate g (%)	323 (59)	270 (59)
Fat g (%)	60 (24)	49 (24)
Protein g (%)	94 (17)	77 (17)
Cholesterol mg	45	31
Sodium mg	2,473	2,310
Chromium mcg	254	224

Saturday

BREAKFAST

4 ounces fresh orange juice (F: omit)
½ cup Nutri-Grain wheat flakes and ½ cup sugar-free corn flakes with 1 banana, 6 ounces skim milk, and 1 tablespoon molasses or 1 tablespoon chopped dates (F: ½ banana)

LUNCH

1 serving tuna salad ✪ in 1 whole wheat pita bread
1 baked sweet potato with ¼ cup unsweetened applesauce and ½ teaspoon cinnamon (F: omit)

SNACK

1 high-chromium muffin (F: omit)
1 apple
2 whole wheat pretzels

DINNER (OUT)

1 serving shrimp cocktail *or* 1 serving oysters or clams on half shell
1 serving polenta, plain or with red sauce

1 serving sautéed broccoli raab or sautéed arugula
salad of mixed greens with 2 tablespoons Italian dressing
¼ melon and ½ cup berries *or* 1 serving sorbet
1 beer *or* 1 glass wine (optional)

Nutritional Information (PER DAY)

	MALE	FEMALE
Calories	2,028	1,611
Carbohydrate g (%)	340 (63)	247 (58)
Fat g (%)	54 (22)	49 (25)
Protein g (%)	81 (15)	71 (17)
Cholesterol mg	227	183
Sodium mg	1,486	1,136
Chromium mcg	214	188

WEEK 2

Sunday

BREAKFAST

4 ounces fresh orange juice
1 serving cracked wheat cereal ✪ with 6 ounces skim milk, ½ banana, and 1 teaspoon molasses *or* 1 tablespoon chopped dates

LUNCH

1 ounce low-fat cheese grilled with tomato on 1 Pritikin English muffin
1 package American Grain rice snacks (F: omit)
1 apple (F: omit)

SNACK

4 cups air-popped popcorn with 1 tablespoon grated Parmesan cheese and Vegit

2 high-chromium gingers ✪
1 pear

DINNER

4 ounces amaranth pasta with 2 servings red clam sauce ✪ (F: 2 ounces pasta, 1 serving sauce)
1 serving succotash ✪
salad of romaine lettuce, celery, mushrooms, onions, and carrots with 2 tablespoons vinaigrette dressing ✪

Nutritional Information (PER DAY)

	MALE	FEMALE
Calories	2,082	1,571
Carbohydrate g (%)	342 (63)	254 (62)
Fat g (%)	56 (23)	43 (24)
Protein g (%)	74 (14)	59 (14)
Cholesterol mg	35	21
Sodium mg	1,117	806
Chromium mcg	259	188

Monday

BREAKFAST

½ cup Kashi pilaf made with ½ cup apple juice and ½ cup water and served with 6 ounces skim milk, 1 teaspoon molasses, 1 tablespoon chopped dates *or* a sprinkle of Mueslix
1 slice whole grain toast with 1 teaspoon butter and 1 tablespoon apple butter (F: omit)

LUNCH

1 high-chromium muffin ✪
1 apple
2 cups salad of lettuce, onion, tomato, celery, mushroom, and ½ avocado with 1 tablespoon olive oil and vinegar to taste

SNACK

1 Twinfast shake ✪
½ package American Grain rice snacks

DINNER

2 servings shrimp creole ✪ (Save leftovers for Tuesday lunch.) (F: 1 serving)
1 baked sweet potato with ½ cup unsweetened applesauce and ½ teaspoon cinnamon
2 slices carrot cake ✪ (F: 1 slice)

Nutritional Information (PER DAY)

	MALE	FEMALE
Calories	2,066	1,556
Carbohydrate g (%)	333 (61)	252 (61)
Fat g (%)	52 (22)	42 (23)
Protein g (%)	93 (17)	66 (16)
Cholesterol mg	288	162
Sodium mg	1,834	1,224
Chromium mcg	254	201

Tuesday

BREAKFAST

2 ounces shredded low-fat Swiss cheese melted on 1 Pritikin English muffin (F: 1 ounce cheese, ½ muffin)
¼ melon
1 banana (F: omit banana)

LUNCH

1 serving leftover shrimp creole (see Monday)
1 baked potato with ¼ avocado and Hot Cha Cha! salsa

SNACK

1 high-chromium muffin ✪

4 cups air-popped popcorn with 1 tablespoon grated Parmesan cheese and Vegit

DINNER

2 servings lima casserole ✪

4 ounces whole wheat pasta with 2 servings Nitza's tomato sauce ✪ and 1 additional tablespoon olive oil (Save leftover sauce for Friday dinner.) (F: 2 ounces pasta, 1 serving sauce)

1 ear corn on the cob *or* 1 serving spinach sauté ✪

Nutritional Information (PER DAY)

	MALE	FEMALE
Calories	2,152	1,669
Carbohydrate g (%)	319 (59)	257 (60)
Fat g (%)	94 (17)	72 (17)
Protein g (%)	56 (23)	43 (23)
Cholesterol mg	171	165
Sodium mg	1,713	1,235
Chromium mcg	232	194

Wednesday

BREAKFAST

½ cup sugar-free corn flakes and ½ cup unsweetened Nutri-Grain wheat flakes with 6 ounces skim milk, ½ banana, 1 teaspoon molasses *or* 1 tablespoon chopped dates

LUNCH (OUT)

1 bowl vegetable soup

1 baked potato with 1 tablespoon cocktail sauce (F: add ¼ avocado)

2 ounces turkey with 2 teaspoons mayonnaise, lettuce, and tomato on 2 slices whole wheat bread (F: omit)
1 beer *or* 1 glass wine (optional) (F: omit)

SNACK
1 high-chromium muffin ✪
4 cups air-popped popcorn with 1 tablespoon grated Parmesan cheese, 1 teaspoon brewer's yeast, and Vegit

DINNER
3 ounces grilled tuna
1 serving grilled eggplant ✪
1 serving Casbah tabouly served with 2 teaspoons olive oil and 2 teaspoons balsamic vinegar (Save leftovers for Thursday lunch.)
1 serving frozen shake ✪
2 New Morning honey graham crackers (F: omit)

Nutritional Information (PER DAY)

	MALE	FEMALE
Calories	2,095	1,696
Carbohydrate g (%)	299 (57)	262 (59)
Fat g (%)	60 (26)	48 (24)
Protein g (%)	92 (17)	72 (16)
Cholesterol mg	147	94
Sodium mg	1,727	1,530
Chromium mcg	214	188

Thursday

BREAKFAST
Casbah breakfast cup
1 banana

LUNCH

½ serving leftover Casbah tabouly (see Wednesday), 1 serving half-the-fat hummus ✪, and tomato in 1 whole wheat pita bread

1 serving Golden Couscous tomato minestrone soup (F: omit)

SNACK

4 cups air-popped popcorn with Vegit (for F only)

1 pear (F: omit)

DINNER

1½ servings killer chromium chili ✪ topped with ½ avocado (F: 1 serving chili, ¼ avocado) (Save leftover chili for Friday lunch.)

1 cup cooked short grain brown rice (F: ½ cup)

1 cup green beans, steamed

2 servings Linn's cole slaw ✪ *or* ½ sweet baked potato

Nutritional Information (PER DAY)

	MALE	FEMALE
Calories	2,075	1,573
Carbohydrate g (%)	331 (61)	243 (59)
Fat g (%)	57 (24)	45 (25)
Protein g (%)	83 (15)	64 (16)
Cholesterol mg	33	23
Sodium mg	1,617	840
Chromium mcg	257	212

Friday

BREAKFAST

1 serving cracked wheat cereal ✪ with ½ cup nonfat yogurt, ½ cup unsweetened applesauce, 1 banana, and 1 tablespoon chopped dates (F: omit banana)

LUNCH

1 serving leftover chili (see Thursday) stuffed in a baked potato and topped with 1 ounce melted low-fat cheese and Hot Cha Cha! salsa (F: ½ serving chili on corn tortilla, omit potato)

SNACK

1 high-chromium muffin ✪
1 apple

DINNER

2 ounces amaranth pasta with 1 serving Nitza's tomato sauce ✪ and 1 additional tablespoon olive oil
2 servings rice salad ✪ (F: 1 serving)
1 slice apple spice cake ✪

Nutritional Information (PER DAY)

	MALE	FEMALE
Calories	2,059	1,566
Carbohydrate g (%)	321 (60)	242 (60)
Fat g (%)	60 (25)	45 (25)
Protein g (%)	79 (15)	60 (15)
Cholesterol mg	66	56
Sodium mg	1,300	1,094
Chromium mcg	265	208

Saturday

BREAKFAST (BRUNCH)

1 serving genuine Austin omelette ✪
1 serving hash brown potatoes ✪ (F: omit)
¼ honeydew melon
½ cup blueberries

SNACK

1 pickle wrapped in ½ ounce sliced Alpine Lace or other low-fat Swiss cheese with mustard

1 whole wheat pita bread toasted to chips
1 serving Fromage Blanc–Vegit dip ✪
1 Christopher's Chewie (F: omit)

DINNER

4 turkey kabobs ✪ (F: omit turkey, use 1 tablespoon less olive oil in recipe)
1 serving curried Waldorf salad ✪
1 serving baked rhubarb ✪
1 beer *or* 1 glass wine (optional)
1 cup nonfat frozen yogurt (commercial brand)

Nutritional Information (PER DAY)

	MALE	FEMALE
Calories	2,075	1,485
Carbohydrate g (%)	320 (59)	233 (60)
Fat g (%)	62 (26)	44 (25)
Protein g (%)	86 (16)	60 (15)
Cholesterol mg	276	229
Sodium mg	2,237	2,185
Chromium mcg	248	201

WEEK 3

Sunday

BREAKFAST

3 buckwheat pancakes ✪ *or* 3 pancakes made from Hodgson Mill buttermilk pancake mix using 2 egg whites and 1 cup skim milk, cooked on a nonstick surface, and topped with 2 tablespoons Fromage Blanc and 1 tablespoon molasses *or* maple syrup (F: 2 pancakes)
½ banana
½ cup strawberries

LUNCH

2 ounces low-fat skim cheese grilled with tomato on 1 Pritikin English muffin (F: ½ oz. cheese) *or* fresh tomato sandwich ✪

1 pear (F: omit)

SNACK

4 cups air-popped popcorn with 1 tablespoon grated Parmesan cheese, 1 teaspoon brewer's yeast, and Vegit

1 apple *or* 1 high-chromium ginger ✪

DINNER

3 ounces lean hamburger with 1 tablespoon ketchup from Laurel's Kitchen ✪, onion, mustard, and pickles on 1 whole wheat bun

1½ servings perfect potato salad ✪ (F: 1 serving)

1 package American Grain rice snacks

1 beer *or* 1 glass wine (optional)

Nutritional Information (PER DAY)

	MALE	FEMALE
Calories	2,058	1,586
Carbohydrate g (%)	318 (60)	246 (61)
Fat g (%)	56 (23)	44 (23)
Protein g (%)	87 (17)	68 (17)
Cholesterol mg	221	172
Sodium mg	1,481	1,155
Chromium mcg	220	200

Monday

BREAKFAST

1 serving cracked wheat cereal ✪ with ½ cup plain nonfat yogurt, ½ cup unsweetened applesauce, mixed with 2 teaspoons Sorrell Ridge conserve and 1 teaspoon cinnamon

1 banana (F: omit)

LUNCH (OUT)

1 bowl gumbo (no sausage), mushroom barley, or noncreamy vegetable-based soup
spinach salad with mushrooms and 2 tablespoons Italian dressing (no egg or bacon)
2 large Vienna-type breadsticks (F: omit)

SNACK

⅓ cup Fromage Blanc–Vegit dip ✪ with 1 whole wheat mini-pita bread toasted to chips

DINNER

2 slices vegetable pizza ✪ (F: 1 slice) (Save leftovers for Tuesday lunch.)
1 serving corn salad ✪
1 serving frozen shake ✪
1 New Morning honey graham cracker *or* 1 high-chromium ginger ✪

Nutritional Information (PER DAY)

	MALE	FEMALE
Calories	2,055	1,530
Carbohydrate g (%)	327 (61)	235 (58)
Fat g (%)	60 (25)	49 (27)
Protein g (%)	73 (14)	58 (14)
Cholesterol mg	38	25
Sodium mg	2,206	1,190
Chromium mcg	239	213

Tuesday

BREAKFAST

1 sliced banana with 1 teaspoon high-chromium spread and 1 teaspoon molasses
1 Alvarado Street Bakery sprouted wheat bagel with 1 tablespoon Fromage Blanc thickened
1 pear (F: omit)

LUNCH

1 slice leftover vegetable pizza (see Monday)
1 serving Golden Couscous tomato minestrone *or* 1 cup noncreamy, vegetable-based soup (take-out)

SNACK

1 Christopher's Chewie with dates
1 apple

DINNER

2 servings Tuscan white bean salad ✪ with 1 additional tablespoon olive oil (F: 1 serving)
1 serving grilled eggplant ✪
2 fresh tomato sandwiches ✪ (F: 1 sandwich)

Nutritional Information (PER DAY)

	MALE	FEMALE
Calories	2,082	1,640
Carbohydrate g (%)	327 (61)	260 (62)
Fat g (%)	61 (25)	47 (25)
Protein g (%)	76 (14)	55 (13)
Cholesterol mg	45	29
Sodium mg	1,961	1,678
Chromium mcg	212	203

Wednesday

BREAKFAST

1 high-chromium muffin ✪ with 1 teaspoon molasses
½ banana

LUNCH

1 serving tuna salad ✪, ¼ slivered avocado, and chopped fresh tomato in 1 whole wheat pita bread

SNACK

1 orange

DINNER

1 cup Ambrosino's Manhattan clam chowder ✪
1 serving Casbah tabouly served with 1 tablespoon olive oil and 2 tablespoons balsamic vinegar
2 servings spaghetti alla puttanesca ✪ (F: 1 serving)

Nutritional Information (PER DAY)

	MALE	FEMALE
Calories	2,105	1,599
Carbohydrate g (%)	345 (63)	258 (62)
Fat g (%)	52 (22)	41 (22)
Protein g (%)	82 (15)	65 (16)
Cholesterol mg	99	99
Sodium mg	1,881	1,606
Chromium mcg	211	198

Thursday

BREAKFAST

1 Casbah breakfast cup (F: omit)
1 Pritikin English muffin with 1 teaspoon butter and 2 teaspoons apple butter
¼ honeydew melon (for F only)

LUNCH (OUT)

1 cup cream of mushroom soup
2 kasha varnishkas (F: 1 varnishka)
pickles with mustard

SNACK

1 high-chromium muffin ✪
1 Christopher's Chewie with dates

DINNER

3 ounces lean, skinless turkey breast grilled with barbecue sauce ✪
2 servings grilled broccoli ✪
1 baked sweet potato with ½ cup unsweetened applesauce and ½ teaspoon cinnamon
1 slice Richard Bourclon sourdough rye with 1 tablespoon Fromage Blanc–Vegit dip ✪

Nutritional Information (PER DAY)

	MALE	FEMALE
Calories	2,166	1,593
Carbohydrate g (%)	340 (61)	255 (61)
Fat g (%)	61 (24)	42 (23)
Protein g (%)	84 (15)	67 (16)
Cholesterol mg	204	179
Sodium mg	2,900	2,823
Chromium mcg	233	203

Friday

BREAKFAST

1 serving cracked wheat cereal ✪ with ¼ cup nonfat yogurt, ½ cup unsweetened applesauce, 2 teaspoons Sorrell Ridge conserve, and ½ teaspoon cinnamon
1 Pritikin English muffin with 1 tablespoon high-chromium spread ✪

LUNCH (OUT)

1 bowl minestrone (F: 1 cup)
1 serving lobster or crab salad
¼ honeydew melon
½ cup strawberries

SNACK

1 whole wheat pita bread toasted to chips
½ avocado with Hot Cha Cha! salsa

DINNER

4 ounces whole wheat pasta with 2 servings tomato zucchini sauce ✪ and 2 tablespoons grated Parmesan cheese *or* with 1 serving peanut sauce ✪ (F: 2 ounces pasta, 1 serving sauce)
½ Grain Dance whole wheat pizza shell with 2 ounces shredded skim-milk mozzarella cheese (F: ⅓ pizza, 1 ounce cheese)
salad of mixed greens, mushrooms, and tomatoes with 1 tablespoon vinaigrette dressing ✪

Nutritional Information (PER DAY)

	MALE	FEMALE
Calories	2,161	1,636
Carbohydrate g (%)	322 (59)	239 (58)
Fat g (%)	58 (24)	49 (26)
Protein g (%)	92 (17)	67 (16)
Cholesterol mg	37	20
Sodium mg	2,100	2,176
Chromium mcg	209	225

Saturday

BREAKFAST (BRUNCH)

1 cup Shredded Wheat 'N Bran, ¼ cup Mueslix, and ¼ cup Fiber One with 4 ounces skim milk, 1 banana, and 1 tablespoon molasses (optional)
1 Alvarado Street Bakery sprouted wheat bagel with sliced sweet onion and 1 tablespoon Fromage Blanc (F: ½ bagel)
¼ cantaloupe

SNACK

½ avocado with Hot Cha Cha! salsa

2 ounces low-fat Swiss cheese melted on 2 corn tortillas (F: 1 ounce cheese, 1 tortilla)

DINNER

salad of red lettuce, watercress, potatoes, white onion, and tomatoes with 1 tablespoon vinaigrette dressing ✪

3 ounces cold grilled salmon steak ✪ (Save leftovers for Sunday lunch.)

1 serving baked rhubarb ✪

1 slice carrot cake ✪ with ½ cup Élan frozen dessert (F: omit)

2 Beer shandys (½ bottle beer: ½ bottle diet ginger ale; makes 2 servings), root beer, or lemonade

Nutritional Information (PER DAY)

	MALE	FEMALE
Calories	2,104	1,560
Carbohydrate g (%)	337 (61)	252 (61)
Fat g (%)	59 (23)	46 (24)
Protein g (%)	84 (15)	62 (15)
Cholesterol mg	56	46
Sodium mg	950	694
Chromium mcg	200	171

WEEK 4

Sunday

BREAKFAST

2 pancakes made from Hodgson Mill buttermilk pancake mix using 2 egg whites and 1 cup skim milk, cooked on a nonstick surface, and topped with 1 tablespoon maple syrup

¼ honeydew melon
½ cup blueberries

LUNCH

2½ ounces leftover salmon (see Saturday) on 2 slices whole grain bread
1 Christopher's Chewie with dates (F: omit)

DINNER

2 servings black beans ✪ with 1 ounce low-fat cheese, melted, and salsa (Save leftovers for Monday dinner.) (F: omit cheese)
2 servings cajun rice ✪ (F: 1 serving) (Save leftovers for Monday dinner.)
1 baked potato with 2 tablespoons Fromage Blanc–Vegit dip ✪

Nutritional Information (PER DAY)

	MALE	FEMALE
Calories	2,049	1,542
Carbohydrate g (%)	326 (59)	236 (57)
Fat g (%)	69 (26)	51 (27)
Protein g (%)	78 (14)	68 (16)
Cholesterol mg	129	129
Sodium mg	860	747
Chromium mcg	219	174

Monday

BREAKFAST

¾ cup Shredded Wheat 'N Bran and ¼ cup Fiber One with 4 ounces skim milk, 1 tablespoon chopped dates (F: omit)
1 high-chromium muffin ✪
½ cup nonfat yogurt mixed with Sorrell Ridge conserve (for F only)

LUNCH (OUT)

1 steamed artichoke with 2 tablespoons Italian dressing
3 ounces fish fillet broiled or poached with herbs, lemon, and wine
½ cup fresh fruit *or* 1 cup sorbet

SNACK

1 apple
1 pear (F: omit)
4 cups air-popped popcorn with 1 teaspoon brewer's yeast and Vegit

DINNER

2 servings leftover black bean and rice pizza ✪ using 1 serving each leftover black beans and cajun rice (see Sunday) (F: 1 serving pizza) (Save leftovers for Tuesday lunch.)
1 baked sweet potato with ½ cup applesauce and ½ teaspoon cinnamon
salad of mixed greens, mushrooms, tomatoes, and onion with 1 tablespoon vinaigrette dressing ✪

Nutritional Information (PER DAY)

	MALE	FEMALE
Calories	2,000	1,631
Carbohydrate g (%)	324 (60)	263 (61)
Fat g (%)	62 (26)	47 (25)
Protein g (%)	73 (14)	61 (14)
Cholesterol mg	131	123
Sodium mg	1,134	1,053
Chromium mcg	197	182

Tuesday

BREAKFAST

1 serving cracked wheat cereal ✪ with ½ cup nonfat yogurt mixed with ½ cup unsweetened applesauce,

½ banana, and 2 teaspoons Sorrell Ridge conserve, and ½ teaspoon cinnamon (F: omit banana)

LUNCH

1 serving leftover black bean and rice pizza (see Monday)
2 cups cantaloupe chunks (take-out)

SNACK

1 apple *or* 1 orange
1 whole wheat pita bread toasted to chips with 2 tablespoons sugar-free apple butter
3 whole walnuts

DINNER

2 servings whole wheat fettucini with zucchini and smoked salmon ✪ (F: 1 serving)
salad of dark greens, mushrooms, and 1 tablespoon vinaigrette dressing ✪
1 cup steamed Brussels sprouts

Nutritional Information (PER DAY)

	MALE	FEMALE
Calories	2,081	1,597
Carbohydrate g (%)	335 (62)	259 (62)
Fat g (%)	57 (24)	46 (24)
Protein g (%)	76 (14)	57 (14)
Cholesterol mg	35	22
Sodium mg	917	667
Chromium mcg	202	181

Wednesday

BREAKFAST

½ cup unsweetened corn flakes and ½ cup Nutri-Grain wheat flakes with 6 ounces skim milk and ½ banana

½ Pritikin English muffin with 2 teaspoons Sorrell Ridge conserve and 1 tablespoon high-chromium spread ✪ (high-chromium spread for F only)

LUNCH

1 cup vegetable soup (take-out)
1 high-chromium muffin ✪ with 1 tablespoon sugar-free apple butter

SNACK

½ avocado with Green Mountain salsa (F: ¼ avocado)
1 corn tortilla toasted to chips
4 cups air-popped popcorn with Vegit (F: omit)

DINNER

1 serving high-chromium meat loaf ✪ with Worcestershire sauce (F: ½ serving)
4 ounces whole wheat pasta with 2 servings Nitza's tomato sauce ✪ (F: 2 ounces pasta, 1 serving sauce) (Save leftover pasta for Thursday dinner and leftover sauce for Friday dinner.)
salad of mixed greens, tomatoes, peppers, and carrots and 2 tablespoons vinaigrette dressing ✪

Nutritional Information (PER DAY)

	MALE	FEMALE
Calories	2,089	1,578
Carbohydrate g (%)	321 (60)	242 (60)
Fat g (%)	53 (23)	43 (24)
Protein g (%)	94 (17)	65 (16)
Cholesterol mg	140	94
Sodium mg	1,668	1,462
Chromium mcg	230	210

Thursday

BREAKFAST

1 Casbah breakfast cup
1 Alvarado Street bakery sprouted wheat bagel with 2 teaspoons Sorrell Ridge conserve (F: omit)

LUNCH

1 bowl legume-based soup (take-out)
1 high-chromium muffin ✪ with 1 tablespoon de-oiled peanut butter (F: omit peanut butter)
1 apple

SNACK

½ serving half-the-fat hummus ✪ with 1 whole wheat pita bread toasted to chips
4 cups air-popped popcorn with Vegit (F: omit)

DINNER

1 serving flexible frittata made with 2 ounces leftover whole wheat pasta (see Wednesday) ✪, topped with 2 tablespoons ready-made pesto mixed with 1 ounce Fromage Blanc
1 serving grilled broccoli ✪ with ½ pound mushrooms added to recipe
1 baked potato with 1 teaspoon butter (F: omit butter)

Nutritional Information (PER DAY)

	MALE	FEMALE
Calories	2,137	1,524
Carbohydrate g (%)	337 (62)	236 (60)
Fat g (%)	58 (24)	44 (25)
Protein g (%)	78 (14)	59 (15)
Cholesterol mg	170	160
Sodium mg	1,511	995
Chromium mcg	234	194

Friday

BREAKFAST

¾ cup Shredded Wheat 'N Bran, ¼ cup Fiber One, and ¼ cup Mueslix with 6 ounces skim milk, ½ banana, and 1 tablespoon chopped dates

LUNCH (OUT)

2 ounces thinly sliced roast beef with 1 teaspoon mayonnaise, horseradish, lettuce, and tomato on 2 slices rye bread

1 cup sauerkraut *or* 1 pickle

SNACK

2 whole wheat pretzels

2 peaches

DINNER

2 servings polenta ✪ with 2 servings leftover Nitza's tomato sauce (see Wednesday) (F: 1 serving polenta, 1 serving sauce) (Save leftover polenta for Saturday dinner.)

salad of dark greens, fennel, mushrooms, and ½ ounce slivered Parmesan cheese with 2 tablespoons vinaigrette dressing ✪

1 serving frozen shake ✪

1 beer *or* 1 glass wine (optional) (F: omit)

Nutritional Information (PER DAY)

	MALE	FEMALE
Calories	2,151	1,599
Carbohydrate g (%)	330 (59)	254 (60)
Fat g (%)	67 (25)	44 (24)
Protein g (%)	88 (16)	70 (16)
Cholesterol mg	66	66
Sodium mg	1,888	1,588
Chromium mcg	211	207

Saturday

BREAKFAST

½ cup Kashi pilaf made with ½ cup apple juice and ½ cup water and served with 6 ounces skim milk, 1 banana, ¼ cup Mueslix, and 4 chopped walnuts (F: omit banana)

LUNCH

⅔ cup Fromage Blanc–Vegit dip ✪ with broccoli, carrots, chilled potatoes, or whole wheat pita bread toasted to chips

DINNER

2 servings split pea and rosemary soup ✪ with 1 tablespoon de-oiled ready-made pesto (Save leftovers for Monday lunch.)

1 serving potato pizza ✪ on Grain Dance whole wheat pizza shell

1 serving grilled leftover polenta (see Friday) (F: omit)

1 root beer float made with sugar-free IBC root beer and 2 ounces Élan coffee frozen dessert (F: omit)

1 beer *or* 1 glass wine (optional)

Nutritional Information (PER DAY)

	MALE	FEMALE
Calories	2,120	1,619
Carbohydrate g (%)	339 (61)	244 (58)
Fat g (%)	62 (24)	52 (25)
Protein g (%)	88 (16)	70 (17)
Cholesterol mg	36	31
Sodium mg	1,020	855
Chromium mcg	220	195

WEEK 5

Sunday

BREAKFAST

3 pancakes made from Hodgson Mill buttermilk pancake mix using 2 egg whites, 1 cup skim milk, prepared with 1 tablespoon canola oil, cooked on a nonstick surface, and topped with 1 tablespoon Fromage Blanc and 1 tablespoon maple syrup (F: 2 pancakes, prepared in 2 teaspoons canola oil)
¼ honeydew melon
½ cup strawberries

LUNCH

3 cucumber sandwiches made with watercress, 2 tablespoons low-fat mayonnaise ✪, and lots of black pepper each on 1 thin slice of whole grain bread
1 package of American Grain rice snacks

SNACK

1 apple
4 cups air-popped popcorn with 1 tablespoon grated Parmesan cheese and Vegit

DINNER

2 servings killer chromium chili ✪ (F: 1 serving) (Save some for Monday dinner.)
1½ cups roasted new potatoes with 1 tablespoon olive oil and 1 teaspoon minced fresh rosemary
1 cup steamed zucchini, plain or with salsa

Nutritional Information (PER DAY)

	MALE	FEMALE
Calories	2,020	1,590
Carbohydrate g (%)	326 (62)	264 (64)

Fat g (%)	54 (23)	42 (23)
Protein g (%)	81 (15)	55 (13)
Cholesterol mg	185	119
Sodium mg	1,556	1,158
Chromium mcg	226	187

Monday

BREAKFAST

1 high-chromium muffin with 2 teaspoons Sorrell Ridge marmalade

1 banana with 1 tablespoon chopped almonds and 1 tablespoon molasses

LUNCH

1 serving leftover split pea and rosemary soup (see Saturday)

1 baked potato with salsa or Vieux Carre seafood sauce

2 whole grain rolls (F: omit)

SNACK

2 whole wheat pretzels

4 cups air-popped popcorn with 1 tablespoon grated Parmesan cheese, 1 teaspoon brewer's yeast, and Vegit

DINNER

1 serving flexible frittata made with ½ serving leftover killer chromium chili (see Sunday) and 1½ ounces shredded low-fat cheese ✪

1 serving grilled eggplant ✪

1 cup cooked short grain brown rice made with 2 cups chicken broth, 1 tablespoon olive oil, dash cinnamon and nutmeg and topped with 1 tablespoon grated Parmesan cheese (F: omit)

1 serving frozen shake ✪

Nutritional Information (PER DAY)

	MALE	FEMALE
Calories	2,152	1,621
Carbohydrate g (%)	331 (59)	245 (58)
Fat g (%)	64 (26)	47 (25)
Protein g (%)	84 (15)	71 (17)
Cholesterol mg	172	172
Sodium mg	1,557	1,163
Chromium mcg	218	195

Tuesday

BREAKFAST

1 high-chromium muffin ✪ broken into chunks with 6 ounces skim milk, 1 banana, and 1 teaspoon molasses *or* with ½ cup nonfat yogurt, ½ cup unsweetened applesauce, and 1 teaspoon cinnamon

LUNCH (OUT)

1 bowl noncreamy soup
1 steamed artichoke with 2 tablespoons Italian dressing (F: omit)
1 serving Caesar salad *or* 3 ounces fish fillet, grilled or poached with wine, lemon, and herbs
2 breadsticks (F: 1 breadstick)

SNACK

1 apple
4 cups air-popped popcorn with 1 teaspoon Brewer's yeast and Vegit

DINNER

2 servings Tuscan white bean salad ✪ (F: 1 serving) (Save leftovers for Wednesday lunch.)
1 fresh tomato sandwich ✪
1 Fantastic Foods Nature's Burger made with 1 table-

spoon brewer's yeast and 5 dashes low-sodium Worcestershire sauce on 1 Pritikin English muffin with ½ ounce Alpine Lace Swiss cheese, ketchup from Laurel's Kitchen ✪, and mustard

Nutritional Information (PER DAY)

	MALE	FEMALE
Calories	2,056	1,594
Carbohydrate g (%)	297 (57)	241 (60)
Fat g (%)	63 (27)	43 (24)
Protein g (%)	85 (16)	63 (16)
Cholesterol mg	75	61
Sodium mg	2,303	1,730
Chromium mcg	210	196

Wednesday

BREAKFAST

¾ cup Shredded Wheat 'N Bran, ¼ cup Fiber One, and 2 tablespoons wheat bran with 4 ounces skim milk, 1 tablespoon chopped dates, and ½ banana

1 Alvarado Street Bakery sprouted wheat bagel with 2 teaspoons sugar-free apple butter and 1 teaspoon butter (F: ½ bagel, omit apple butter)

LUNCH

1 cup leftover Tuscan white bean salad (see Tuesday), diced tomatoes, extra basil, ½ ounce shredded low-fat mozzarella, and ¼ slivered avocado in 1 whole wheat pita bread

1 pear

SNACK

1 high-chromium muffin ✪ with 1 tablespoon de-oiled peanut butter (F: omit peanut butter)

1 apple

DINNER

3 ounces grilled swordfish with ½ cup mushrooms and ½ cup peppers sautéed in 2 teaspoons olive oil (Save leftover fish for Thursday dinner.)
2 servings Fantastic Foods quick pilaf made with no oil (F: 1 serving)
1 stick Panda licorice (F: omit)

Nutritional Information (PER DAY)

	MALE	FEMALE
Calories	2,004	1,526
Carbohydrate g (%)	332 (62)	246 (59)
Fat g (%)	54 (23)	44 (24)
Protein g (%)	81 (15)	69 (17)
Cholesterol mg	117	117
Sodium mg	1,886	1,385
Chromium mcg	222	197

Thursday

BREAKFAST

mixture of ¾ cup Shredded Wheat 'N Bran and ½ cup sugar-free corn flakes, with 6 ounces skim milk, 1 banana, and 1 tablespoon chopped dates (F: 1 cup mixture, ½ banana)

LUNCH

1 cup Golden Couscous curried lentil soup
1 high-chromium muffin ✪

SNACK

1 large frozen nonfat yogurt (take-out)

DINNER

2 servings Pizsoy pizza (F: 1 serving) (Save leftovers for Friday lunch.)

3 ounces amaranth pasta with 2 servings red or white clam sauce using leftover swordfish (see Wednesday) ✪ (F: 2 ounces pasta, 1 serving sauce)
salad of romaine lettuce and mushrooms with 2 tablespoons vinaigrette dressing ✪
1 glass wine (optional)

Nutritional Information (PER DAY)

	MALE	FEMALE
Calories	2,081	1,615
Carbohydrate g (%)	345 (62)	270 (62)
Fat g (%)	59 (23)	45 (23)
Protein g (%)	86 (15)	63 (15)
Cholesterol mg	82	69
Sodium mg	2,352	1,990
Chromium mcg	219	183

Friday

BREAKFAST
1 Casbah breakfast cup
2 slices Food for Life seven-grain sprouted cinnamon raisin bread with 1 tablespoon sugar-free apple butter and 2 tablespoons skim-milk ricotta cheese (F: omit)

LUNCH
1 serving leftover Pizsoy pizza (see Thursday)
1 cup chicken noodle soup (take-out)

SNACK
1 Christopher's Chewie with dates *or* 2 high-chromium gingers ✪
1 apple with 1 tablespoon de-oiled peanut butter

DINNER (OUT)

1 bowl minestrone with 1 tablespoon grated Parmesan cheese (F: 1 cup, no cheese)
1 serving risotto with red or mushroom sauce
1 serving spinach with garlic and oil
¼ cantaloupe *or* 1 serving sorbet
1 glass wine (optional)

or

1 shrimp cocktail with salsa
1 serving seafood paella
salad with touch of guacamole
house fruit dessert
1 glass wine or Sangria (optional)

Nutritional Information (PER DAY)

	MALE	FEMALE
Calories	1,977	1,560
Carbohydrate g (%)	313 (61)	259 (62)
Fat g (%)	61 (25)	50 (26)
Protein g (%)	68 (13)	48 (13)
Cholesterol mg	28	7
Sodium mg	1,647	1,337
Chromium mcg	183	162

Saturday

BREAKFAST

6 ounces fresh orange juice (F: omit)
1 serving hash brown potatoes ✪ with ketchup from Laurel's Kitchen ✪
¼ honeydew melon or cantaloupe

LUNCH

1 Alvarado Street Bakery sprouted wheat bagel with 2 tablespoons de-oiled peanut butter, 1 tablespoon high-chromium spread, and 1 slice sweet onion

SNACK

1 whole wheat pita bread toasted to chips
½ avocado with Hot Cha Cha! salsa (F: ¼ avocado)

DINNER

1 serving corn meal scallops ✪
2 servings whole wheat noodles with peanut sauce ✪ (F: 1 serving)
1 serving grilled broccoli ✪
1 slice apple spice cake ✪ *or* carrot cake ✪

Nutritional Information (PER DAY)

	MALE	FEMALE
Calories	2,143	1,610
Carbohydrate g (%)	343 (63)	253 (61)
Fat g (%)	52 (21)	40 (22)
Protein g (%)	88 (16)	70 (17)
Cholesterol mg	45	45
Sodium mg	1,329	1,127
Chromium mcg	187	171

WEEK 6

Sunday

BREAKFAST (BRUNCH)

3 slices French toast ✪, cooked in 2 teaspoons canola oil and topped with 2 tablespoons maple syrup and 2 teaspoons butter (F: 2 slices French toast, 1 tablespoon syrup)
fruit compote of ¼ cantaloupe, 1 banana, ½ cup blueberries, 1 pear

SNACK

4 cups air-popped popcorn with 1 teaspoon Brewer's yeast and Vegit

1 stick Panda licorice *or* 1 high-chromium ginger ✪

DINNER

3 ounces high-chromium meat loaf ✪ (Save leftovers for Tuesday lunch.)

1 cup steamed Brussels sprouts

2 servings rice salad ✪ with 1 teaspoon olive oil (F: 1 serving) (Save leftovers for Monday lunch.)

1 slice apple spice cake ✪ with 1 tablespoon skim-milk ricotta cheese

Nutritional Information (PER DAY)

	MALE	FEMALE
Calories	2,028	1,608
Carbohydrate g (%)	318 (58)	260 (59)
Fat g (%)	61 (25)	46 (24)
Protein g (%)	92 (17)	75 (17)
Cholesterol mg	109	103
Sodium mg	1,275	993
Chromium mcg	221	200

Monday

BREAKFAST

1 cup Nutri-Grain wheat flakes and 2 tablespoons wheat bran with 4 ounces skim milk, 1 sliced peach, and 1 tablespoon chopped dates

1 slice Food for Life seven-grain sprouted cinnamon raisin bread with 1 tablespoon de-oiled peanut butter and 2 teaspoons Sorrell Ridge conserve (F: omit)

LUNCH

1½ servings leftover rice salad (see Sunday) and ¼ slivered avocado in 1 whole wheat pita bread (F: 1 serving rice salad)

SNACK

1 high-chromium muffin ✪ with 1 tablespoon sugar-free apple butter
1 banana (F: ½ banana)

DINNER

3 ounces grilled salmon with lemon and herbs
½ pound mushrooms mixed with ¾ cup fresh or frozen peas and sautéed in 1 tablespoon olive oil
1 baked sweet potato with ½ cup unsweetened applesauce and ½ teaspoon cinnamon (Make extra potatoes for Tuesday dinner.)
1 serving frozen shake (F: omit)
1 high-chromium ginger (F: omit)

Nutritional Information (PER DAY)

	MALE	FEMALE
Calories	2,082	1,511
Carbohydrate g (%)	327 (59)	237 (58)
Fat g (%)	63 (26)	47 (26)
Protein g (%)	82 (15)	64 (16)
Cholesterol mg	88	88
Sodium mg	1,339	1,030
Chromium mcg	218	176

Tuesday

BREAKFAST

1 high-chromium muffin ✪ broken into chunks
½ cup nonfat yogurt mixed with ½ cup unsweetened applesauce, 2 teaspoons Sorrell Ridge conserve, and ½ teaspoon cinnamon

LUNCH

2 oz serving leftover high-chromium meat loaf (see Sunday) with Worcestershire sauce, tomato, and romaine lettuce in 1 whole wheat pita bread *or* on 2 thin slices whole grain bread

2 cups melon chunks (take-out)

SNACK

1 slice apple spice cake ✪

2 Chico-San popcorn cakes with 1 tablespoon high-chromium spread ✪

DINNER

4 ounces whole wheat pasta with 2 servings sweet potato sauce ✪ (F: 2 ounces pasta, 1 serving sauce)

2 servings spinach sauté ✪

2 roasted red peppers with 2 tablespoons vinaigrette dressing ✪

Nutritional Information (PER DAY)

	MALE	FEMALE
Calories	2,071	1,632
Carbohydrate g (%)	335 (61)	259 (59)
Fat g (%)	58 (24)	49 (25)
Protein g (%)	87 (16)	70 (16)
Cholesterol mg	95	94
Sodium mg	1,338	1,125
Chromium mcg	218	198

Wednesday

BREAKFAST

¾ cup Shredded Wheat 'N Bran, ¼ cup Fiber One, and ¼ cup Mueslix with 4 ounces skim milk and 1 banana

LUNCH

2 slices whole grain bread with 1 tablespoon de-oiled peanut butter and 3 dried figs
1 apple

SNACK

1 high-chromium muffin ✪
4 cups air-popped popcorn with 1 tablespoon grated Parmesan cheese and Vegit

DINNER

1 serving Jaclyn's mushroom barley soup with 1 tablespoon de-oiled pesto
1 serving winter wheat shrimp salad ✪ with 1 tablespoon olive oil
2 ounces whole wheat pasta with quicker tomato sauce ✪ topped with 2 tablespoons grated Parmesan cheese (F: omit)
1 serving grilled broccoli ✪

Nutritional Information (PER DAY)

	MALE	FEMALE
Calories	2,032	1,591
Carbohydrate g (%)	321 (59)	266 (61)
Fat g (%)	61 (25)	42 (23)
Protein g (%)	87 (16)	71 (16)
Cholesterol mg	281	271
Sodium mg	1,662	1,383
Chromium mcg	218	210

Thursday

BREAKFAST

⅓ cup rolled oats and ⅓ cup wheat bran, cooked in 1⅓ cups water and served with ½ banana and 1 tablespoon chopped dates

LUNCH

1 Alvarado Street Bakery sprouted wheat bagel with 1 sliced cucumber, 1 tablespoon mayonnaise, tomato, and sprouts

1 package American Grain rice snacks (F: omit)

SNACK

2 plums

4 cups air-popped popcorn with 1 tablespoon grated Parmesan cheese and Vegit

DINNER

1½ servings pasta with scallops, peas, and vodka ✪ (F: 1 serving)

salad of romaine lettuce, mushrooms, cucumbers, tomatoes, carrots, celery, and ¼ avocado with 2 tablespoons vinaigrette dressing (F: omit avocado)

1 serving chromium crostini ✪

Nutritional Information (PER DAY)

	MALE	FEMALE
Calories	2,022	1,596
Carbohydrate g (%)	316 (58)	258 (59)
Fat g (%)	64 (26)	47 (25)
Protein g (%)	86 (16)	68 (16)
Cholesterol mg	70	49
Sodium mg	1,138	824
Chromium mcg	203	190

Friday

BREAKFAST

8 ounces fresh orange juice (F: omit)

1 serving cracked wheat cereal ✪ with ½ cup plain nonfat yogurt and 1 tablespoon chopped dates

1 Pritikin English muffin grilled with 1 ounce skim-milk mozzarella cheese (F: omit)

LUNCH

1 cup whole wheat couscous Casbah mushroom tofu soup
1 high-chromium muffin ✪ with 1 tablespoon de-oiled peanut butter (F: omit peanut butter)

SNACK

1 Christopher's Chewie with dates

DINNER (OUT)

1 bowl chili (any variety)
1 baked potato with cocktail sauce (F: ½ baked potato)
3 cups salad bar (include any vegetables not fried, creamed or mixed with cheese) with 1½ tablespoons dressing

or

3 ounces poached or grilled fish
1 cup steamed vegetables
1 baked potato with salsa or cocktail sauce *or* 1 serving rice with salsa or cocktail sauce
1 beer *or* 1 glass wine (optional)

Nutritional Information (PER DAY)

	MALE	FEMALE
Calories	2,071	1,576
Carbohydrate g (%)	330 (60)	255 (59)
Fat g (%)	63 (26)	49 (26)
Protein g (%)	83 (15)	61 (14)
Cholesterol mg	146	129
Sodium mg	1,322	1,021
Chromium mcg	217	191

Saturday

BREAKFAST (BRUNCH)

8 ounces fresh orange juice
1 serving huevos rancheros ✪
½ honeydew melon (F: ¼ melon)
½ cup blueberries

SNACK

2 Crispini crackers
½ avocado with Green Mountain salsa
4 cups air-popped popcorn with 1 teaspoon brewer's yeast and Vegit
1 pear

DINNER

2 servings mushroom risotto ✪ (F: 1 serving)
3 dried figs with a 1-ounce piece of Parmesan cheese
¾ cup steamed peas (fresh or frozen) with 2 tablespoons skim-milk ricotta cheese
2 servings grilled broccoli
1 root beer float made with sugar-free IBC root beer and 4 ounces Élan coffee frozen dessert

Nutritional Information (PER DAY)

	MALE	FEMALE
Calories	2,056	1,526
Carbohydrate g (%)	319 (59)	233 (58)
Fat g (%)	60 (25)	48 (27)
Protein g (%)	86 (16)	61 (15)
Cholesterol mg	51	24
Sodium mg	1,472	813
Chromium mcg	214	170

GROUP II

WEEK I

Sunday

BREAKFAST (BRUNCH)

1 serving genuine Austin omelette ✪
1 Pritikin English muffin with 1 tablespoon sugar-free apple butter
1 serving hash brown potatoes ✪ (F: omit)
¼ honeydew melon *or* ½ cup berries

SNACK

1 high-chromium muffin ✪ with 2 teaspoons Sorrell Ridge conserve or marmalade
4 dates with 1 tablespoon high-chromium spread ✪
2 peaches

DINNER

4 ounces whole wheat pasta with 2 servings red or white clam sauce ✪ (F: 2 ounces pasta, 1 serving sauce)
2 servings corn meal pizza shell ✪ *or* Grain Dance whole wheat pizza shell with 2 servings tomato zucchini sauce ✪ (Save leftovers for Monday lunch.)
1 serving spinach sauté ✪

Nutritional Information (PER DAY)

	MALE	FEMALE
Calories	2,385	1,852
Carbohydrate g (%)	404 (65)	311 (64)
Fat g (%)	55 (20)	44 (20)

Protein g (%)	97 (15)	80 (16)
Cholesterol mg	295	282
Sodium mg	1,856	1,680
Chromium mcg	224	218

Monday

BREAKFAST

1 ounce wheatgrass juice, fresh or Perfect Foods frozen

2 servings cracked wheat cereal ✪ with 6 ounces skim milk, 1 banana, and 1 tablespoon chopped dates (F: 1 serving)

1 Alvarado Street Bakery sprouted wheat bagel with 1 tablespoon sugar-free apple butter and 1 tablespoon de-oiled peanut butter (F: omit peanut butter)

LUNCH

1 serving leftover pizza with tomato zucchini sauce (see Sunday)

1 cup legume-based soup (take-out) *or* Casbah whole wheat couscous tofu mushroom soup

1 oat bran muffin (take-out) *or* 2 high-chromium gingers ✪ (F: omit)

SNACK

1 Twinfast shake ✪

4 cups air-popped popcorn with Vegit (F: omit)

DINNER (OUT)

mixed pepper salad and mushroom antipasto with 1 tablespoon Italian dressing

1 bowl minestrone or pasta e fagioli with 1 tablespoon grated Parmesan cheese (F: 1 cup soup)

1 slice whole wheat bread with little or no butter

1 serving pappardelle ai funghi (noodles with mushroom sauce) *or* 1 serving gnocchi with red sauce

or

3 ounces fish fillet grilled with garlic and wine
1 serving broccoli raab *or* sautéed spinach
1 glass wine *or* 1 beer (optional)
1 serving Campari or grapefruit sorbet

Nutritional Information (PER DAY)

	MALE	FEMALE
Calories	2,371	1,799
Carbohydrate g (%)	388 (64)	300 (64)
Fat g (%)	58 (21)	41 (19)
Protein g (%)	95 (16)	72 (16)
Cholesterol mg	13	10
Sodium mg	2,784	2,120
Chromium mcg	251	236

Tuesday

BREAKFAST

1 ounce wheatgrass juice, fresh or Perfect Foods frozen
1 Pritikin English muffin with 2 teaspoons Sorrell Ridge conserve and 1 tablespoon de-oiled peanut butter (F: omit peanut butter)
¾ cup Shredded Wheat 'N Bran, ¼ cup Fiber One, ¼ cup Mueslix, and 1 tablespoon wheat germ with 6 ounces skim milk, 1 banana, and 1 tablespoon chopped dates

LUNCH

1 serving tuna salad ✪ in 1 whole wheat pita bread
1 cup de-oiled ratatouille (take-out)
2 cups cantaloupe chunks (take-out)

SNACK

4 cups air-popped popcorn with Vegit (F: omit)

⅔ cup Fromage Blanc–Vegit dip ✪ with 1 whole wheat pita bread toasted to chips

DINNER

1½ servings stir-fried chicken with chromium-rich vegetables ✪ with 1 tablespoon mixture hot sesame oil and peanut oil (F: 1 serving)

1½ servings lima casserole ✪ (F: 1 serving)

1½ jalapeno corn muffins ✪ (F: 1 muffin)

Nutritional Information (PER DAY)

	MALE	FEMALE
Calories	2,404	1,818
Carbohydrate g (%)	405 (64)	313 (64)
Fat g (%)	55 (19)	40 (19)
Protein g (%)	107 (17)	78 (17)
Cholesterol mg	71	53
Sodium mg	1,457	1,378
Chromium mcg	231	178

Wednesday

BREAKFAST

1 ounce wheatgrass juice, fresh or Perfect Foods frozen

¾ cup Shredded Wheat 'N Bran, ¼ cup Fiber One, and ¼ cup Mueslix with 6 ounces skim milk, 1 banana, and 1 tablespoon chopped dates (F: ½ banana)

1 slice Food for Life seven-grain sprouted cinnamon raisin bread with 2 teaspoons Sorrell Ridge conserve and 1 tablespoon de-oiled peanut butter (F: omit peanut butter)

LUNCH

1 serving curried chicken and rice salad ✪ on 2 slices whole grain bread
1 pear (F: omit)

SNACK

2 whole wheat pretzels *or* 2 high-chromium gingers ✪
3 dried figs
1 apple *or* 1 Twinfast shake ✪

DINNER

1 serving minestrone alla Burrini ✪ (Save leftovers for Friday dinner.)
1 ounce whole wheat elbow pasta mixed with 1 cup cooked Kashi pilaf, 3 tablespoons de-oiled pesto, and 2 ounce Fromage Blanc (F: ½ ounce pasta, ½ cup Kashi pilaf, 2 tablespoons pesto, 1 ounce Fromage Blanc)
2½ cups steamed, chilled mixed vegetables (broccoli, cauliflower, and others) with 2 tablespoons vinaigrette dressing ✪

Nutritional Information (PER DAY)

	MALE	FEMALE
Calories	2,417	1,800
Carbohydrate g (%)	422 (66)	316 (65)
Fat g (%)	53 (19)	39 (19)
Protein g (%)	101 (16)	76 (16)
Cholesterol mg	62	26
Sodium mg	1,127	962
Chromium mcg	238	221

Thursday

BREAKFAST

1 Casbah breakfast cup

1 banana, split and filled with 1 tablespoon high-chromium spread ✪ and 1 tablespoon molasses

LUNCH

1 serving Casbah tabouly with chopped tomato, 1 tablespoon olive oil, and 2 tablespoons balsamic vinegar in a whole wheat pita bread

1 serving cold sesame noodles (take-out) (F: omit)

2 cups cantaloupe chunks (take-out)

SNACK

1 high-chromium muffin ✪ with 2 teaspoons Sorrell Ridge marmalade

1 apple

DINNER

1 serving Jaclyn's mushroom barley soup

2 servings Pizsoy pizza (F: 1 serving)

1 baked sweet potato topped with ½ cup unsweetened applesauce and ½ teaspoon cinnamon

1 medium nonfat frozen yogurt (commercial)

Nutritional Information (PER DAY)

	MALE	FEMALE
Calories	2,323	1,796
Carbohydrate g (%)	402 (65)	325 (68)
Fat g (%)	58 (21)	40 (19)
Protein g (%)	88 (14)	61 (13)
Cholesterol mg	48	48
Sodium mg	1,849	1,524
Chromium mcg	214	196

Friday

BREAKFAST

1 ounce wheatgrass juice, fresh or Perfect Foods frozen

¼ cup Nutri-Grain wheat flakes, ½ cup unsweetened cornflakes, and ¼ cup wheat bran with 6 ounces skim milk, 1 banana, and 1 tablespoon chopped dates

1 Pritikin English muffin with 2 tablespoons sugar-free apple butter (F: omit)

LUNCH (OUT)

3 ounces shrimp cocktail

1 baked potato with 1 tablespoon cocktail sauce

2½ cups salad bar selections (three-bean salad, mushrooms, corn relish, any vegetables) with 2 teaspoons oil and vinegar or low-cal dressing

SNACK

½ Twinfast shake ✪

1 Christopher's Chewie with dates

DINNER

2 servings ribollita using leftover minestrone alla Burrini (see Wednesday) ✪ (F: 1 serving)

2 servings acorn squash souffle ✪

2 roasted red peppers ✪ with balsamic vinegar (F: omit)

1 slice apple spice cake ✪ *or* 2 high-chromium gingers ✪

Nutritional Information (PER DAY)

	MALE	FEMALE
Calories	2,355	1,794
Carbohydrate g (%)	400 (63)	311 (64)

Fat g (%)	59 (21)	41 (19)
Protein g (%)	99 (16)	80 (17)
Cholesterol mg	297	293
Sodium mg	1,711	1,310
Chromium mcg	208	182

Saturday

BREAKFAST

3 pancakes made from Hodgson Mill buttermilk pancake mix using 2 egg whites, 2 teaspoons canola oil, and 1 cup skim milk, cooked on a nonstick surface, and topped with 1 tablespoon maple syrup (F: 2 pancakes)
1 banana with 1 tablespoon chopped almonds and 1 tablespoon molasses

LUNCH

1 serving whole wheat noodles with peanut sauce ✪
1 serving shrimp salad ✪ in 1 whole wheat pita bread

SNACK

1 high-chromium muffin ✪
1 pear (F: omit)

DINNER

2 servings killer chromium chili ✪ (F: 1 serving) (Freeze leftovers for lunch week 3.)
1 jalapeno corn muffin ✪
1 baked potato topped with ¼ slivered avocado
1 cup canned mandarin oranges *or* 1 fresh orange

Nutritional Information (PER DAY)

	MALE	FEMALE
Calories	2,338	1,849
Carbohydrate g (%)	400 (67)	312 (65)

Fat g (%)	48 (17)	41 (19)
Protein g (%)	100 (16)	74 (15)
Cholesterol mg	321	355
Sodium mg	1,836	1,437
Chromium mcg	227	176

WEEK 2

Sunday

BREAKFAST (BRUNCH)

1 cup cooked Kashi pilaf made with 1 cup water and 1 cup apple juice and served with 1 sliced banana, 6 ounces skim milk, and 1 tablespoon chopped dates (F: ½ cup Kashi pilaf)
½ Pritikin English muffin with 2 teaspoons sugar-free apple butter (F: omit)
¼ honeydew melon
½ cup berries

LUNCH

1 fresh tomato sandwich ✪
1 package American Grain rice snacks

SNACK

1 high-chromium muffin ✪ with 2 teaspoons Sorrell Ridge conserve
1 apple

DINNER

3 ounces cold grilled salmon (Save leftovers for Monday lunch.)
2 servings rice salad ✪ (F: 1 serving)
1 serving baked rhubarb ✪ with 4 ounces Dole raspberry sorbet and 1 ounce Élan chocolate almond frozen desert

Nutritional Information (PER DAY)

	MALE	FEMALE
Calories	2,350	1,807
Carbohydrate g (%)	411 (66)	319 (67)
Fat g (%)	52 (19)	37 (18)
Protein g (%)	92 (15)	74 (15)
Cholesterol mg	101	101
Sodium mg	1,160	1,015
Chromium mcg	237	188

Monday

BREAKFAST

1 ounce wheatgrass juice, fresh or Perfect Foods frozen

1 serving cracked wheat cereal ✪ with 1 banana, 4 ounces skim milk, and 1 tablespoon molasses

1 slice Food for Life seven-grain sprouted cinnamon raisin toast with 2 teaspoons Sorrell Ridge conserve

LUNCH

2½ ounces leftover grilled salmon (see Sunday) with red lettuce, ½ tomato, and sweet minced onion in a whole wheat pita bread *or* on 2 slices whole grain bread

1 orange

1 beer (optional) (F: omit)

SNACK

1 Christopher's chewie with dates *or* 2 high-chromium gingers ✪ (for F only)

4 cups air-popped popcorn with Vegit

1 apple (F: omit)

DINNER

1 ounce Casbah tabouly with 2 tablespoons olive oil and 2 tablespoons balsamic vinegar

1 serving cold whole wheat noodles with peanut sauce ✪ (F: omit)
1 baked sweet potato with ½ cup unsweetened applesauce mixed with ½ teaspoon cinnamon (F: omit)
1 ear corn on the cob
1 Fantastic Foods Nature's Burger on 1 Pritikin English muffin with 1 ounce low-fat cheese, ketchup from Laurel's Kitchen ✪, and mustard

Nutritional Information (PER DAY)

	MALE	FEMALE
Calories	2,385	1,835
Carbohydrate g (%)	395 (65)	300 (64)
Fat g (%)	55 (20)	39 (19)
Protein g (%)	92 (15)	78 (17)
Cholesterol mg	38	38
Sodium mg	1,444	1,231
Chromium mcg	203	183

Tuesday

BREAKFAST

1 ounce wheatgrass juice
3 egg whites and 1 egg yolk scrambled with Hot Cha Cha! salsa and 1 ounce shredded low-fat Swiss cheese
2 Crispini crackers
8 ounces fresh orange juice

LUNCH

1 Alvarado Street Bakery sprouted wheat bagel with sliced sweet onion, lettuce, tomato, mustard, and sprouts
1 bowl tomato vegetable soup (take-out)

SNACK

1 high-chromium muffin ✪
4 dried figs (F: 2 figs)
2 whole wheat pretzels
1 pear (F: omit)

DINNER

2 servings pasta with braised lentils ✪ (F: 1 serving)
salad of dark green lettuce, mushrooms, carrot, 1 small potato cubed, and onion with 2 tablespoons vinaigrette dressing ✪

Nutritional Information (PER DAY)

	MALE	FEMALE
Calories	2,309	1,830
Carbohydrate g (%)	370 (65)	283 (63)
Fat g (%)	49 (19)	42 (21)
Protein g (%)	93 (16)	74 (16)
Cholesterol mg	350	334
Sodium mg	1,933	1,619
Chromium mcg	217	180

Wednesday

BREAKFAST

1 ounce wheatgrass juice
⅓ cup oat bran and ⅓ cup wheat bran, plus 2 tablespoons rye flakes made with 1⅓ cups water served with 6 ounces skim milk, 1 banana, and 1 tablespoon molasses *or* 1 tablespoon chopped dates
½ Pritikin English muffin with 1 tablespoon sugar-free apple butter (F: omit)

LUNCH

1 serving Golden Couscous tomato minestrone soup
1 ounce Casbah tabouly with sprouts, tomatoes, 1 tea-

spoon olive oil, and 1 teaspoon balsamic vinegar in 1 whole wheat pita bread

1 high-chromium muffin ✪

SNACK

¼ avocado with Green Mountain salsa
2 Chico-San popcorn cakes
1 pear (F: omit)

DINNER

1 serving corn bread "fried" chicken ✪ (F: ½ serving) (Save leftovers for Thursday dinner.)
1 serving baked beans ✪
1 baked potato with 1 tablespoon de-oiled pesto (F: omit)
1 cup zucchini sautéed in 1 tablespoon olive oil with garlic, dash red pepper flakes, and 3 plum tomatoes

Nutritional Information (PER DAY)

	MALE	FEMALE
Calories	2,372	1,829
Carbohydrate g (%)	413 (64)	323 (65)
Fat g (%)	54 (19)	43 (19)
Protein g (%)	109 (17)	83 (16)
Cholesterol mg	135	90
Sodium mg	2,170	1,946
Chromium mcg	247	227

Thursday

BREAKFAST

8 ounces fresh orange juice (F: omit)
¾ cup Shredded Wheat 'N Bran, ¼ cup Fiber One, and ¼ cup Mueslix with 6 ounces skim milk, and 1 banana

LUNCH (OUT)

4 oysters or clams on the half shell *or* 1 serving shrimp cocktail
3 cups salad bar selections (three-bean salad, mushrooms, corn relish, any vegetables) with 2 tablespoons diet dressing
1 slice bread
1 beer *or* 1 glass wine (optional)

SNACK

4 cups air-popped popcorn with Vegit
1 apple

DINNER

½ serving leftover corn bread "fried" chicken (see Wednesday)
1 cup cooked short grain brown rice mixed with 6 ounces fresh, cooked mushrooms (F: ¾ cup rice)
3 small new potatoes grilled in 2 teaspoons olive oil and ½ teaspoon fresh rosemary
1 cup Health Valley black bean soup, mixed with 3 tablespoons rice and spooned on a corn tortilla (F: omit)
1 jalapeno corn muffin ✪
1 slice apple spice cake (F: omit)

Nutritional Information (PER DAY)

	MALE	FEMALE
Calories	2,258	1,772
Carbohydrate g (%)	401 (68)	301 (65)
Fat g (%)	49 (17)	44 (20)
Protein g (%)	88 (15)	74 (15)
Cholesterol mg	104	104
Sodium mg	1,582	1,122
Chromium mcg	215	197

Friday

BREAKFAST

½ cup unsweetened corn flakes and ½ cup Nutri-Grain wheat flakes with 6 ounces skim milk, 1 banana, and 1 tablespoon chopped dates
1 Pritikin English muffin with 2 teaspoons sugar-free apple butter

LUNCH

1 cup vegetarian chili stuffed in a baked potato with salsa (take-out)
1 serving Golden Couscous curried lentil soup

SNACK

1 apple *or* 2 peaches
1 Christopher's Chewie with dates (F: omit)
1 fruit-flavored nonfat yogurt (F: omit)
1 New Morning honey graham cracker (F: omit)

DINNER (OUT)

¼ cantaloupe
1 bowl minestrone (F: omit)
1 serving pasta in red clam sauce
1 cup spinach sautéed in oil
1 cup strawberries with zabaglione

Nutritional Information (PER DAY)

	MALE	FEMALE
Calories	2,412	1,854
Carbohydrate g (%)	446 (69)	332 (68)
Fat g (%)	49 (17)	39 (18)
Protein g (%)	88 (14)	69 (14)
Cholesterol mg	73	63
Sodium mg	2,062	1,562
Chromium mcg	207	206

Saturday

BREAKFAST

2 servings potato pancakes ✪ with ¼ cup unsweetened applesauce *or* 2 tablespoons sugar-free apple butter mixed with 2 tablespoons skim-milk ricotta cheese
¼ honeydew melon
½ cup berries

LUNCH

1 serving tuna salad ✪ with ½ slivered avocado and chopped tomato in 1 whole wheat pita bread *or* on 2 slices whole grain bread
8 ounces sugar-free lemonade

SNACK

1 high-chromium muffin with 2 teaspoons Sorrell Ridge conserve

DINNER

2 servings pasta primavera ✪ with 1 teaspoon additional olive oil (F: 1 serving) (Save leftovers for Sunday dinner.)
2 servings acorn squash souffle ✪ (F: 1 serving) (Save leftovers for Sunday brunch.)
1 baked sweet potato
1 slice carrot cake ✪ *or* 1 high-chromium ginger (F: omit)

Nutritional Information (PER DAY)

	MALE	FEMALE
Calories	2,343	1,801
Carbohydrate g (%)	435 (68)	326 (67)
Fat g (%)	49 (17)	40 (19)
Protein g (%)	94 (15)	69 (14)

Cholesterol mg	265	161
Sodium mg	1,913	1,476
Chromium mcg	249	221

WEEK 3

Sunday

BREAKFAST (BRUNCH)

4 egg whites and 1 egg yolk scrambled with ½ green pepper, ½ onion, parsley, basil, and black pepper in nonstick skillet and served on a toasted corn tortilla
1 serving hash brown potatoes ✪
1 serving leftover acorn squash soufflé (see Saturday)

SNACK

1 Alvarado Street Bakery sprouted wheat bagel with 2 tablespoons high-chromium spread and 4 dried figs (F: omit)
4 cups air-popped popcorn with Vegit
1 apple and 1 pear *or* orange

DINNER

2 ounces roast chicken prepared with red wine and sage and stuffed and 2 servings leftover pasta primavera (see Saturday) (Save leftover chicken for Monday lunch.)
salad of dark greens, romaine lettuce, mushrooms, and tomato with 2 tablespoons vinaigrette dressing ✪
1 baked sweet potato (Bake an extra potato for Monday lunch.)
1 New Morning honey graham cracker with 1 tablespoon sugar-free apple butter *or* 1 high-chromium ginger ✪

Nutritional Information (PER DAY)

	MALE	FEMALE
Calories	2,355	1,851
Carbohydrate g (%)	412 (66)	323 (65)
Fat g (%)	49 (17)	40 (18)
Protein g (%)	107 (17)	87 (17)
Cholesterol mg	470	470
Sodium mg	1,445	951
Chromium mcg	228	208

Monday

BREAKFAST

8 ounces fresh orange juice

¾ cup Shredded Wheat 'N Bran, ¼ cup Fiber One, and ¼ cup Mueslix with 4 ounces skim milk, 1 banana, and 1 tablespoon chopped dates

LUNCH

1 serving curried chicken salad and rice salad (substitute sweet potato chunks for rice) ✪ in 1 whole wheat pita bread (F: omit pita)

2 cups melon chunks (take-out)

SNACK

1 baked potato with ½ slivered avocado and Hot Cha Cha! salsa

2 whole wheat pretzels

DINNER

2 servings winter wheat, corn, and cheese casserole ✪ (F: 1 serving) (Save leftovers for Tuesday dinner.)

2 cups stewed Del Monte tomatoes (unsalted)

1 serving milk-soaked haddock ✪

2 cups watermelon chunks

1 serving carrot cake topped with 2 tablespoons prune whip ✪ (F: omit)

Nutritional Information (PER DAY)

	MALE	FEMALE
Calories	2,344	1,776
Carbohydrate g (%)	421 (67)	326 (67)
Fat g (%)	47 (17)	36 (17)
Protein g (%)	101 (16)	76 (16)
Cholesterol mg	152	141
Sodium mg	1,968	1,383
Chromium mcg	241	181

Tuesday

BREAKFAST

1 serving cracked wheat cereal ✪ with 4 ounces skim milk, 1 banana, and 1 tablespoon molasses *or* 1 tablespoon chopped dates

1 Pritikin English muffin with 2 tablespoons prune whip ✪

LUNCH (OUT)

1 steamed artichoke with 1 tablespoon dressing

Caesar salad

1 slice bread (F: omit)

1 beer *or* 1 glass wine (optional)

SNACK

4 cups air-popped popcorn with Vegit

1 serving frozen nonfat yogurt

1 pear (F: omit)

1 apple (F: omit)

DINNER

1 serving flexible frittata using 1 cup leftover winter wheat, corn, and cheese casserole (see Monday) ✪

1 serving spaghetti alla puttanesca ✪

2 cups steamed broccoli

Nutritional Information (PER DAY)

	MALE	FEMALE
Calories	2,267	1,816
Carbohydrate g (%)	370 (64)	305 (65)
Fat g (%)	59 (21)	48 (21)
Protein g (%)	89 (15)	64 (14)
Cholesterol mg	123	8
Sodium mg	1,756	1,310
Chromium mcg	231	184

Wednesday

BREAKFAST

½ cup Kashi pilaf made with ½ cup apple juice and ½ cup water and served with ½ cup unsweetened applesauce, ½ cup nonfat yogurt, ½ teaspoon cinnamon, 2 teaspoons Sorrell Ridge conserve, and 1 sliced banana

2 slices Food for Life seven-grain sprouted cinnamon raisin bread with 2 tablespoons prune whip ✪ (F: omit)

LUNCH

½ serving killer chromium chili (frozen week 1 on Saturday) with shredded lettuce, diced tomato, and ½ slivered avocado in 1 whole wheat pita bread

2 cups watermelon chunks

SNACK

1 high-chromium muffin ✪

1 Christopher's Chewie with dates (F: omit)

DINNER (OUT)

1 cup Manhattan clam chowder (F: omit)

relish tray selections (pickles, hot peppers, corn relish)

½ pound lobster, broiled or steamed
salad of mixed greens and croutons with 2 tablespoons house dressing
2 slices bread
1 baked potato with cocktail sauce
1 serving sorbet *or* 1 serving fresh fruit

Nutritional Information (PER DAY)

	MALE	FEMALE
Calories	2,327	1,845
Carbohydrate g (%)	397 (65)	304 (63)
Fat g (%)	50 (18)	44 (20)
Protein g (%)	101 (17)	85 (17)
Cholesterol mg	180	177
Sodium mg	2,080	1,736
Chromium mcg	247	207

Thursday

BREAKFAST

1 Casbah breakfast cup
1 banana (F: omit)

LUNCH

2 ounces lean white turkey with mustard, tomato, lettuce, and sprouts on 1 cracked wheat, rye, or sprouted wheat bagel
1 package American Grain rice snacks
1 pickle

SNACK

1 high-chromium muffin ✪
1 pat butter
2 teaspoons Sorrell Ridge conserve

DINNER

1 serving minestrone alla Burrini ✪ with 1 tablespoon de-oiled pesto (Save leftovers for Friday dinner.)
2 servings whole wheat noodles with peanut sauce ✪ (F: 1 serving) (Save leftovers for Friday lunch.)
1 baked sweet potato with ½ cup unsweetened applesauce and ½ teaspoon cinnamon
1 beer *or* 1 glass of wine (optional) (F: omit)

Nutritional Information (PER DAY)

	MALE	FEMALE
Calories	2,435	1,841
Carbohydrate g (%)	413 (66)	312 (65)
Fat g (%)	56 (19)	38 (18)
Protein g (%)	97 (15)	80 (17)
Cholesterol mg	125	125
Sodium mg	2,098	1,848
Chromium mcg	198	182

Friday

BREAKFAST

1 high-chromium muffin ✪ with 2 tablespoons sugar-free apple butter and 2 tablespoons high-chromium spread ✪ (F: omit apple butter and high-chromium spread)
½ cup nonfat yogurt with ½ cup unsweetened applesauce, ½ teaspoon cinnamon, 2 teaspoons Sorrell Ridge conserves, and 1 sliced banana (F: omit banana)

LUNCH

1 serving leftover whole wheat noodles with peanut sauce (see Thursday)
1 serving mushroom barley soup, Jaclyn's or take-out
1 pear

SNACK

4 dried figs
4 cups air-popped popcorn with Vegit

DINNER

2 servings ribollita using leftover minestrone alla Burrini (see Thursday) ✪ (F: 1 serving)
4 turkey kabobs ✪
1 serving succotash ✪ *or* salad of dark greens and mushrooms with 2 tablespoons vinaigrette dressing ✪

Nutritional Information (PER DAY)

	MALE	FEMALE
Calories	2,315	1,800
Carbohydrate g (%)	390 (64)	301 (64)
Fat g (%)	58 (22)	42 (20)
Protein g (%)	85 (14)	73 (16)
Cholesterol mg	100	97
Sodium mg	1,324	1,085
Chromium mcg	233	199

Saturday

BREAKFAST

½ cup Kashi pilaf made with ½ cup apple juice and ½ cup water and served with ½ cup unsweetened applesauce, 2 teaspoons Sorrell Ridge conserve, 1 sliced banana, and 1 tablespoon chopped dates (F: ½ banana)
1 slice whole grain bread with 1 tablespoon unsweetened apple butter

LUNCH

2 cups cooked long grain brown rice with 2 servings sweet potato sauce ✪ (F: 1 cup rice, 1 serving sauce)
1 pear (F: omit)

SNACK

1 whole wheat pita bread toasted to chips
½ avocado with Green Mountain salsa

DINNER

1 serving winter wheat shrimp salad ✪
1 serving potato and broccoli pizza ✪

Nutritional Information (PER DAY)

	MALE	FEMALE
Calories	2,378	1,836
Carbohydrate g (%)	411 (68)	310 (67)
Fat g (%)	47 (18)	35 (17)
Protein g (%)	85 (14)	75 (16)
Cholesterol mg	240	240
Sodium mg	1,009	943
Chromium mcg	221	197

WEEK 4

Sunday

BREAKFAST

3 slices French toast ✪ made in a nonstick skillet with 1 teaspoon canola oil and served with 2 tablespoons maple syrup
¼ honeydew melon
1 cup strawberries

LUNCH

1 serving egg salad, made with 4 hard-boiled egg whites, 2 tablespoons low-fat mayonnaise ✪, 4 teaspoons diced bread & butter chips sweet pickles,

and black pepper, with chopped tomato in one whole wheat pita bread

1 baked sweet potato with ½ cup applesauce and ½ teaspoon cinnamon (F: ½ sweet potato)

SNACK

1 pear

4 cups air-popped popcorn with Vegit

DINNER

1 serving Jaclyn's breaded cauliflower with dip of 2 tablespoons rice vinegar and 2 tablespoons low-sodium Worcestershire sauce

3 servings corn meal pizza ✪ topped with 2 servings Nitza's tomato sauce ✪ (F: omit) (Save leftovers for Monday dinner.)

2 servings mushroom risotto ✪

large salad of romaine lettuce, tomatoes, cucumbers, and mushrooms with 2 tablespoons vinaigrette dressing ✪

1 New Morning honey graham cracker (for F only)

1 stick Panda licorice (F: omit)

Nutritional Information (PER DAY)

	MALE	FEMALE
Calories	2,350	1,815
Carbohydrate g (%)	380 (63)	301 (63)
Fat g (%)	57 (22)	45 (21)
Protein g (%)	92 (15)	78 (16)
Cholesterol mg	16	13
Sodium mg	2,113	1,711
Chromium mcg	253	201

Monday

BREAKFAST

¾ cup Shredded Wheat 'N Bran, ¼ cup Fiber One, and ¼ cup Mueslix with 6 ounces skim milk, 1 banana, and 1 tablespoon chopped dates

2 slices Food for Life seven-grain sprouted cinnamon raisin bread with 3 teaspoons Sorrell Ridge conserve (F: omit)

LUNCH

1 Alvarado Street Bakery sprouted wheat bagel with lettuce, tomato, onion, and 2 tablespoons high-chromium spread ✪

2 cups melon chunks (take-out)

SNACK

1 high-chromium muffin ✪

1 apple

DINNER

1 serving flexible frittata using 1 cup leftover mushroom risotto (see Sunday) ✪ with 1 serving leftover Nitza's tomato sauce (see Sunday) (F: ½ serving risotto)

1½ servings corn salad ✪ (F: 1 serving)

1 head steamed broccoli

1 serving frozen shake ✪

Nutritional Information (PER DAY)

	MALE	FEMALE
Calories	2,350	1,808
Carbohydrate g (%)	397 (64)	314 (65)
Fat g (%)	57 (21)	43 (21)
Protein g (%)	89 (14)	70 (15)

Cholesterol mg	162	160
Sodium mg	1,737	1,451
Chromium mcg	288	238

Tuesday

BREAKFAST

1 serving cracked wheat cereal ✪ with ½ cup nonfat yogurt, ½ teaspoon cinnamon, and 2 teaspoons molasses (for F only)
1 Casbah breakfast cup (F: omit)
1 sliced banana with 2 teaspoons high-chromium spread ✪ (for F only)
1 Pritikin English muffin with 2 tablespoons high-chromium spread (F: omit)

LUNCH

1 bowl vegetable soup (take-out)
1 high-chromium muffin ✪
1 pear

SNACK

1 apple
2 whole wheat pretzels
4 cups air-popped popcorn with Vegit

DINNER (OUT)

1 appetizer serving pasta marinara
4 ounces salmon, grilled with wine and herbs
1 baked potato with marinara sauce
2 slices bread (F: omit)
1 serving salad with 2 tablespoons house Italian dressing
1 cup raspberries or other fresh fruit
1 beer *or* 1 glass wine (optional)

Nutritional Information (PER DAY)

	MALE	FEMALE
Calories	2,388	1,842
Carbohydrate g (%)	386 (63)	299 (64)
Fat g (%)	60 (21)	45 (20)
Protein g (%)	92 (15)	74 (16)
Cholesterol mg	100	101
Sodium mg	1,469	906
Chromium mcg	244	194

Wednesday

BREAKFAST

1 Casbah breakfast cup
1 banana (F: omit)

LUNCH (TAKE-OUT OR OUT)

1 serving cold sesame noodles (F: ¾ serving)
1 serving steamed vegetables with shrimp and 2 tablespoons spicy garlic or black bean sauce
1 orange (F: omit)

SNACK

2 ounces wheatgrass juice
2 plums *or* 1 apple
1 high-chromium muffin ✪

DINNER

2 servings Pizsoy pizza (F: 1 serving)
2 servings Fantastic Foods Shells 'n Curry (follow package directions, omitting oil) or 2 servings Fantastic Foods Tofu Scrambler
1 baked sweet potato with ½ cup unsweetened applesauce and ½ teaspoon cinnamon (Make four extra sweet potatoes for Thursday dinner.)
1 slice apple spice cake ✪

Nutritional Information (PER DAY)

	MALE	FEMALE
Calories	2,361	1,840
Carbohydrate g (%)	414 (64)	319 (64)
Fat g (%)	57 (20)	45 (20)
Protein g (%)	106 (16)	80 (16)
Cholesterol mg	126	126
Sodium mg	3,223	1,566
Chromium mcg	251	207

Thursday

BREAKFAST

1 cup Nutri-Grain wheat flakes and ¼ cup wheat bran with 6 ounces skim milk, 1 banana, and 1 tablespoon molasses

1 Pritikin English muffin with 2 teaspoons Sorrell Ridge marmalade and 1 tablespoon high-chromium spread ✪ (F: omit)

LUNCH (OUT)

1 bowl noncreamy soup (F: 1 cup)

1 steamed artichoke with 2 tablespoons Italian dressing (F: 1 tablespoon) or steamed vegetable

1 Caesar salad

1 cup berries *or* ¼ melon

SNACK

4 cups air-popped popcorn with Vegit

1 apple

DINNER

1½ servings split pea and rosemary soup ✪ (F: 1 serving)

2 ounces whole wheat pasta with 1 serving sweet potato sauce ✪ (Save leftovers for Friday lunch.)

2 roasted peppers ✪
1 slice whole grain bread with 2 ounces Fromage Blanc–Vegit dip ✪

Nutritional Information (PER DAY)

	MALE	FEMALE
Calories	2,334	1,828
Carbohydrate g (%)	398 (66)	330 (68)
Fat g (%)	57 (21)	42 (19)
Protein g (%)	81 (13)	62 (13)
Cholesterol mg	10	10
Sodium mg	1,842	1,394
Chromium mcg	252	206

Friday

BREAKFAST

4 ounces fresh orange juice
1 banana with ⅓ cup nonfat yogurt mixed with 2 teaspoons de-oiled peanut butter and 2 teaspoons molasses (F: omit)
1 ounce shredded low-fat mozzarella cheese melted on 1 Alvarado Street Bakery sprouted wheat bagel

LUNCH

1½ servings leftover pasta with sweet potato sauce (see Thursday) (F: 1 serving)
1 high-chromium muffin ✪ with 1 tablespoon high-chromium spread ✪
1 pear

SNACK

1 Christopher's Chewie with dates (F: omit)
2 whole wheat pretzels
4 cups air-popped popcorn with Vegit

DINNER

2 servings black beans ✪ (Save leftovers for Saturday brunch.)
1 serving cajun rice ✪
1 serving spinach sauté ✪

Nutritional Information (PER DAY)

	MALE		FEMALE	
Calories	2,341		1,789	
Carbohydrate g (%)	403	(64)	300	(64)
Fat g (%)	63	(22)	44	(21)
Protein g (%)	87	(14)	72	(15)
Cholesterol mg	67		65	
Sodium mg	1,341		1,259	
Chromium mcg	253		229	

Saturday

BREAKFAST (BRUNCH)

1 serving huevos rancheros using leftover black beans (see Friday) ✪
2 toasted corn tortillas with Hot Cha Cha! salsa
¼ honeydew melon

SNACK

1 slice apple spice cake ✪

DINNER

2 servings cooked brown rice with 3 servings primavera sauce (see pasta primavera ✪) (F: 1 serving rice, 1 serving sauce) (Save leftovers for Sunday dinner.)
2 ounces swordfish chunks (see turkey kabob variation using swordfish)
1 serving Casbah tabouly with 1 tablespoon olive oil and 2 teaspoons balsamic vinegar

1 baked acorn squash with 1 tablespoon apple juice concentrate

Nutritional Information (PER DAY)

	MALE	FEMALE
Calories	2,309	1,867
Carbohydrate g (%)	410 (67)	322 (65)
Fat g (%)	50 (19)	44 (20)
Protein g (%)	89 (15)	75 (15)
Cholesterol mg	42	41
Sodium mg	1,070	932
Chromium mcg	187	186

WEEK 5

Sunday

BREAKFAST

2 cups sliced fruit (including peaches, banana, grapes) topped with 1 cup Altadena lemon nonfat yogurt, whipped with ¼ teaspoon freshly grated ginger

1 high-chromium muffin ✪ broken into chunks with 4 ounces skim milk and 1 tablespoon molasses

LUNCH

1 serving perfect potato salad ✪ with diced tomato in 1 whole wheat pita bread

1 pear (F: omit)

SNACK

4 cups air-popped popcorn with Vegit

2 Crispini crackers (F: omit)

DINNER

2 ounces roast chicken with 2 servings high-chromium stuffing ✪ (F: 1 ounce chicken) (Save leftovers for Monday lunch.)
1 serving leftover brown rice with primavera sauce (see Saturday)
2 tomatoes grilled with 2 tablespoons olive oil (F: 1 tomato, 1 tablespoon olive oil)
1 glass wine (optional)
1 slice apple spice cake ✪ (F: ½ slice)

Nutritional Information (PER DAY)

	MALE	FEMALE
Calories	2,399	1,821
Carbohydrate g (%)	408 (64)	320 (66)
Fat g (%)	61 (21)	44 (19)
Protein g (%)	96 (15)	74 (15)
Cholesterol mg	142	118
Sodium mg	2,030	1,511
Chromium mcg	261	230

Monday

BREAKFAST

1 cup Nutri-Grain wheat flakes and ¼ cup wheat bran with 4 ounces skim milk, 1 banana, and 1 tablespoon molasses
½ Pritikin English muffin with 1 tablespoon de-oiled peanut butter and 2 teaspoons Sorrell Ridge conserve

LUNCH

1 serving Casbah mushroom tofu soup (F: omit)
1 serving curried chicken and rice salad using leftover chicken (see Sunday) ✪ with ¼ slivered avocado on 1 whole wheat pita bread

SNACK

2 plums (for F only)
1 orange
4 cups air-popped popcorn with Vegit

DINNER

2 servings zuppa di verdure ✪ with 1 tablespoon grated Parmesan cheese and 1 tablespoon de-oiled ready-made pesto (Save leftovers for Wednesday dinner.) (F: omit)
2 servings acorn squash souffle ✪ (F: 1 serving)
1 jalapeno corn muffin ✪

Nutritional Information (PER DAY)

	MALE	FEMALE
Calories	2,423	1,867
Carbohydrate g (%)	426 (65)	337 (66)
Fat g (%)	53 (18)	41 (18)
Protein g (%)	107 (16)	78 (15)
Cholesterol mg	159	98
Sodium mg	1,743	1,292
Chromium mcg	229	167

Tuesday

BREAKFAST

8 ounces fresh orange juice (F: omit)
1 poached egg on 1 Pritikin English muffin

LUNCH

1 bowl legume-based soup (take-out)
1 high-chromium muffin ✪ with 2 teaspoons Sorrell Ridge conserve
1 cup cantaloupe chunks (take-out)

SNACK

4 cups air-popped popcorn with Vegit
4 dates with 1 tablespoon de-oiled peanut butter (F: 2 teaspoons peanut butter)
1 pear

DINNER

1 serving winter wheat shrimp salad ✪ with ½ avocado and diced tomato (Save leftovers for Wednesday lunch.)
1 serving Grain Dance whole wheat pizza shell topped with 2 servings grilled eggplant ✪ with rosemary and 1 ounce feta cheese (F: omit pizza shell, 1 serving eggplant, omit feta)
1 baked sweet potato with ½ cup unsweetened applesauce and ½ teaspoon cinnamon
2 New Morning honey graham crackers
1 cup blueberries (F: omit)

Nutritional Information (PER DAY)

	MALE	FEMALE
Calories	2,305	1,825
Carbohydrate g (%)	380 (65)	292 (63)
Fat g (%)	52 (20)	43 (21)
Protein g (%)	90 (15)	77 (17)
Cholesterol mg	562	537
Sodium mg	1,697	1,069
Chromium mcg	213	167

Wednesday

BREAKFAST

1 Twinfast shake made with ½ banana ✪
1 high-chromium muffin ✪ with 2 teaspoons Sorrell Ridge conserve

LUNCH

½ serving leftover winter wheat shrimp salad (see Tuesday) with diced tomato and sprouts in 1 whole wheat pita bread

1 serving Golden Couscous tomato minestrone soup

SNACK

1 Christopher's Chewie with dates

1 apple

4 cups air-popped popcorn with Vegit

DINNER

2 servings ribollita made with leftover zuppa di verdure (see Monday) ✪ (F: 1 serving)

1 serving Casbah tabouly with 2 tablespoons olive oil and 1 tablespoon balsamic vinegar (Save leftovers for Thursday lunch.)

4 dried figs (F: omit)

1 serving frozen shake ✪

Nutritional Information (PER DAY)

	MALE	FEMALE
Calories	2,370	1,780
Carbohydrate g (%)	417 (66)	308 (66)
Fat g (%)	54 (19)	38 (18)
Protein g (%)	90 (14)	77 (16)
Cholesterol mg	160	157
Sodium mg	2,237	1,988
Chromium mcg	250	239

Thursday

BREAKFAST

¾ cup Shredded Wheat 'N Bran, ¼ cup Fiber One, and ¼ cup Mueslix with 6 ounces skim milk and 1 tablespoon chopped dates

1 banana, split and filled with 1 tablespoon de-oiled peanut butter

LUNCH

1 serving half-the-fat hummus ✪, 1 serving leftover Casbah tabouly (see Wednesday), and chopped tomato in 1 whole wheat pita bread (F: 1 ounce hummus)
1 cup mushroom barley soup (take-out) (F: omit)
1 apple

SNACK

1 high-chromium muffin ✪
1 Christopher's Chewie with dates (F: omit)
1 peach (F: omit)

DINNER

4 ounces lean select (not prime or choice) beef, broiled or sautéed in nonstick skillet with 1 sliced green pepper and 1 diced onion (F: 3 ounces)
1½ servings mushroom risotto ✪ (F: 1 serving)
1 baked acorn squash with 1 tablespoon apple juice concentrate

Nutritional Information (PER DAY)

	MALE	FEMALE
Calories	2,367	1,863
Carbohydrate g (%)	340 (63)	319 (63)
Fat g (%)	62 (22)	49 (22)
Protein g (%)	99 (15)	76 (15)
Cholesterol mg	148	122
Sodium mg	1,388	1,127
Chromium mcg	237	181

Friday

BREAKFAST

8 ounces fresh orange juice (F: omit)

⅓ cup rolled oats, ⅓ cup wheat bran, and 1 banana, cooked in 1⅓ cups water and served with 2 tablespoons chopped dates and 2 teaspoons molasses (F: ½ banana)

LUNCH

1½ ounces white meat turkey with 2 thin slices avocado, tomato, sprouts, and mustard on 1 Alvarado Street Bakery sprouted wheat bagel

1 pear (F: omit)

SNACK

2 Crispini crackers with 2 fresh or dried figs (F: 1 cracker)

DINNER (OUT)

1 bowl vegetable broth soup

1 serving cold sesame noodles

1 serving steamed vegetables with tofu (F: omit)

1 serving spicy vegetable and oyster or shrimp dish (mix with steamed vegetables)

1 serving orange slices or other fresh fruit

2 fortune cookies (F: omit)

Nutritional Information (PER DAY)

	MALE	FEMALE
Calories	2,394	1,801
Carbohydrate g (%)	422 (65)	311 (64)
Fat g (%)	52 (18)	41 (19)
Protein g (%)	111 (17)	83 (17)
Cholesterol mg	67	67
Sodium mg	2,179	2,023
Chromium mcg	230	199

Saturday

BREAKFAST

1 serving Kashi pilaf made with ½ cup apple juice and ½ cup water, served with 4 ounces skim milk, 1 banana, 1 teaspoon molasses, and 1 tablespoon chopped dates
8 ounces fresh orange juice (F: omit)

LUNCH

1 serving tuna salad ✪ topped with ¼ slivered avocado in 1 whole wheat pita bread (F: omit avocado)
1 package American Grain rice snacks
1 pear

SNACK

8 to 10 almonds
1 Chico-San corn cake with 1 tablespoon sugar-free apple butter
1 baked potato with ¼ slivered avocado (F: omit)

DINNER

1 serving pasta with scallops, peas, and vodka ✪
2 servings lima casserole ✪ (F: 1 serving)
salad of lettuce, mushrooms, and water chestnuts with 1 tablespoon vinaigrette dressing ✪

Nutritional Information (PER DAY)

	MALE	FEMALE
Calories	2,334	1,775
Carbohydrate g (%)	404 (66)	309 (67)
Fat g (%)	51 (18)	35 (17)
Protein g (%)	92 (15)	77 (17)
Cholesterol mg	57	57
Sodium mg	1,202	1,160
Chromium mcg	219	169

WEEK 6

Sunday

BREAKFAST

1 serving Fantastic Foods tofu scrambler using 2 egg whites with 2 thin avocado slices and Green Mountain salsa rolled in a flour tortilla

1 Pritikin English muffin toasted with 1 ounce shredded skim-milk mozzarella cheese

LUNCH

1 Alvarado Street Bakery sprouted wheat bagel with tomato, lettuce, onion, and mustard

1 pear (F: omit)

1 peach (for F only)

SNACK

1 serving frozen shake ✪

DINNER

2 cups new potatoes roasted with rosemary and 1 tablespoon olive oil (F: 1 cup potatoes)

2 servings killer chromium chili ✪ (F: 1 serving) (Save leftovers for Monday dinner.)

1 ear corn on the cob

1 baked acorn squash with 1 tablespoon apple juice concentrate

1 baked banana with 1 tablespoon chocolate syrup

Nutritional Information (PER DAY)

	MALE	FEMALE
Calories	2,339	1,832
Carbohydrate g (%)	409 (66)	313 (65)
Fat g (%)	48 (18)	40 (19)
Protein g (%)	104 (17)	80 (16)

Cholesterol mg	54	35
Sodium mg	1,668	1,361
Chromium mcg	246	170

Monday

BREAKFAST

⅓ cup rolled oats and ⅓ cup oat bran cooked with 1⅓ cups water, ½ diced apple, 2 teaspoons vanilla, ½ teaspoon cinnamon, and ½ sliced banana and served with 2 tablespoons Mueslix

LUNCH

1 bowl legume-based soup (take-out)
1 high-chromium muffin ✪ with 2 teaspoons Sorrell Ridge conserve
2 cups cantaloupe chunks (take-out)

SNACK

1 ounce wheatgrass juice
4 cups air-popped popcorn with 1 teaspoon brewer's yeast and Vegit
2 figs (F: omit)

DINNER

1 serving flexible frittata made with ½ serving leftover killer chromium chili (see Sunday), 1½ ounces shredded low-fat cheese, and ¼ avocado ✪ (F: omit avocado)
1½ servings whole wheat noodles with peanut sauce ✪ (F: 1 serving)
1 serving Casbah nutty pilaf

Nutritional Information (PER DAY)

	MALE	FEMALE
Calories	2,322	1,839
Carbohydrate g (%)	375 (64)	297 (65)

Fat g (%)	49 (19)	36 (18)
Protein g (%)	99 (17)	79 (17)
Cholesterol mg	175	165
Sodium mg	1,653	1,394
Chromium mcg	216	177

Tuesday

BREAKFAST

1 Casbah breakfast cup
1 banana (F: omit)

LUNCH (OUT)

1 bowl mushroom barley soup
1 serving kasha varnishkas
2 ounces white meat turkey with tomato, onion, mustard, and pickle on 2 slices whole wheat bread
1 beer (optional) (F: omit)

SNACK

1 ounce wheatgrass
2 cups melon chunks
1 Christopher's Chewie with dates (F: omit)

DINNER

2 servings black beans ✪ with Hot Cha Cha! salsa (F: 1 serving) (Save leftovers for Wednesday dinner.)
1 cup cooked brown rice made in low-sodium chicken broth with grated Parmesan cheese (F: ½ cup)
salad of mushrooms, tomatoes, onions, and 1 per serving corn tortilla toasted to chips with 1 serving avocado dressing ✪

Nutritional Information (PER DAY)

	MALE	FEMALE
Calories	2,356	1,821
Carbohydrate g (%)	412 (65)	308 (63)
Fat g (%)	61 (21)	45 (21)
Protein g (%)	88 (14)	79 (16)
Cholesterol mg	50	50
Sodium mg	2,217	2,182
Chromium mcg	206	196

Wednesday

BREAKFAST

⅔ cup rolled oats cooked with 1 banana, 1⅓ cups water, ½ diced apple, 1 teaspoon vanilla, 1 teaspoon cinnamon, and 1 tablespoon chopped dates (F: ½ banana)

1 slice Food for Life seven-grain sprouted cinnamon raisin bread with 1 tablespoon sugar-free apple butter (F: omit)

LUNCH

1 serving frozen nonfat yogurt

1 high-chromium muffin ✪

SNACK

1 pear

4 cups air-popped popcorn with 1 teaspoon brewer's yeast and Vegit

1 stick Panda licorice

DINNER

1 serving Jaclyn's split pea soup

2 servings black bean and rice pizza ✪ (F: 1 serving) (Save leftovers for Thursday lunch.)

3 ounces turkey (white meat) grilled with barbecue sauce ✪ (F: 2 ounces turkey)
2 grilled tomatoes with 1 tablespoon olive oil

Nutritional Information (PER DAY)

	MALE	FEMALE
Calories	2,385	1,826
Carbohydrate g (%)	390 (63)	306 (64)
Fat g (%)	57 (21)	40 (19)
Protein g (%)	102 (16)	79 (17)
Cholesterol mg	135	101
Sodium mg	1,012	890
Chromium mcg	241	193

Thursday

BREAKFAST

8 ounces fresh orange juice (F: omit)
1 high-chromium muffin ✪ broken into chunks with 4 ounces skim milk, 1 sliced banana, and 2 teaspoons molasses

LUNCH

1 serving leftover black bean and rice pizza (see Wednesday)
1 serving Golden Couscous tomato minestrone

SNACK

1 Christopher's Chewie with dates
4 cups air-popped popcorn with 1 teaspoon brewer's yeast and Vegit
2 plums

DINNER

4 ounces grilled salmon with lemon and dill (F: 3 ounces salmon) (Save leftover for Friday lunch.)

4 ounces amaranth pasta with 8 ounces mushrooms sautéed in 1 tablespoon olive oil and 3 cloves garlic, topped with 1 tablespoon grated Parmesan cheese and black pepper (F: 2 ounces pasta, 2 teaspoons oil)
1 baked sweet potato with ½ cup unsweetened applesauce and ½ teaspoon cinnamon

Nutritional Information (PER DAY)

	MALE	FEMALE
Calories	2,306	1,869
Carbohydrate g (%)	388 (65)	319 (65)
Fat g (%)	50 (19)	40 (19)
Protein g (%)	98 (16)	78 (16)
Cholesterol mg	117	100
Sodium mg	1,378	1,288
Chromium mcg	254	215

Friday

BREAKFAST
1 Casbah breakfast cup
1 banana

LUNCH
2 ounces leftover salmon (see Thursday) on 2 slices whole grain bread
1 baked potato with Hot Cha Cha! salsa
1 pear

DINNER (OUT)
1 serving antipasto of marinated mushrooms and roasted peppers (F: omit)
1 bowl pasta e fagioli (F: 1 cup)
1 serving pasta with red clam sauce (F: ½ serving)
2 slices bread (F: omit)
1 serving asparagus with lemon

1 serving sorbet *or* ¼ melon
1 glass wine (optional)

Nutritional Information (PER DAY)

	MALE	FEMALE
Calories	2,316	1,762
Carbohydrate g (%)	392 (64)	290 (63)
Fat g (%)	54 (19)	47 (21)
Protein g (%)	102 (17)	75 (16)
Cholesterol mg	328	228
Sodium mg	1,718	1,511
Chromium mcg	224	192

Saturday

BREAKFAST (BRUNCH)

6 ounces fresh orange juice
1 serving huevos rancheros ✪
3 peaches and 1 banana with ½ cup Altadena lemon nonfat yogurt whipped with 1 teaspoon freshly grated ginger (F: omit banana)

SNACK

1 whole wheat pita bread toasted to chips with Green Mountain salsa
1 apple

DINNER

1 serving hash brown potatoes ✪
2 servings shellfish risotto ✪ (follow mushroom risotto recipe ✪ substituting 1 pound shellfish for mushrooms) (F: 1 serving)
2 servings Grain Dance whole wheat pizza shell baked with 1 tablespoon olive oil and 3 minced cloves garlic (F: 1 serving)

1 serving grilled vegetable (follow grilled eggplant recipe ✪)
2 New Morning honey graham crackers

Nutritional Information (PER DAY)

	MALE	FEMALE
Calories	2,392	1,823
Carbohydrate g (%)	392 (64)	298 (64)
Fat g (%)	61 (22)	47 (22)
Protein g (%)	87 (14)	66 (14)
Cholesterol mg	141	136
Sodium mg	1,618	1,256
Chromium mcg	259	195

GROUP III

WEEK 1

Sunday

BREAKFAST (BRUNCH)

4 ounces fresh orange juice (F: omit)
3 pancakes made from Hodgson Mill buttermilk pancake mix using 2 egg whites and 1½ cups skim milk, cooked on a nonstick surface with 2 teaspoons canola oil, and topped with 2 tablespoons molasses *or* maple syrup
1 Alvarado Street Bakery sprouted wheat bagel with 2 ounces Fromage Blanc, 2 ounces smoked salmon, and 1 sweet onion
¼ honeydew melon or cantaloupe with mint or lime

SNACK

AM: 1 high-chromium muffin ✪
1 package American Grain rice snacks
1 pear (F: omit)

PM: 1 slice apple spice cake (F: omit)

DINNER

4 ounces quinoa pasta and 1 serving sauce with 2 servings seafood sauce ✪ (F: 2 ounces pasta)
2 servings grilled broccoli ✪ (F: 1 serving)
1 baked sweet potato with ½ cup unsweetened applesauce and ½ teaspoon cinnamon
2 chromium crostini ✪ (F: 1 crostini)
1 serving frozen shake ✪

Nutritional Information (PER DAY)

	MALE	FEMALE
Calories	2,761	2,086
Carbohydrate g (%)	481 (67)	355 (65)
Fat g (%)	56 (18)	43 (18)
Protein g (%)	111 (15)	91 (17)
Cholesterol mg	241	241
Sodium mg	2,688	2,462
Chromium mcg	239	200

Monday

BREAKFAST

2 servings cracked wheat cereal ✪ with 6 ounces skim milk, 1 banana, and ¼ cup Mueslix (F: 1 serving)
2 slices Food for Life seven-grain sprouted cinnamon raisin bread with 1 tablespoon Sorrell Ridge conserve

LUNCH

1 bowl vegetarian chili (take-out)
1 orange

SNACK

AM: 1 high-chromium muffin ✪
PM: 1 ounce Perfect Foods frozen wheatgrass juice
1 apple

DINNER

1½ servings high-chromium meat loaf ✪ (F: 1 serving)
2 servings whipped buttermilk potatoes ✪ (F: 1 serving)
2 ears corn on the cob (F: 1 ear)
1 serving Casbah tabouly with 1 tablespoon olive oil and 2 tablespoons balsamic vinegar (F: 2 tablespoons olive oil)

Nutritional Information (PER DAY)

	MALE	FEMALE
Calories	2,768	2,099
Carbohydrate g (%)	480 (64)	369 (65)
Fat g (%)	68 (20)	49 (19)
Protein g (%)	125 (16)	90 (16)
Cholesterol mg	209	161
Sodium mg	1,743	1,493
Chromium mcg	297	252

Tuesday

BREAKFAST

¼ cup millet porridge, ¼ cup rolled or ¼ cup rye flakes oats, and ¼ cup wheat bran cooked with 1½ cups water and topped with 1 tablespoon sunflower seeds, 1 sliced banana, 1 tablespoon chopped dates, and 1 tablespoon molasses

LUNCH

3 cups salad bar selections (excluding mayonnaise- and oil-based foods, such as macaroni salad and marinated vegetables) with 2 tablespoons Italian dressing

1 baked potato with salsa or cocktail sauce

SNACK

AM: 1 Alvarado Street Bakery sprouted wheat bagel with 1 tablespoon sugar-free apple butter
1 orange

PM: 2 whole wheat pretzels *or* 2 high-chromium gingers ✪
1 ounce wheatgrass juice
3 dried figs

DINNER

1½ servings corn bread "fried" chicken ✪ (F: 1 serving) (Save leftovers for Wednesday lunch.)

1½ jalapeno corn muffins ✪ (F: 1 muffin)

1 baked acorn squash with 1 tablespoon apple juice concentrate

1 serving nonfat yogurt dessert ✪ topped with 1 crumbled New Morning honey graham cracker (F: omit)

Nutritional Information (PER DAY)

	MALE	FEMALE
Calories	2,753	2,115
Carbohydrate g (%)	496 (66)	376 (65)
Fat g (%)	57 (17)	46 (18)
Protein g (%)	130 (17)	99 (17)
Cholesterol mg	136	88
Sodium mg	1,144	879
Chromium mcg	247	210

Wednesday

BREAKFAST

½ cup oatmeal cooked with 1 cup water, 1 teaspoon vanilla, 1 teaspoon cinnamon, 1 diced pear, and 1 banana (F: omit pear)

2 slices Food for Life seven-grain sprouted cinnamon raisin bread with 4 teaspoons Sorrell Ridge conserve and 1 teaspoon butter

LUNCH

1 serving leftover corn bread "fried" chicken (see Tuesday)

1 serving Golden Couscous tomato minestrone soup

SNACK

AM: 2 apples

PM: 1 ounce wheatgrass juice
2 whole wheat pretzels
4 cups air-popped popcorn with Vegit
1 stick Panda licorice (F: ½ stick)

DINNER

2 servings pasta primavera ✪ (F: 1 serving)

2 servings high-chromium salad ✪ with 2 teaspoons olive oil and ¼ slivered avocado (F: 1 serving)

1 baked sweet potato with ½ cup unsweetened applesauce and ½ teaspoon cinnamon

½ high-chromium muffin ✪ broken into chunks and topped with 3 ounces Élan coffee frozen dessert

Nutritional Information (PER DAY)

	MALE	FEMALE
Calories	2,820	2,066
Carbohydrate g (%)	502 (66)	351 (65)
Fat g (%)	56 (17)	44 (18)

Protein g (%)	132 (17)	94 (17)
Cholesterol mg	277	172
Sodium mg	1,845	1,341
Chromium mcg	225	176

Thursday

BREAKFAST

1 serving Diet-Fuel (F: omit)

½ cup Nutri-Grain wheat flakes and ½ cup corn flakes with 4 ounces skim milk, 1 banana, 1 tablespoon molasses, and 1 tablespoon chopped dates

1 Pritikin English muffin with 2 ounces low-fat Swiss cheese

LUNCH

1 serving half-the-fat hummus ✪ with diced tomatoes and ¼ slivered avocado in 1 whole wheat pita bread

1 cup legume-based soup (take-out) *or* 1 serving Golden Couscous curried lentil soup

SNACK

AM: 1 Alvarado Street Bakery sprouted wheat bagel with 1 tablespoon sugar-free apple butter (F: omit)
1 orange

PM: 1 ounce wheatgrass juice
1 Christopher's Chewie with dates (F: omit)
2 peaches *or* 1 cup melon chunks (for F only)

DINNER

1 serving killer chromium chili ✪ (Freeze leftovers for lunch next Tuesday.)

1 serving Pizsoy pizza

1 ear corn on the cob with 1 teaspoon butter (F: omit)

1 baked potato topped with salsa and ¼ slivered avocado (F: omit avocado)
salad of lettuce, mushrooms, tomatoes, and carrot with 1 tablespoon vinaigrette dressing ✪ (for F only)
½ stick Panda licorice (F: omit)

Nutritional Information (PER DAY)

	MALE	FEMALE
Calories	2,763	2,047
Carbohydrate g (%)	471 (65)	348 (65)
Fat g (%)	58 (18)	45 (19)
Protein g (%)	119 (16)	84 (16)
Cholesterol mg	34	23
Sodium mg	2,879	2,294
Chromium mcg	250	189

Friday

BREAKFAST
8 ounces fresh orange juice (F: omit)
¾ cup Nutri-Grain biscuits and ¼ cup Fiber One with 4 ounces skim milk, 1 banana, and ¼ cup Mueslix
1 high-chromium muffin ✪ with 1 tablespoon sugar-free apple butter

LUNCH
1 serving Diet-Fuel
1 Pritikin English muffin with tomato and ¼ slivered avocado

SNACK
AM: 1 pear
PM: 1 ounce wheatgrass juice

1 apple with 1 tablespoon de-oiled peanut butter (F: omit)
4 cups air-popped popcorn with Vegit

DINNER

2 servings zuppa di verdure ✪ (Save leftovers for Sunday dinner.)
2 Fantastic Foods Nature's Burgers with ketchup from Laurel's Kitchen ✪ and 1 tablespoon low-sodium Worcestershire sauce in one whole wheat pita bread (F: 1 burger)
2 servings Kashi pilaf, chilled and mixed with tomato, mushroom, lettuce, onions, ¼ avocado, and 3 tablespoons vinaigrette dressing ✪ (F: 1 serving Kashi pilaf 2 tablespoons vinaigrette)

Nutritional Information (PER DAY)

	MALE	FEMALE
Calories	2,783	2,004
Carbohydrate g (%)	493 (67)	355 (66)
Fat g (%)	63 (19)	45 (19)
Protein g (%)	102 (14)	79 (15)
Cholesterol mg	46	46
Sodium mg	1,842	1,309
Chromium mcg	269	227

Saturday

BREAKFAST (BRUNCH)

4 ounces fresh orange juice
1 poached egg
2 slices whole wheat sprouted toast
2 cups melon chunks and berries
2 servings hash brown potatoes ✪ (F: 1 serving)

SNACK

1 high-chromium muffin ✪ with 2 tablespoons sugar-free apple butter (F: omit apple butter)
1 pear
3 servings Linn's cole slaw ✪ (F: omit)
1 slice low-fat Swiss cheese rolled around a sweet pickle (F: omit cheese)
1 banana

DINNER (OUT)

1 lean hamburger on whole wheat bun (or bread) with grilled mushrooms, peppers, lettuce, tomatoes, pickle
1 serving French fries (F: omit)
1 bowl legume-based soup
2 cups steamed zucchini or other vegetable
salad of mixed greens with 2 tablespoons low-cal dressing
1 beer (optional)

Nutritional Information (PER DAY)

	MALE	FEMALE
Calories	2,806	2,056
Carbohydrate g (%)	460 (63)	336 (63)
Fat g (%)	77 (22)	55 (21)
Protein g (%)	109 (15)	84 (16)
Cholesterol mg	426	391
Sodium mg	2,181	1,980
Chromium mcg	243	216

WEEK 2

Sunday

BREAKFAST (BRUNCH)

1 serving Diet-Fuel (F: omit)
¾ cup Shredded Wheat 'N Bran and ¼ cup Nutri-Grain wheat flakes with 6 ounces skim milk, 1 banana, and ¼ cup Mueslix
½ melon
2 slices Food for Life seven-grain sprouted cinnamon raisin bread with 2 tablespoons prune whip ✪

SNACK

2 apples, sliced, with 4 teaspoons high-chromium spread ✪
4 cups air-popped popcorn with Vegit
or
1 whole wheat pita bread toasted to chips with 2 ounces Fromage Blanc–Vegit dip ✪

DINNER

2 servings ribollita using leftover zuppa di verdure (see Friday) ✪ (F: 1½ servings)
2 servings acorn squash souffle ✪
2 roasted red peppers ✪ with 1½ tablespoons vinaigrette dressing ✪ (F: 1 tablespoon dressing)
5 figs (F: omit)
2 New Morning honey graham crackers *or* 2 high-chromium gingers ✪ (F: omit)

Nutritional Information (PER DAY)

	MALE	FEMALE
Calories	2,759	2,079
Carbohydrate g (%)	483 (67)	377 (68)
Fat g (%)	58 (18)	44 (18)

Protein g (%)	109 (15)	73 (13)
Cholesterol mg	137	135
Sodium mg	1,433	1,068
Chromium mcg	266	180

Monday

BREAKFAST

1 ounce wheatgrass juice
4 ounces fresh orange juice
¾ cup Shredded Wheat 'N Bran, ¼ cup Fiber One, and ¼ cup Mueslix with 6 ounces skim milk, 1 banana, and 1 tablespoon molasses
1 Alvarado Street Bakery sprouted wheat bagel toasted with 1½ ounces shredded skim-milk mozzarella cheese (F: omit)

LUNCH

1 serving Diet-Fuel
1 high-chromium muffin ✪ with 2 tablespoons deoiled peanut butter
1 pear

SNACK

AM: 1 Christopher's Chewie with dates
1 orange
PM: 2 whole wheat pretzels *or* 2 high-chromium gingers ✪
3 ounces Élan vanilla frozen dessert

DINNER

2 servings pasta with braised lentils ✪ (F: 1 serving)
1 cup fresh or frozen green peas, steamed and sautéed with 4 ounces mushrooms in 2 teaspoons olive oil and served with 1 teaspoon butter

1 baked sweet potato with ½ cup unsweetened applesauce with ½ teaspoon cinnamon

Nutritional Information (PER DAY)

	MALE	FEMALE
Calories	2,783	2,095
Carbohydrate g (%)	462 (64)	362 (65)
Fat g (%)	63 (20)	49 (20)
Protein g (%)	122 (17)	86 (15)
Cholesterol mg	121	81
Sodium mg	2,107	1,279
Chromium mcg	250	232

Tuesday

BREAKFAST

8 ounces fresh orange juice (F: omit)

2 servings cracked wheat cereal ✪ with ½ cup nonfat yogurt mixed with ½ cup applesauce, 1 tablespoon chopped dates, and 1 tablespoon molasses (F: 1 serving cereal)

1 Pritikin English muffin with 1 tablespoon sugar-free apple butter and 1 tablespoon de-oiled peanut butter

LUNCH

1 serving leftover killer chromium chili (frozen, see Thursday) stuffed in a baked potato and topped with salsa and ½ ounce shredded low-fat cheese

SNACK

AM: 1 ounce wheatgrass juice
1 orange

PM: 1 stick Panda licorice
1 pear

DINNER

2 servings Jaclyn's mushroom barley soup (F: 1 serving)
1 serving Fantastic Foods tofu scrambler
3 servings Pizsoy pizza (F: 2 servings)
salad of romaine lettuce, mushrooms, celery, and onions with 1 tablespoon vinaigrette dressing ✪
1 slice orange peanut bread ✪ topped with 1½ tablespoons Sorrell Ridge marmalade (F: omit)

Nutritional Information (PER DAY)

	MALE	FEMALE
Calories	2,726	2,010
Carbohydrate g (%)	485 (65)	350 (64)
Fat g (%)	59 (18)	45 (19)
Protein g (%)	123 (17)	94 (17)
Cholesterol mg	21	21
Sodium mg	2,293	1,665
Chromium mcg	270	225

Wednesday

BREAKFAST

1 serving Kashi pilaf made with ½ cup apple juice and ½ cup water, served with ½ cup unsweetened applesauce mixed with ½ cup nonfat yogurt and 1 tablespoon molasses (Save leftover Kashi pilaf for Thursday breakfast.)
2 slices whole wheat toast with 1 tablespoon Sorrell Ridge conserve (F: omit)

LUNCH (OUT)

3 ounces turkey club with lettuce, tomatoes, sprouts, mustard or low-calorie dressing, and pickle with 2 tablespoons mayonnaise on 3 slices whole wheat or rye bread
1 bowl Manhattan clam chowder or minestrone

SNACK

AM: 1 high-chromium muffin ✪ with 2 teaspoons Sorrell Ridge conserve
1 ounce wheatgrass juice

PM: 5 dried figs
1 banana

DINNER

1 serving John's scallops ✪
2 servings whole wheat noodles with 2 servings peanut sauce ✪ (F: 1 serving each)
1 baked acorn squash with 1 tablespoon apple juice concentrate
1 serving frozen shake ✪ (F: omit)

Nutritional Information (PER DAY)

	MALE	FEMALE
Calories	2,746	2,087
Carbohydrate g (%)	462 (66)	338 (64)
Fat g (%)	53 (17)	44 (18)
Protein g (%)	117 (17)	93 (18)
Cholesterol mg	171	170
Sodium mg	2,129	1,517
Chromium mcg	220	180

Thursday

BREAKFAST

8 ounces fresh orange juice
1 serving leftover Kashi pilaf (see Wednesday) with ½ cup nonfat yogurt, ½ cup unsweetened applesauce, and 1 tablespoon molasses

LUNCH (OUT)

1 Caesar salad
1 baked potato with cocktail sauce
1 serving sorbet

SNACK

AM: 1 Christopher's Chewie with dates (F: omit)
PM: 1 high-chromium muffin ✪

DINNER

2 servings minestrone alla Burrini ✪ (F: 1 serving)
2 servings whole wheat fettucini with zucchini and smoked salmon ✪ (F: 1 serving)
1 tomato roasted in 1 tablespoon olive oil, topped with 2 teaspoons grated Parmesan cheese
1 slice orange peanut bread

Nutritional Information (PER DAY)

	MALE	FEMALE
Calories	2,713	2,034
Carbohydrate g (%)	456 (64)	345 (64)
Fat g (%)	63 (20)	48 (20)
Protein g (%)	117 (16)	83 (16)
Cholesterol mg	107	76
Sodium mg	1,849	1,449
Chromium mcg	260	208

Friday

BREAKFAST

4 ounces fresh orange juice
⅔ cup rolled oats cooked with 1½ cups water, 1 cubed apple, 1 sliced banana, 1 teaspoon vanilla, ½ teaspoon cinnamon, and topped with ¼ cup Mueslix
1 Pritikin English muffin with 2 teaspoons Sorrell Ridge conserve

LUNCH (OUT)

1½ servings cold sesame noodles (F: 1 serving)
1 serving mixed vegetables with shrimp or oysters in garlic or black bean sauce
1 fortune cookie

SNACK

AM: 2 cups melon chunks (take-out)
PM: 1 Christopher's Chewie with dates (F: omit)
4 cups air-popped popcorn with Vegit

DINNER

3 ounces grilled swordfish prepared with 6 ounces mushrooms, 2 teaspoons olive oil, ½ teaspoon rosemary, and black pepper (Save leftovers for Saturday dinner.)
2 servings corn salad (F: 1 serving)
2 peaches *or* 1 pear
½ stick Panda licorice (F: omit)

Nutritional Information (PER DAY)

	MALE	FEMALE
Calories	2,756	2,120
Carbohydrate g (%)	459 (63)	351 (63)
Fat g (%)	72 (22)	52 (21)
Protein g (%)	110 (15)	93 (17)
Cholesterol mg	156	154
Sodium mg	1,449	1,136
Chromium mcg	260	190

Saturday

BREAKFAST (BRUNCH)

4 ounces fresh orange juice (F: omit)
1 serving genuine Austin omelette ✪
2 apples, sliced, with lemon
½ jalapeno corn muffin ✪

SNACK

2 slices orange peanut bread with 2 teaspoons Sorrell Ridge marmalade (F: 1 serving)

1 stick Panda licorice
4 cups air-popped popcorn with Vegit

DINNER

4 ounces amaranth or whole wheat pasta with 2 servings red or white clam sauce substituting leftover swordfish (see Friday) for clams ✪ (F: 2 ounces pasta, 1 serving sauce) (Save leftover sauce for Sunday lunch.)
2 servings succotash ✪ (F: 1 serving)
2 fresh tomato sandwiches ✪ (F: 1 sandwich)
1 beer *or* 1 glass wine (optional) (F: omit)

Nutritional Information (PER DAY)

	MALE		FEMALE	
Calories	2,781		2,061	
Carbohydrate g (%)	461	(64)	338	(63)
Fat g (%)	65	(20)	50	(21)
Protein g (%)	112	(15)	87	(16)
Cholesterol mg	254		251	
Sodium mg	2,043		1,604	
Chromium mcg	239		189	

WEEK 3

Sunday

BREAKFAST

4 ounces fresh orange juice
3 buckwheat pancakes ✪, cooked in 2 teaspoons canola oil and topped with 2 tablespoons maple syrup
1 Alvarado Street Bakery sprouted wheat bagel with

1 ounce smoked salmon, 1 ounce Fromage Blanc, and 1 slice sweet onion (F: omit)
½ honeydew melon (F: ¼ melon)
½ cup berries

LUNCH

1 baked potato topped with 1 serving leftover swordfish sauce (see Saturday)
2 servings Pizsoy pizza (F: 1 serving) (Save leftovers for Monday lunch.)

SNACK

AM: 1 apple
PM: 4 cups air-popped popcorn with Vegit
1 whole wheat pita bread toasted to chips with ¼ slivered avocado

DINNER

2 servings split pea and rosemary soup ✪ (F: 1 serving) (Save leftovers for Monday lunch.)
1 serving milk-soaked haddock ✪
1 ear corn on the cob *or* 1 cup stewed tomatoes (unsalted)
1 high-chromium muffin ✪ broken into chunks and topped with 2 ounces Élan coffee or chocolate frozen dessert (F: ½ muffin)

Nutritional Information (PER DAY)

	MALE	FEMALE
Calories	2,818	2,072
Carbohydrate g (%)	484 (65)	358 (65)
Fat g (%)	62 (18)	47 (19)
Protein g (%)	127 (17)	85 (16)
Cholesterol mg	323	293
Sodium mg	2,550	1,501
Chromium mcg	240	186

Monday

BREAKFAST

4 ounces fresh orange juice (F: omit)
1 serving cracked wheat cereal ✪ with ½ cup nonfat yogurt mixed with ½ cup unsweetened applesauce, 1 banana, 1 tablespoon sunflower seeds, and 1 tablespoon molasses
1 Pritikin English muffin with 1 ounce Fromage Blanc mixed with 1 tablespoon Sorrel Ridge conserve

LUNCH

1 serving leftover Pizsoy pizza (see Sunday)
1 serving leftover split pea and rosemary soup (see Sunday) with 1 tablespoon wheat bran and 1 tablespoon grated Parmesan cheese

SNACK

AM: 1 ounce wheatgrass juice
1 high-chromium muffin ✪
PM: 1 pear (F: omit)

DINNER

4 ounces pasta with 2 servings lima and pesto sauce ✪ (F: 1 serving) (Save leftovers for Tuesday dinner.)
2 servings Isadore's bulgur salad ✪
2 cups diced zucchini sautéed in 1 tablespoon olive oil, minced garlic, and black pepper
1 serving soft frozen yogurt in a waffle cone (F: omit)

Nutritional Information (PER DAY)

	MALE	FEMALE
Calories	2,763	2,069
Carbohydrate g (%)	478 (66)	361 (65)
Fat g (%)	60 (19)	48 (19)
Protein g (%)	115 (16)	85 (15)

Cholesterol mg	85	64
Sodium mg	1,713	1,324
Chromium mcg	272	241

Tuesday

BREAKFAST

8 ounces fresh orange juice
½ cup rolled oats and ¼ cup wheat bran or rye flakes prepared in 1½ cups water cooked with 1 sliced banana, 1 diced apple, 1 teaspoon vanilla, ½ teaspoon cinnamon, served with 1 tablespoon chopped dates, and 1 tablespoon molasses
1 high-chromium muffin ✪ (F: omit)

LUNCH (OUT)

1 bowl tomato or legume-based soup
3 ounces fish fillet prepared with herbs, lemon, and wine
1 serving steamed asparagus with 1 tablespoon house dressing
1 cup sorbet *or* 1 cup berries
1 glass wine (optional) (F: omit)

SNACK

AM: 1 cup melon chunks (take-out)
1 ounce wheatgrass juice
PM: 2 ounces half-the-fat hummus ✪ with 2 whole wheat pita breads toasted to chips (F: 1 pita, same hummus) (Save leftovers for Wednesday lunch.)

DINNER

1 serving flexible frittata made with 1 serving leftover lima and pesto sauce (see Monday) ✪

2 servings Fantastic Foods Shells 'N Curry* (F: omit)
1 baked sweet potato with ½ cup unsweetened applesauce and ½ teaspoon cinnamon
salad of romaine lettuce, mushrooms, tomato, and onion with 1½ tablespoons vinaigrette dressing ✪
1 stick Panda licorice (F: omit)

Nutritional Information (PER DAY)

	MALE	FEMALE
Calories	2,781	2,110
Carbohydrate g (%)	467 (64)	357 (65)
Fat g (%)	68 (21)	47 (19)
Protein g (%)	115 (16)	87 (16)
Cholesterol mg	216	172
Sodium mg	2,180	1,908
Chromium mcg	216	172

Wednesday

BREAKFAST

8 ounces fresh orange juice (F: omit)
3 egg whites scrambled with 1 teaspoon de-oiled ready-made pesto and 1 teaspoon grated Parmesan cheese in a nonstick skillet
1 Alvarado Street Bakery sprouted wheat bagel with 1 ounce Fromage Blanc mixed with 2 teaspoons Sorrell Ridge blueberry conserve

LUNCH

2 ounces leftover half-the-fat hummus (see Tuesday) with sprouts, lettuce, and diced tomatoes in 1 whole wheat pita bread
1 bowl legume-based soup (take-out) *or* 1 serving Golden Couscous curried lentil soup

*Follow directions on package omitting oil.

SNACK

AM: 1 pear

PM: 1 high-chromium muffin ✪

1 apple

DINNER

2 servings cajun rice ✪ with 3½ ounces Holland's Pride mussels in cocktail sauce (F: 1½ servings rice) (Save leftover rice for Thursday lunch.)

3 servings Jaclyn's mushrooms with dipping sauce of 3 tablespoons low-sodium Worcestershire sauce and 3 tablespoons rice vinegar (F: omit)

1 serving grilled broccoli and/or cauliflower ✪ served cool with lemon juice and balsamic vinegar

2 slices whole wheat or rye bread with 1 ounce Fromage Blanc–Vegit dip ✪ (F: 1 slice)

Nutritional Information (PER DAY)

	MALE	FEMALE
Calories	2,785	2,025
Carbohydrate g (%)	476 (64)	331 (64)
Fat g (%)	76 (20)	45 (19)
Protein g (%)	115 (15)	88 (17)
Cholesterol mg	255	255
Sodium mg	2,708	2,355
Chromium mcg	286	207

Thursday

BREAKFAST

¾ cup Shredded Wheat 'N Bran, ¼ cup Fiber One, and ¼ cup Mueslix with 6 ounces skim milk, 1 banana, and 1 tablespoon chopped dates

2 slices Food for Life seven-grain sprouted cinnamon

raisin bread with 2 teaspoons Sorrell Ridge conserve (F: 1 slice)

LUNCH

1 bowl legume-based soup (take-out) (F: 1 cup)
1 serving leftover cajun rice (see Wednesday)

SNACK

AM: 2 cups melon chunks (take-out) *or* 2 high-chromium gingers ✪
PM: 1 serving Diet-Fuel

DINNER

4 ounces quinoa pasta with 4 tablespoons ready-made de-oiled pesto mixed with 2 ounces Fromage Blanc (make extra for Friday) (F: 2 ounces pasta, 2 tablespoons pesto, 1 ounce Fromage Blanc)
2 Fantastic Foods Nature's Burgers made with 1 tablespoon low-sodium Worcestershire sauce and 1 tablespoon brewer's yeast and served on 1 Pritikin English muffin with 1½ ounces low-fat Swiss cheese and ketchup from Laurel's Kitchen ✪ (F: 1 burger, 1 ounce cheese)
1 baked potato with ¼ slivered avocado and Hot Cha Cha! salsa

Nutritional Information (PER DAY)

	MALE	FEMALE
Calories	2,836	2,054
Carbohydrate g (%)	448 (63)	335 (64)
Fat g (%)	70 (22)	51 (21)
Protein g (%)	113 (16)	81 (16)
Cholesterol mg	52	33
Sodium mg	1,588	1,070
Chromium mcg	266	185

Friday

BREAKFAST

1 serving Kashi pilaf made with ½ cup apple juice and ½ cup water and served with 6 ounces skim milk, 1 banana, and 1 tablespoon molasses

2 slices whole grain bread with 1 tablespoon sugar-free apple butter (F: 2 tablespoons)

LUNCH (OUT)

1 bowl gumbo (no sausage) or Manhattan clam chowder

1 serving crab or lobster salad

1 baked potato with cocktail sauce

SNACK

AM: 2 peaches

PM: 1 Christopher's Chewie with dates

1 pear (F: omit)

DINNER

3 ounces roast chicken in red wine and sage (do not eat chicken skin), stuffed with 1 serving leftover 2 ounces pasta and 2 ounces pesto or served on the side (see Thursday) (F: ½ serving pasta) (Save leftover chicken for Saturday lunch.)

2 servings curried Waldorf salad ✪ (F: 1 serving) (Save leftovers for Saturday lunch.)

1½ cups Casbah nutty pilaf (F: ½ cup)

3 dried figs (F: omit)

Nutritional Information (PER DAY)

	MALE	FEMALE
Calories	2,776	2,099
Carbohydrate g (%)	476 (68)	349 (66)
Fat g (%)	57 (18)	41 (18)

Protein g (%)	100 (14)	86 (16)
Cholesterol mg	125	123
Sodium mg	1,501	1,477
Chromium mcg	200	178

Saturday

BREAKFAST

4 ounces fresh orange juice
3 pancakes made from Hodgson Mill buttermilk pancake mix with 2 egg whites and 1½ cups skim milk, cooked on a nonstick surface with 1 tablespoon canola oil, and served with 2 tablespoons maple syrup
1 Pritikin English muffin with 2 tablespoons prune whip ✪
½ honeydew melon with lime (F: ¼ melon)

LUNCH

2 servings curried chicken and rice salad made with leftover roast chicken (see Friday) mixed with 2 servings leftover curried Waldorf salad (see Friday) with shredded lettuce in 2 whole wheat pita breads (F: 1 serving curried salad, 1 serving Waldorf salad, 1 pita)

SNACK

4 cups air-popped popcorn with Vegit
1 banana, split and filled with 1 tablespoon almond butter (F: omit)

DINNER

1 serving winter wheat shrimp salad ✪ with ½ slivered avocado (F: ¼ avocado)
1 serving killer chromium chili ✪ (F: ½ serving) (Save leftovers for Monday lunch.)

1 baked sweet potato with ½ cup unsweetened applesauce and ½ teaspoon cinnamon
1 slice orange peanut bread ✪ with 2 teaspoons Sorrell Ridge marmalade (for F only)

Nutritional Information (PER DAY)

	MALE	FEMALE
Calories	2,756	2,104
Carbohydrate g (%)	452 (63)	350 (64)
Fat g (%)	63 (20)	43 (18)
Protein g (%)	125 (17)	97 (18)
Cholesterol mg	430	395
Sodium mg	1,807	1,513
Chromium mcg	238	169

WEEK 4

Sunday

BREAKFAST

3 slices French toast ✪, cooked in 1 tablespoon canola oil and topped with 2 tablespoons maple syrup
½ cup rolled oats cooked in 1 cup water with 1 sliced banana, 1 diced apple, 1 teaspoon vanilla, and 1 teaspoon cinnamon and served with 1 tablespoon molasses

LUNCH (OUT OR TAKE-OUT)

1 bowl mushroom barley soup
1 serving kasha varnishkas
2 ounces lean roast beef with horseradish and pickle *or* ½ cup sauerkraut on 2 slices rye bread

DINNER

1 serving whipped buttermilk potatoes ✪ (F: omit)
3 servings black beans ✪ (F: 1 serving) (Save leftovers for Monday dinner.)
1½ cups cooked short grain brown rice with salsa (F: 1 cup) (Save leftovers for Monday dinner.)
salad of romaine lettuce, chopped onion, tomatoes, and 3 olives with 1 ounce avocado dressing ✪

Nutritional Information (PER DAY)

	MALE	FEMALE
Calories	2,728	2,102
Carbohydrate g (%)	487 (67)	358 (65)
Fat g (%)	56 (17)	47 (19)
Protein g (%)	113 (16)	86 (16)
Cholesterol mg	59	58
Sodium mg	2,624	2,500
Chromium mcg	245	251

Monday

BREAKFAST

1 Casbah breakfast cup
2 slices Food for Life seven-grain sprouted cinnamon raisin bread with 4 teaspoons Sorrell Ridge conserve mixed with 2 ounces Fromage Blanc (F: 2 teaspoons conserve, omit Fromage Blanc)

LUNCH

1 serving leftover killer chromium chili (see Saturday) with Green Mountain salsa and/or tomato chunks in 1 whole wheat pita bread
1 baked potato

SNACK

AM: 1 apple
1 high-chromium muffin ✪

PM: 4 cups air-popped popcorn with Vegit
1 pear (F: omit)

DINNER

2 servings black bean and rice pizza ✪ (F: 1 serving pizza)

1 serving Casbah tabouly with 1 tablespoon olive oil and 2 tablespoons balsamic vinegar

1 serving acorn squash souffle ✪ (Save leftovers for Tuesday lunch.)

Nutritional Information (PER DAY)

	MALE	FEMALE
Calories	2,773	2,057
Carbohydrate g (%)	466 (64)	348 (65)
Fat g (%)	68 (21)	49 (21)
Protein g (%)	104 (14)	72 (14)
Cholesterol mg	150	70
Sodium mg	1,577	1,321
Chromium mcg	265	194

Tuesday

BREAKFAST

2 servings cracked wheat cereal ✪ with ½ cup plain nonfat yogurt mixed with ½ cup unsweetened applesauce and 1 tablespoon molasses (F: 1 serving cereal)

1 Alvarado Street Bakery sprouted wheat bagel with 1 tablespoon de-oiled peanut butter and 2 teaspoons Sorrell Ridge marmalade

LUNCH

1 bowl legume- or tomato-based soup (take-out)
1 high-chromium muffin ✪ with 2 teaspoons almond butter (F: omit almond butter)
5 dried figs *or* 1 serving leftover acorn squash souffle (see Monday) (F: omit)

SNACK

AM: 1 plum, 1 pear, and 1 apple
PM: 1 tomato with ½ slivered avocado
2 Crispini crackers (F: omit)

DINNER (OUT)

6 oysters or clams on the half-shell
condiment tray selections including pickles and corn relish
½ pound lobster, broiled or steamed (no butter)
1 baked potato with cocktail sauce
1 cup steamed vegetables
1 ear corn on the cob
1 slice bread (F: omit)
1 cup strawberries with 3 tablespoons whipped cream (F: omit cream)
1 glass wine (optional)

Nutritional Information (PER DAY)

	MALE	FEMALE
Calories	2,788	2,077
Carbohydrate g (%)	460 (65)	340 (65)
Fat g (%)	61 (19)	44 (18)
Protein g (%)	113 (16)	94 (18)
Cholesterol mg	260	198
Sodium mg	2,597	1,982
Chromium mcg	244	196

Wednesday

BREAKFAST

¾ cup Shredded Wheat 'N Bran, ¼ cup Fiber One, and ¼ cup Mueslix with 6 ounces skim milk, 1 banana, and 1 tablespoon chopped dates

1 Alvarado Street Bakery sprouted wheat bagel with 2 tablespoons sugar-free apple butter

LUNCH

2 ounces half-the-fat hummus ✪ with chopped tomatoes, cucumbers, and ¼ slivered avocado in 1 whole wheat pita bread

1 cup legume-based soup (take-out) *or* 1 serving Golden Couscous tomato minestrone

SNACK

AM: 1 ounce wheatgrass juice
1 apple
1 Christopher's Chewie with dates (F: omit)

PM: 1 high-chromium muffin ✪

DINNER

1 serving high-chromium meat loaf ✪ (Save leftovers for Thursday lunch.)

2½ ounces whole wheat pasta (F: 1½ ounces)

½ cup peas and 2 cups summer squash, steamed and sautéed in 2 tablespoons olive oil and 1 clove garlic and served on top of pasta (F: omit peas)

1 serving hash brown potatoes ✪

1 serving frozen shake ✪ (for F only)

Nutritional Information (PER DAY)

	MALE	FEMALE
Calories	2,781	2,077
Carbohydrate g (%)	480 (64)	382 (67)

Fat g (%)	70 (21)	39 (15)
Protein g (%)	113 (15)	101 (18)
Cholesterol mg	140	141
Sodium mg	2,136	2,095
Chromium mcg	254	207

Thursday

BREAKFAST

4 ounces fresh orange juice

1 banana, split and filled with ½ tablespoon de-oiled peanut butter mixed with 1 tablespoon molasses (F: omit peanut butter)

⅔ cup rolled oats cooked with 1 diced apple, 1 teaspoon vanilla, ½ teaspoon cinnamon, and 1½ cups water

LUNCH

½ serving leftover high-chromium meat loaf (see Wednesday) with barbecue sauce or 1 tablespoon low-sodium Worcestershire sauce, Romaine lettuce, and ¼ avocado on 2 slices whole grain bread

1 bowl legume- or tomato-based soup (take-out) (F: omit)

SNACK

AM: 2 plums
1 pear

PM: 1 high-chromium muffin ✪
2 whole wheat pretzels

DINNER

1 serving corn bread "fried" chicken made with 1 teaspoon additional olive oil ✪

2 servings winter wheat, corn, and cheese casserole ✪ (F: 1 serving) (Save leftovers for Friday dinner.)

1 baked sweet potato with ½ cup unsweetened applesauce and ½ teaspoon cinnamon
3 servings Linn's cole slaw ✪ (F: omit)
1 stick Panda licorice (F: ½ stick)

Nutritional Information (PER DAY)

	MALE	FEMALE
Calories	2,801	2,068
Carbohydrate g (%)	463 (63)	353 (64)
Fat g (%)	60 (19)	44 (18)
Protein g (%)	131 (18)	102 (18)
Cholesterol mg	190	179
Sodium mg	1,505	1,109
Chromium mcg	248	174

Friday

BREAKFAST

1 serving Kashi pilaf made with ½ cup apple juice and ½ cup water and topped with 1 sliced banana and 1 tablespoon molasses
2 slices whole grain bread with 1 tablespoon Sorrell Ridge conserve

LUNCH (OUT)

1 slice bread
3 ounces fish fillet grilled with lemon, wine, and herbs
spinach salad (with no egg yolks and no bacon) with 1 tablespoon olive oil, lemon juice or vinegar, and pepper
¼ melon *or* 1 cup berries

SNACK

AM: 1 high-chromium muffin ✪ with 2 teaspoons Sorrell Ridge conserve

PM: 2 New Morning honey graham crackers with 2 tablespoons sugar-free apple butter

DINNER

1 serving flexible frittata made with 2 servings leftover winter wheat, corn, and cheese casserole (see Thursday) ✪ (F: 1 serving casserole)
2 cups red potatoes, roasted
2 cups steamed broccoli
3 servings Jaclyn's cauliflower with dipping sauce of 2 tablespoons rice vinegar mixed with 2 tablespoons low-sodium Worcestershire sauce (F: 1 serving)
1 slice Grain Dance whole wheat pizza shell baked with 1 clove minced garlic on top (F: omit)
1 slice apple spice cake ✪ (F: omit)

Nutritional Information (PER DAY)

	MALE	FEMALE
Calories	2,784	2,038
Carbohydrate g (%)	483 (64)	347 (64)
Fat g (%)	63 (19)	47 (20)
Protein g (%)	129 (17)	91 (17)
Cholesterol mg	215	214
Sodium mg	2,171	1,531
Chromium mcg	286	237

Saturday

BREAKFAST (BRUNCH)

1 serving Huevos rancheros ✪
1 serving fruit salad (1 cup melon chunks, 1 sliced plum, 1 sliced banana, 1 sliced pear, 2 tablespoons diced prunes) with ½ cup lemon nonfat yogurt whipped with 1 teaspoon freshly grated ginger

SNACK

PM: 1 high-chromium muffin ✪
1 package American Grain rice snacks (F: omit)

DINNER

2 servings whole wheat noodles with peanut sauce ✪
1 serving grilled eggplant ✪
2 Fantastic Foods Nature's Burgers made with 1 tablespoon brewer's yeast and 1 tablespoon low-sodium Worcestershire sauce and served with 1 ounce shredded low-fat Swiss cheese, 1 slice tomato, and 1 slice onion on a toasted Alvarado Street Bakery sprouted wheat bagel
1 baked potato stuffed with 2 servings Fantastic Foods refried beans (F: omit)

Nutritional Information (PER DAY)

	MALE	FEMALE
Calories	2,755	2,024
Carbohydrate g (%)	476 (67)	343 (66)
Fat g (%)	50 (16)	40 (18)
Protein g (%)	119 (17)	88 (17)
Cholesterol mg	77	77
Sodium mg	2,874	1,690
Chromium mcg	262	184

WEEK 5

Sunday

BREAKFAST

8 ounces fresh orange juice (F: omit)
3 slices French toast ✪, cooked in 1 tablespoon canola oil and topped with 2 tablespoons maple syrup or molasses

1 serving fruit salad (½ honeydew melon in chunks, ½ cup berries, 1 sliced banana, 1 tablespoon chopped dates, and 3 tablespoon slivered almonds)

LUNCH

1 serving Fantastic Foods tofu scrambler (made according to package directions substituting water for oil) rolled in 1 flour tortilla and topped with ¼ slivered avocado
1 baked potato with Hot Cha Cha! salsa

SNACK

1 slice carrot cake ✪
1 pear

DINNER

2 servings shrimp creole ✪ (F: 1 serving) (Save leftovers for Monday lunch.)
2 baked acorn squash with 2 tablespoons apple juice concentrate (F: 1 squash)
1 cup steamed green peas
salad of lettuce, tomatoes, mushrooms, and onions with 1 tablespoon vinaigrette dressing ✪ (F: omit)
½ stick Panda licorice

Nutritional Information (PER DAY)

	MALE	FEMALE
Calories	2,730	2,017
Carbohydrate g (%)	475 (66)	341 (64)
Fat g (%)	59 (18)	46 (20)
Protein g (%)	112 (16)	84 (16)
Cholesterol mg	233	118
Sodium mg	2,254	1,828
Chromium mcg	246	178

Monday

BREAKFAST

8 ounces fresh orange juice (F: 4 ounces)
1 Casbah breakfast cup
1 Alvarado Street Bakery sprouted wheat bagel with 2 teaspoons Sorrell Ridge conserve (F: omit)

LUNCH

1 serving leftover shrimp creole (see Sunday) stuffed in a baked potato (F: ½ serving)
1 serving Casbah whole wheat couscous mushroom tofu soup

SNACK

AM: 1 cup melon chunks (take-out)
PM: 1 high-chromium muffin ✪ with 2 tablespoons sugar-free apple butter
4 cups air-popped popcorn with Vegit

DINNER

3 ounces roast chicken (no skin) (Save leftovers for Tuesday lunch.)
2 servings high-chromium stuffing ✪ (F: 1 serving)
2 servings mushroom risotto ✪ (F: 1 serving) (Save leftovers for Tuesday lunch.)
1 tomato grilled with ½ teaspoon olive oil
1 serving carrot cake ✪ topped with 2 ounces Élan vanilla frozen dessert

Nutritional Information (PER DAY)

	MALE	FEMALE
Calories	2,808	2,049
Carbohydrate g (%)	460 (64)	333 (63)
Fat g (%)	62 (18)	46 (19)
Protein g (%)	127 (18)	95 (18)

Cholesterol mg	245	183
Sodium mg	2,127	1,410
Chromium mcg	277	214

Tuesday

BREAKFAST

¼ cup millet porridge, ¼ cup rye flakes, and 4 tablespoons wheat bran cooked in 1¼ cups water with 1 sliced banana, 1 tablespoon chopped dates, 1 teaspoon vanilla, and ½ teaspoon cinnamon

2 slices Food for Life seven-grain sprouted cinnamon raisin bread with 1 tablespoon prune whip ✪

LUNCH

1 serving curried chicken and rice salad made with leftover chicken and risotto (see Monday) ✪ on 2 slices whole grain bread

1 apple

SNACK

AM: 1 pear (F: omit)

PM: 1 high-chromium muffin ✪ broken into chunks with 2 ounces Élan coffee frozen dessert

DINNER

4 ounces whole wheat pasta with 2 servings lima and pesto sauce ✪ (F: 2 ounces pasta, 1 serving sauce.)

2 servings corn salad ✪ (F: 1 serving)

1 baked sweet potato with ½ cup unsweetened applesauce and ½ teaspoon cinnamon

Nutritional Information (PER DAY)

	MALE	FEMALE
Calories	2,754	2,041
Carbohydrate g (%)	485 (66)	374 (69)

Fat g (%)	66 (20)	42 (17)
Protein g (%)	99 (14)	77 (14)
Cholesterol mg	89	83
Sodium mg	1,553	1,224
Chromium mcg	260	222

Wednesday

BREAKFAST

1 serving cracked wheat cereal ✪ with ½ cup nonfat yogurt mixed with ½ cup unsweetened applesauce and 1 tablespoon molasses

1 Pritikin English muffin toasted with ½ ounce shredded skim-milk mozzarella cheese

LUNCH (OUT OR TAKE-OUT)

1 bowl vegetable soup

2½ ounces white meat turkey with lettuce, tomatoes, sprouts, mustard or low-calorie dressing, and pickle on 3 slices whole wheat or rye bread (thin slices if possible)

SNACK

1 package American Grain rice snacks

2 apples

DINNER

2 servings spaghetti alla puttanesca ✪ (F: 1 serving)

1 baked potato stuffed with 2 ounces half-the-fat hummus ✪

1 serving grilled broccoli ✪ with 2 teaspoons additional olive oil

1 high-chromium crostini ✪ (F: omit)

½ slice carrot cake ✪ (F: omit)

Nutritional Information (PER DAY)

	MALE	FEMALE
Calories	2,763	2,072
Carbohydrate g (%)	451 (65)	337 (65)
Fat g (%)	61 (20)	43 (19)
Protein g (%)	106 (15)	84 (16)
Cholesterol mg	71	71
Sodium mg	2,780	2,350
Chromium mcg	246	181

Thursday

BREAKFAST

8 ounces fresh orange juice (F: omit)
1 Casbah breakfast cup
1 banana

LUNCH (OUT)

1 serving spinach salad (no bacon) with 2 tablespoons low-cal dressing
3 ounces fish fillet grilled in wine, herbs, and lemon
1 cup cooked rice (F: omit)
1 baked potato with cocktail sauce

SNACK

2 cups melon chunks (take-out)
½ high-chromium muffin ✪

DINNER

2 servings minestrone alla Burrini ✪ (Save leftovers for Saturday dinner.)
2 servings winter wheat salad without shrimp ✪ (F: 1 serving)
1 baked acorn squash with 1 tablespoon apple juice concentrate

2 New Morning honey graham crackers with 1 tablespoon sugar-free apple butter

Nutritional Information (PER DAY)

	MALE		FEMALE	
Calories	2,769		2,084	
Carbohydrate g (%)	484	(66)	351	(64)
Fat g (%)	56	(17)	45	(19)
Protein g (%)	120	(16)	101	(18)
Cholesterol mg	127		127	
Sodium mg	1,591		1,418	
Chromium mcg	228		207	

Friday

BREAKFAST

8 ounces fresh orange juice

⅓ cup rolled oats, ¼ cup oat bran, and 3 tablespoons wheat bran prepared in 1½ cups water cooked with 1 sliced banana, 1 tablespoon chopped dates, 2 tablespoons slivered almonds, 1 teaspoon vanilla, and ½ teaspoon cinnamon

LUNCH

1 serving Diet-Fuel

1 high-chromium muffin ✪ with 2 teaspoons Sorrell Ridge conserve

1 stick Panda licorice (F: omit)

SNACK

2 whole wheat pretzels

1 apple

1 pear

4 cups air-popped popcorn with Vegit

DINNER

2 servings split pea and rosemary soup ✪ (F: 1 serving)
3 servings vegetable pizza ✪ (F: 2 servings)
2 roasted red peppers ✪ with 1 tablespoon vinaigrette dressing ✪ (F: omit)
1 baked sweet potato with ½ cup unsweetened applesauce and ½ teaspoon cinnamon
1 ear corn on the cob (F: omit)
1 root beer float made with IBC root beer and 2 ounces Élan coffee frozen dessert

Nutritional Information (PER DAY)

	MALE	FEMALE
Calories	2,749	2,051
Carbohydrate g (%)	468 (64)	361 (66)
Fat g (%)	71 (21)	47 (19)
Protein g (%)	102 (14)	78 (15)
Cholesterol mg	87	74
Sodium mg	1,679	1,334
Chromium mcg	254	207

Saturday

BREAKFAST (BRUNCH)

1 serving Kashi pilaf made with ½ cup apple juice and ½ cup water and served with 6 ounces skim milk, 1 banana, 1 tablespoon chopped dates, and 1 tablespoon almonds (Make extra Kashi pilaf for Sunday breakfast.)
2 slices Food for Life seven-grain sprouted cinnamon raisin bread with 1 tablespoon de-oiled peanut butter and 2 tablespoons sugar-free apple butter (F: omit peanut butter)
¼ honeydew melon or cantaloupe

SNACK

1 ounce wheatgrass juice
1 serving Diet-Fuel
4 cups air-popped popcorn with Vegit

DINNER

3 servings ribollita made with leftover minestrone (see Thursday) ✪ (F: 2 servings)
2 servings acorn squash souffle ✪ (F: 1 serving)
salad of sliced tomato, sliced cucumber, sliced pimento, and sliced onion with 1 tablespoon vinaigrette dressing ✪
1 frozen nonfat yogurt (F: omit)
1 beer (optional)

Nutritional Information (PER DAY)

	MALE	FEMALE
Calories	2,723	2,059
Carbohydrate g (%)	438 (64)	341 (65)
Fat g (%)	66 (21)	46 (19)
Protein g (%)	109 (15)	79 (15)
Cholesterol mg	17	9
Sodium mg	1,186	764
Chromium mcg	207	177

WEEK 6

Sunday

BREAKFAST

1 serving leftover Kashi pilaf (see Saturday) with 4 ounces skim milk, 1 banana, 1 tablespoon chopped dates, and 1 tablespoon molasses
2 servings potato pancakes ✪ (F: 1 serving)

LUNCH

1 serving tuna salad ✪ in 1 whole wheat pita bread
1 package American Grain rice snacks

SNACK

4 cups air-popped popcorn with Vegit
1 pear (F: omit)

DINNER

1 serving high-chromium meat loaf ✪ (Save leftovers for Monday lunch.)
2 servings cajun rice ✪ (F: 1 serving)
1 serving Casbah tabouly with 2 tablespoons olive oil and 2 tablespoons balsamic vinegar (F: 1 tablespoon olive oil) (Save leftovers for Monday lunch.)
3 ounces Élan chocolate almond frozen dessert with 1 New Morning honey graham cracker (F: omit graham cracker)

Nutritional Information (PER DAY)

	MALE	FEMALE
Calories	2,730	2,115
Carbohydrate g (%)	465 (66)	356 (64)
Fat g (%)	64 (20)	55 (20)
Protein g (%)	100 (14)	92 (16)
Cholesterol mg	117	117
Sodium mg	1,634	1,482
Chromium mcg	234	192

Monday

BREAKFAST

¼ cup rolled oats, ¼ cup oat bran, and 3 tablespoons wheat bran cooked with 1½ cups water, 1 sliced banana, 1 teaspoon vanilla, and 1 teaspoon cinnamon and served with ¼ cup Mueslix

1 Alvarado Street Bakery sprouted wheat bagel with 1 tablespoon Sorrell Ridge conserve

LUNCH

2 ounces half-the-fat hummus ✪ and 1 serving leftover tabouly (see Sunday) with ¼ slivered avocado in 1 whole wheat pita bread

2 peaches or plums *or* 4 figs (F: omit)

or

1 serving leftover high-chromium meat loaf (see Sunday) with Worcestershire sauce on 2 slices whole grain bread

SNACK

1 ounce wheatgrass juice

1 package American Grain rice snacks

1 apple

2 whole wheat pretzels (F: omit)

DINNER

1½ servings corn meal scallops ✪ (F: 1 serving)

2 servings Casbah nutty pilaf (F: 1 serving)

2 servings spinach sauté ✪ (F: 1 serving)

1 slice apple spice cake ✪ with 2 ounces Élan frozen dessert

Nutritional Information (PER DAY)

	MALE	FEMALE
Calories	2,770	2,073
Carbohydrate g (%)	491 (67)	370 (67)
Fat g (%)	56 (17)	42 (17)
Protein g (%)	119 (16)	87 (16)
Cholesterol mg	92	63
Sodium mg	1,931	1,592
Chromium mcg	199	168

Tuesday

BREAKFAST

8 ounces fresh orange juice
1 high-chromium muffin ✪

LUNCH (OUT OR TAKE-OUT)

1 bowl Manhattan clam chowder or vegetable soup
2 ounces white meat turkey with 1 tablespoon mayonnaise on 2 slices whole wheat or rye bread (thin slices if possible)
pickles

SNACK

2 cups melon chunks (take-out)
1 whole wheat pita bread toasted to chips with 2 ounces Fromage Blanc–Vegit dip ✪

DINNER

2 servings Jaclyn's mushroom barley (F: 1 serving)
2 servings polenta ✪ with 2 servings Nitza's tomato sauce ✪ (Save leftovers for Wednesday dinner.)
2 ounces whole wheat pasta with 1 cup squash, steamed and sautéed in 1 tablespoon olive oil with garlic and pepper (F: omit)
salad of mixed greens, mushrooms, tomato, and carrot with 2 tablespoons low-calorie dressing
1 slice apple spice cake ✪ (F: omit)

Nutritional Information (PER DAY)

	MALE	FEMALE
Calories	2,729	2,051
Carbohydrate g (%)	438 (64)	322 (63)
Fat g (%)	64 (20)	45 (20)
Protein g (%)	103 (15)	87 (17)
Cholesterol mg	106	106

Sodium mg	2,459	2,182
Chromium mcg	263	198

Wednesday

BREAKFAST

8 ounces fresh orange juice (F: omit)
1 serving cracked wheat cereal ✪ with ½ cup nonfat yogurt mixed with ½ cup unsweetened applesauce, 1 tablespoon molasses, and ¼ cup Mueslix
1 banana, split and filled with 1 tablespoon de-oiled peanut butter and 1 tablespoon chopped almonds

LUNCH

1 serving Casbah whole wheat couscous mushroom tofu soup
1 high-chromium muffin ✪ with 1 tablespoon sugar-free apple butter

SNACK

1 Christopher's Chewie with dates (F: omit)
1 apple
1 pear
2 plums

DINNER

2 servings vegetable pizza ✪ (F: 1 serving) (Save leftovers for Thursday lunch.)
1 serving flexible frittata made with 1 serving leftover polenta (see Tuesday) ✪ with 2 servings leftover Nitza's tomato sauce (see Tuesday)
1½ cups stewed tomatoes (unsalted)

Nutritional Information (PER DAY)

	MALE	FEMALE
Calories	2,752	2,065
Carbohydrate g (%)	461 (65)	349 (65)

Fat g (%)	70 (22)	50 (21)
Protein g (%)	94 (13)	73 (14)
Cholesterol mg	194	169
Sodium mg	2,367	1,717
Chromium mcg	279	232

Thursday

BREAKFAST

4 ounces fresh orange juice (F: omit)
3 egg whites scrambled with 3 tablespoons skim-milk ricotta cheese, basil, 1 tablespoon grated Parmesan cheese, black pepper, and Green Mountain salsa
1 Pritikin English muffin with 1 tablespoon Sorrell Ridge conserve

LUNCH

1 cup split pea soup (take-out) (F: omit)
1 serving leftover vegetable pizza (see Wednesday) salad bar selections (bean salad, hard-boiled egg whites, dark greens, and vegetables with 1 tablespoon low-cal or olive oil and vinegar dressing)

SNACK

AM: 1 orange
1 banana
PM: 4 cups air-popped popcorn with Vegit

DINNER

4 ounces quinoa pasta with 2 servings sweet potato sauce ✪ (F: 3 ounces pasta)
2 servings succotash ✪ (F: omit)
1 jalapeno corn muffin ✪
2 roasted red peppers ✪ cucumber, and onion with balsamic vinegar

Nutritional Information (PER DAY)

	MALE	FEMALE
Calories	2,778	2,055
Carbohydrate g (%)	460 (65)	337 (64)
Fat g (%)	64 (20)	49 (21)
Protein g (%)	106 (15)	80 (15)
Cholesterol mg	39	37
Sodium mg	1,666	1,552
Chromium mcg	246	180

Friday

BREAKFAST

8 ounces fresh orange juice (F: omit)
1 Casbah breakfast cup
2 slices Food for Life seven-grain sprouted cinnamon raisin bread with 2 tablespoons prune whip ✪

LUNCH (OUT)

1 shrimp cocktail
1 baked potato with cocktail sauce
1 serving steamed asparagus with 1 tablespoon dressing
1 slice bread
1 serving house salad with 2 tablespoons low-cal Italian dressing

SNACK

AM: 1 banana
PM: 1 high-chromium muffin ✪
1 Christopher's Chewie with dates (F: omit)

DINNER

2 servings whole wheat fettucine with zucchini and smoked salmon ✪ (F: 1 serving)
1½ cups shredded cabbage, braised in ½ cup chicken

broth, ½ teaspoon honey, black pepper, and 1 teaspoon caraway seeds

1 jalapeno corn muffin ✪

Nutritional Information (PER DAY)

	MALE	FEMALE
Calories	2,759	2,056
Carbohydrate g (%)	460 (65)	334 (63)
Fat g (%)	60 (19)	47 (20)
Protein g (%)	117 (16)	93 (17)
Cholesterol mg	242	229
Sodium mg	2,163	1,601
Chromium mcg	250	217

Saturday

BREAKFAST (BRUNCH)

4 ounces fresh orange juice

4 servings potato pancakes ✪ with 1 cup unsweetened applesauce (F: 2 servings, ½ cup applesauce)

¼ honeydew melon with lime

1 jalapeno corn muffin ✪

SNACK

1 apple

1 pear

1 stick Panda licorice

DINNER

1 serving grilled lobster tail ✪

1 cup cooked brown rice with diced onion, chopped tomato, ¼ slivered avocado, and Hot Cha Cha! salsa on 1 toasted corn tortilla

2 servings corn salad ✪ (F: 1 serving)

2 servings baked rhubarb ✪ (F: 1 serving)

Nutritional Information (PER DAY)

	MALE	FEMALE
Calories	2,795	2,123
Carbohydrate g (%)	466 (64)	354 (64)
Fat g (%)	71 (22)	49 (20)
Protein g (%)	101 (14)	88 (16)
Cholesterol mg	157	157
Sodium mg	1,557	1,321
Chromium mcg	268	211

RECIPES

ACORN SQUASH SOUFFLE

4 medium acorn squash
½ cup soft tofu or 4 ounces Fromage Blanc
1 whole egg
1 egg white
2 teaspoons honey or ¼ cup frozen apple juice concentrate (defrosted)
1 teaspoon melted butter (not essential)
⅛ teaspoon ground allspice
freshly ground black pepper to taste
cinnamon to taste
freshly ground nutmeg to taste
PAM

Preheat oven to 375°. Spray 1-quart baking dish with PAM. Bake acorn squash for 40 minutes. Lower oven temperature to 350°. Cut squash in half and allow to cool. Scoop out seeds and peel. In a large bowl, mash cooled, peeled squash. Add tofu or Fromage Blanc and beat until well blended. In another bowl, beat eggs lightly. Add eggs to squash with remaining ingredients, and mix well. Turn into baking dish. Bake for 30–45 minutes, until appears set and top is slightly browned. Serve sprinkled with additional allspice, cinnamon, and nutmeg.

4 servings

Nutritional Information (PER SERVING)

Calories	190	Cholesterol mg	61
Carbohydrate g (%)	37 (70)	Sodium mg	73
Fat g (%)	3 (13)	Chromium mcg	8
Protein g (%)	9 (17)		

AMBROSINO'S MANHATTAN CLAM CHOWDER

5 baking potatoes, scrubbed and diced
1 pound carrots, scraped and diced
1 32-ounce can whole tomatoes, mashed
3 dozen fresh clams, chopped, with juice
1 tablespoon thyme
black pepper to taste

In a large saucepan, bring 4 quarts of water to a boil. Add potatoes and carrots. Cook for 5 minutes and pour through a colander. In a large soup pot, combine the tomatoes, cooked potatoes and carrots, clams and their juice, thyme, and pepper. Bring to a boil and serve.

2 quarts (freezes beautifully)

Nutritional Information (PER SERVING)

Calories	229	Cholesterol mg	41
Carbohydrate g (%)	35 (59)	Sodium mg	248
Fat g (%)	2 (8)	Chromium mcg	42
Protein g (%)	20 (34)		

APPLE SPICE CAKE

1¾ cups whole wheat flour
¾ cup raw wheat germ
1 teaspoon baking soda
1 heaping teaspoon cinnamon
1 teaspoon ground allspice
½ teaspoon ground cloves
2 egg whites
½ cup water

1 12-ounce can frozen apple juice concentrate (defrosted)
1 cup shredded apples, without skins
¾ cup diced apples, with skins
sliced walnuts or almonds (optional)
PAM

Preheat oven to 350°. Spray a nonstick loaf pan with PAM. In a large mixing bowl, combine dry ingredients. In another bowl, mix egg whites, water, and apple juice concentrate. Add apples and wet ingredients to dry ingredients and mix well. Pour batter into pan, top with walnut or almond slices (optional), and bake for 1 hour or until toothpick comes out clean. Turn out of pan and allow to cool on a wire rack.

8 servings

Nutritional Information (PER SERVING)

Calories	166	Cholesterol mg	0
Carbohydrate g (%)	34 (77)	Sodium mg	118
Fat g (%)	2 (9)	Chromium mcg	18
Protein g (%)	7 (15)		

AVOCADO DRESSING

½ avocado, mashed
1 tablespoon lemon juice
½ cup nonfat yogurt or Fromage Blanc
½ teaspoon chili powder
¼ teaspoon Tabasco

Mix all ingredients.

4 servings

Nutritional Information (PER SERVING)

Calories	68	Cholesterol mg	3
Carbohydrate g (%)	4 (21)	Sodium mg	38
Fat g (%)	5 (58)	Chromium mcg	0
Protein g (%)	4 (21)		

BAKED BEANS

- *2 cups dried red pinto beans or 2 15½-ounce cans pinto or kidney beans, thoroughly rinsed*
- *2 quarts water*
- *1 onion, minced*
- *1 green pepper, chopped*
- *8 ounces tomato sauce (unsalted)*
- *½ teaspoon ground cumin seed*
- *1 tablespoon blackstrap molasses*
- *Vegit and black pepper to taste*

If using dried beans, soak beans overnight or use the quick-soak method (see page 244). Cook for 1 hour 15 minutes, or until tender, in 2 quarts of water. To the prepared or canned beans, add onions, pepper, and tomato sauce, and continue cooking for 15 minutes. Add more water as necessary to keep the beans moist, but most of the liquid should be absorbed by the end of the cooking time. Add cumin, molasses, pepper, and Vegit, mix well, and serve.

4 servings

Nutritional Information (PER SERVING)

Calories	166	Cholesterol mg	0
Carbohydrate g (%)	33 (74)	Sodium mg	22
Fat g (%)	1 (4)	Chromium mcg	13
Protein g (%)	10 (22)		

BAKED RHUBARB

- *2 pounds fresh rhubarb, cut into 1-inch chunks*
- *3 tablespoons sugar or fructose*

Preheat oven to 350°. Cover the bottom of a shallow 4-quart baking dish with the rhubarb chunks. Sprinkle with sugar. Bake for 20 minutes. Excellent served with Dole raspberry sorbet.

4 servings

Nutritional Information (PER SERVING)

Calories	66	Cholesterol mg	0
Carbohydrate g (%)	16 (94)	Sodium mg	4
Fat g (%)	0 (0)	Chromium mcg	13
Protein g (%)	1 (6)		

BARBECUE SAUCE

- 12 *ounces tomato paste (unsalted)*
- ⅓ *cup blackstrap molasses*
- ⅓ *cup red wine vinegar*
- 2 *teaspoons Dijon mustard*
- 1 *teaspoon Tabasco*
- 2 *teaspoons Worcestershire sauce*
- ¼ *cup lemon juice*

In a 4-quart saucepan, mix all ingredients. Heat over medium flame for 20 minutes.

Nutritional Information (PER SERVING)

Calories	16	Cholesterol mg	0
Carbohydrate g (%)	4 (85)	Sodium mg	17
Fat g (%)	0.1 (5)	Chromium mcg	16
Protein g (%)	0.4 (9)		

BEAN PREPARATION

Overnight Method

Put beans in a large pot. Cover with 4 inches of water and leave overnight. Pour beans into a colander to drain off the water and return them to the pot. Cover with 2 inches of water, bring to a boil, reduce heat to medium-low, and cook uncovered until tender but not mushy, 1 hour 15 minutes or more, depending on the type of bean.

Quick-Soak Method

Put beans in a large pot. Cover with 4 inches of water, bring to boil, and boil for 2 minutes. Remove the pot from the heat, cover, and allow to sit for 1 hour. As soon as the hour is up, pour beans into a colander to drain off the water and return them to the pot. Cover with 2 inches of water, bring to a boil, reduce heat to medium-low, and cook uncovered until tender but not mushy, 1 hour 15 minutes or more, depending on the type of bean.

BLACK BEAN AND RICE PIZZA

- 1 *recipe pizza dough (see page 285)* or *use Grain Dance whole wheat pizza shell*
- 2 *tablespoons olive oil*
- 1 *giant sweet Vadalia onion* or *1 small red onion, cut in 1½-inch slices*
- 1 *clove garlic, minced*
- ¾ *cup soaked sun-dried tomatoes*
- 1½ *cups cooked black beans (see below)*
- 1 *cup already cooked brown rice*
- 1 *tablespoon balsamic vinegar*
- 1 *ounce shredded smoked Gruyere cheese*
- *Vegit and black pepper to taste*

Preheat oven to 500°. Prepare pizza dough according to the directions. In a large skillet, sauté the onion in the olive oil until soft. Stir in the garlic and sun-dried tomatoes. Add beans, rice, vinegar, and seasonings, and cook over medium heat until heated through, about 3 minutes. Roll out the dough and lay on a heavy baking sheet or pizza pan. Top with the black bean mixture, leaving an inch border all around, and sprinkle the cheese over the beans. Bake in the top third of the oven for approximately 13 minutes, or until the crust is golden and cheese is melted.

5 servings as side dish, 3 servings as main course

Nutritional Information (PER SERVING)

Calories	321	Cholesterol mg	8
Carbohydrate g (%)	42 (49)	Sodium mg	42
Fat g (%)	15 (39)	Chromium mcg	33
Protein g (%)	11 (12)		

BLACK BEANS

2 cups dried black beans
4 cups water
1 green pepper, diced
1 large onion, diced
1 tablespoon garlic, minced
2 bay leaves
1 tablespoon oregano
2 tablespoons thyme
black pepper to taste
3 tablespoons cider vinegar
1 tablespoon brewer's yeast

In a large pot, soak beans overnight or use the quick-soak method (see page 244). Cover soaked beans with water, approximately 4 cups, bring to a boil, reduce the heat, and simmer covered for 30 minutes. Add the remaining ingredients except vinegar and brewer's yeast and simmer covered for 1 hour, watching to make certain the water doesn't evaporate. Stir in vinegar and brewer's yeast just before serving.

You can use Health Valley canned black bean soup as a substitute for beans cooked this way. It's not as good, but it is helpful if you don't have the time to prepare the recipe.

8 servings

Nutritional Information (PER SERVING)

Calories	166	Cholesterol mg	0
Carbohydrate g (%)	33 (74)	Sodium mg	22
Fat g (%)	1 (4)	Chromium mcg	13
Protein g (%)	10 (22)		

BUCKWHEAT PANCAKES

1 cup buckwheat flour
1 teaspoon baking powder
2 egg whites, lightly beaten
1 cup skim milk
PAM

Combine all the ingredients in the work bowl of a food processor. Pulse 3 or 4 times, just to incorporate the mixture. Do not overblend. Set a nonstick skillet or griddle sprayed with PAM over high heat. Add a few drops of canola oil to pan. Use about 1 teaspoon in all to cook the pancakes. Pour about ¼ cup batter for each pancake. Cook, turning once, until the pancakes are nicely browned on both sides.

6 5-inch pancakes

Nutritional Information (PER SERVING)

Calories	84	Cholesterol mg	4
Carbohydrate g (%)	15 (70)	Sodium mg	93
Fat g (%)	1 (11)	Chromium mcg	4
Protein g (%)	4 (19)		

CAJUN RICE

1 tablespoon (or less) olive oil
2 cups chopped onion
1 clove garlic, minced
1 cup chopped green pepper
2 cups tomato sauce (unsalted)
2 cups white wine or *chicken or vegetable stock*
2 teaspoons cayenne pepper
1 cup sun-dried tomatoes, chopped
1 cup long grain brown rice
Vegit to taste

In a large pot, sauté onions, garlic, and pepper in olive oil until soft. Add remaining ingredients and bring to a boil. Reduce heat and simmer uncovered for 40 minutes until moisture is absorbed.

4 servings

Nutritional Information (PER SERVING)

Calories	340	Cholesterol mg	0
Carbohydrate g (%)	57 (69)	Sodium mg	103
Fat g (%)	10 (23)	Chromium mcg	40
Protein g (%)	7 (7)		

CARROT CAKE

2½ cups whole wheat flour
1 teaspoon baking soda
2½ teaspoons baking powder
1 tablespoon ground cinnamon
2 teaspoons ground ginger
½ teaspoon freshly grated nutmeg
¼ teaspoon ground allspice
¼ cup chopped pecans
¼ cup dark raisins
3 egg whites
1 tablespoon canola oil
1 teaspoon pure vanilla extract
1 6-ounce can frozen unsweetened apple juice concentrate
1 8-ounce can unsweetened crushed pineapple in juice
3 cups carrots, grated
PAM

Preheat oven to 350°. Spray a 9 × 5-inch nonstick loaf pan with PAM. Combine dry ingredients. Combine all the remaining ingredients in a separate bowl and mix well. Mix the wet and dry ingredients until flour disappears. Pour the batter into the prepared pan. Bake for 40 to 45 minutes or until cake begins to pull away from the sides of the pan.

1 loaf (8 slices)

Nutritional Information (PER SERVING)

Calories	160	Cholesterol mg	0
Carbohydrate g (%)	32 (77)	Sodium mg	154
Fat g (%)	2 (11)	Chromium mcg	15
Protein g (%)	5 (12)		

CHEESE SAUCE

- *1 teaspoon butter, unsalted*
- *1 tablespoon whole wheat flour*
- *½ cup Health Valley or Pritikin chicken broth*
- *1 cup skim milk*
- *3.5 ounces low-fat Swiss cheese, cut into chunks*
- *3 tablespoons grated Parmesan cheese*
- *¼ cup fresh or frozen basil, chopped*
- *Vegit and black pepper to taste*

In a saucepan, melt the butter and add the flour, whisking for 1 minute over medium high heat. Gradually add the broth and milk, stirring until the sauce comes to a boil and thickens slightly. Add the cheeses and basil, stirring until blended. Season with pepper and Vegit. Remove from heat and keep covered. Delicious over pasta, rice, vegetables, kashi pilaf, and potatoes.

Enough for 1 pound pasta (1 serving—1 cup)

Nutritional Information (PER SERVING)

Calories	75	Cholesterol mg	4.2
Carbohydrate g (%)	2.8 (15)	Sodium mg	166
Fat g (%)	4.4 (55)	Chromium mcg	0
Protein g (%)	5.5 (30)		

CHICKEN CACCIATORE

- *1 small broiler-fryer, skinned and cut into serving pieces*
- *Vegit or comparable no-salt seasoning*
- *freshly ground black pepper*
- *1½ tablespoons olive oil*

1 medium onion, sliced
1 large clove garlic, minced
1 16-ounce can Italian-style plum tomatoes with juice
1 16-ounce can stewed tomatoes with juice (preferably unsalted)
½ cup white wine
12 ounces whole wheat noodles

Sprinkle chicken pieces with Vegit and pepper. Heat oil in large skillet and brown chicken well on both sides. Remove chicken and set aside. In the same skillet, sauté onion and garlic until softened. Add plum tomatoes with juice, stewed tomatoes with juice, and wine, and bring mixture to a boil. Return chicken pieces to the skillet and reduce the heat. Cover and simmer for about 25 minutes. Cook noodles according to package directions and drain. Transfer noodles to serving dish, arrange chicken over noodles, and serve.

6 servings

Nutritional Information (PER SERVING)

Calories	469	Cholesterol mg	91
Carbohydrate g (%)	51 (44)	Sodium mg	262
Fat g (%)	13 (24)	Chromium mcg	37
Protein g (%)	38 (32)		

CHROMIUM CROSTINI

6 thin slices whole wheat or corn bread
½ cup black olives, pitted and chopped
1 pound fresh mushrooms, diced
1 teaspoon black pepper
1 teaspoon fresh or ⅓ teaspoon dried sage
1 tablespoon olive oil

Preheat oven to 500°. Spray a large cookie sheet with PAM and place the bread slices on the pan. In a food processor, mix olives, mushrooms, pepper, and sage. Drizzle a few drops of olive oil on each bread slice, just enough to moisten. Spread olive-mushroom mixture on top. Bake for 4 to 5 minutes until the edges are golden crispy. Delicious with a bowl of soup.

6 servings

Nutritional Information (PER SERVING)

Calories	104	Cholesterol mg	0
Carbohydrate g (%)	11 (39)	Sodium mg	77
Fat g (%)	6 (50)	Chromium mcg	29
Protein g (%)	3 (11)		

CORN BREAD "FRIED" CHICKEN

1 tablespoon olive oil
3 large cloves garlic, minced
2 large shallots, minced
1 cup parsley, chopped fine
1½ cups corn bread crumbs or ¾ cup corn meal
2 tablespoons grated Parmesan cheese
lots of black pepper (or to taste)
2 egg whites, lightly beaten
4 chicken cutlets, pounded flat

Preheat oven to 425°. In a large skillet, which can later be placed in the oven, sauté garlic, shallots, and parsley in oil over medium heat for about 2 minutes. In a food processor, blend corn bread, Parmesan cheese, and pepper (or simply mix corn meal, cheese, and pepper). Place egg whites in shallow bowl and spread corn mixture on plate. Dip chicken one slice at a time in the egg whites and then in the corn mixture, and add to the skillet. Bake the chicken in the skillet uncovered for 35 minutes until the top is crispy.

4 servings

Nutritional Information (PER SERVING)

Calories	286	Cholesterol mg	87
Carbohydrate g (%)	15 (22)	Sodium mg	165
Fat g (%)	8 (27)	Chromium mcg	33
Protein g (%)	36 (51)		

CORN MEAL PIZZA SHELL

- *3 tablespoons hot water*
- *3 tablespoons skim milk*
- *1¼ teaspoon active dry yeast*
- *pinch of sugar or fructose*
- *1 tablespoon olive oil*
- *3 tablespoons unbleached white flour*
- *½ cup yellow corn meal*
- *PAM*

Combine the water and milk (the mixture should be warm, not hot). Add yeast and sugar and stir to dissolve yeast. Mix in the olive oil and 2 tablespoons white flour and gradually add corn meal, stirring to make a soft workable dough. Add the remaining 1 tablespoon white flour. Turn out onto a lightly floured surface and knead for about 5 minutes. Put the dough into a lightly oiled bowl and turn once to coat entire surface with oil. Cover the bowl and let the dough rise in a warm spot about 30 minutes. Spray pizza pan or baking sheet with PAM. Roll out the dough on a floured surface into a 10-inch round about ⅛ inch thick. Set the dough on the pan. Add topping and bake according to chosen recipe directions.

1 10-inch pizza shell (4 servings)

Nutritional Information (PER SERVING)

Calories	90	Cholesterol mg	1
Carbohydrate g (%)	13 (57)	Sodium mg	20
Fat g (%)	3 (30)	Chromium mcg	13
Protein g (%)	3 (13)		

CORN MEAL SCALLOPS

15 fresh sea scallops
2 cups skim milk
¾ cup corn meal
black pepper to taste
1 tablespoon olive oil

Soak scallops in milk 1 to 6 hours (the longer the better). Mix the pepper and corn meal, and roll scallops in the mixture. Heat olive oil in a skillet, and sauté scallops for a scant 3 minutes on each side. Serve.

4 servings

Nutritional Information (PER SERVING)

Calories	208	Cholesterol mg	57
Carbohydrate g (%)	14 (26)	Sodium mg	286
Fat g (%)	6 (24)	Chromium mcg	14
Protein g (%)	27 (50)		

CORN SALAD

1 package frozen corn, steamed
4 zucchini, washed, diced, and steamed
4 pieces whole grain bread, cut into 1" cubes, preferably stale
1 tomato, cubed
2 ounces pimentos, fresh or canned, rinsed and drained, cut into thin strips
15 Calamata olives, pitted and chopped
½ cup vinaigrette dressing (page 306)

Mix all ingredients in a bowl.

4 servings

Nutritional Information (PER SERVING)

Calories	275	Cholesterol mg	0
Carbohydrate g (%)	33 (44)	Sodium mg	120
Fat g (%)	16 (48)	Chromium mcg	50
Protein g (%)	6 (8)		

CRACKED WHEAT CEREAL

¼ cup Hodgson Mill cracked wheat cereal
½ cup water

In a bowl, mix cereal and water, cover with plastic, and cook in microwave on high for 5 minutes. Or, follow directions on package for stove-top cooking. Serve with skim milk, sliced banana or other fruit, molasses, or chopped dates.

1 serving

Nutritional Information (PER SERVING)

Calories	107	Cholesterol mg	0
Carbohydrate g (%)	24 (82)	Sodium mg	0
Fat g (%)	1 (5)	Chromium mcg	38
Protein g (%)	4 (13)		

CURRIED CHICKEN AND RICE SALAD

2 cups cold, cooked long grain brown rice
1 cup diced cooked chicken
1 cup diced celery
1 apple, peeled, cored, and diced
2 tablespoons minced onion
½ cup diced cucumber
½ cup nonfat yogurt
2 tablespoons Hellman's light mayonnaise
1 teaspoon curry powder
Vegit and black pepper to taste
Romaine lettuce leaves

Mix rice, chicken, celery, apples, onion, and cucumber. In a separate bowl, mix mayonnaise, yogurt, curry powder, pepper, and Vegit. Add dressing to chicken and mix well. Serve on romaine lettuce.

6 servings

Nutritional Information (PER SERVING)

Calories	122	Cholesterol mg	24
Carbohydrate g (%)	17 (55)	Sodium mg	42
Fat g (%)	1 (11)	Chromium mcg	15
Protein g (%)	10 (34)		

CURRIED WALDORF SALAD

4 apples (with skin), cored and cut in chunks
6 large walnuts, shelled and broken into pieces
¼ cup plump raisins
⅓ cup low-fat mayonnaise (page 197)
1 teaspoon curry powder
radicchio leaves

Mix all ingredients. Serve on radicchio.

4 servings

Nutritional Information (PER SERVING)

Calories	137	Cholesterol mg	2
Carbohydrate g (%)	25 (66)	Sodium mg	15
Fat g (%)	4 (26)	Chromium mcg	13
Protein g (%)	3 (8)		

FLEXIBLE FRITTATA (ITALIAN OMELETTE)

10 egg whites
2 egg yolks
1 tablespoon water
5 tablespoons Italian parsley, chopped
1 teaspoon Italian seasonings
1 cup filling (see below)
1–2 tablespoons olive oil
Vegit and black pepper to taste

Fillings

any kind of cooked, puréed, or chopped vegetables
cooked chicken, seafood, lean meat
cooked pasta

low-fat cheese (shredded hard cheese, ricotta, or cottage cheese)
cooked brown rice or leftover rice casserole
cooked beans

Preheat broiler to 500°. In a mixing bowl, beat egg whites and yolks together with water, parsley, and Italian seasonings. Add the filling, Vegit, and pepper to the egg mixture. In a 9-inch heavy skillet, heat the olive oil, tilting the skillet enough so that the oil covers the bottom of the pan. Add the egg mixture, making a ½-inch layer. Cook over low heat without turning or stirring until just set, but still moist on top. Slide the skillet under the broiler for about 4 minutes to finish cooking. Serve plain or with tomato sauce.

4 servings

Nutritional Information (PER SERVING)

Calories	126	Cholesterol mg	111
Carbohydrate g (%)	1 (3)	Sodium mg	112
Fat g (%)	9 (67)	Chromium mcg	15
Protein g (%)	9 (30)		

FRENCH TOAST

4 slices whole grain or corn bread
1 cup skim milk
4 egg whites
black pepper
2 tablespoons maple syrup or molasses
PAM

Soak bread in milk until saturated. Lightly beat egg whites and pepper. Spray a nonstick skillet with PAM and heat. Dip milk-soaked bread in egg whites, covering both sides, and sear in skillet until egg cooks and is golden on the outside, approximately 2 minutes. Top with maple syrup or molasses.

2 servings

Nutritional Information (PER SERVING)

Calories	257	Cholesterol mg	2
Carbohydrate g (%)	44 (68)	Sodium mg	250
Fat g (%)	2 (8)	Chromium mcg	8
Protein g (%)	16 (24)		

FRESH TOMATO SANDWICH

4 slices rye bread
4 cloves garlic, minced
1/3 cup olive oil
4 small fresh tomatoes, sliced thinly
4 teaspoons grated Parmesan cheese

Preheat broiler to 450°. Spread garlic on bread, cover with olive oil and then tomatoes, and top with Parmesan cheese. Bake about 4 minutes.

4 servings

Nutritional Information (PER SERVING)

Calories	109	Cholesterol mg	2
Carbohydrate g (%)	20 (68)	Sodium mg	156
Fat g (%)	2 (15)	Chromium mcg	17
Protein g (%)	5 (17)		

FROMAGE BLANC, THICKENED

1 8-ounce container Fromage Blanc

Pour Fromage Blanc into a jelly bag, or line a bowl with several layers of cheesecloth and pour in Fromage Blanc. Tie the bag or cheesecloth closed and hang from the kitchen faucet to allow Fromage Blanc to drain, or suspend bag or cheesecloth in a large jar or bowl so that moisture can drip through. Drain overnight. The Fromage Blanc will be the consistency of sour cream.

4 2-ounce servings

Nutritional Information (PER SERVING)

Calories	160	Cholesterol mg	20
Carbohydrate g (%)	16 (39)	Sodium mg	280
Fat g (%)	0.4 (2)	Chromium mcg	0
Protein g (%)	24 (59)		

FROMAGE BLANC–VEGIT DIP

1 8-ounce container Fromage Blanc

2 heaping tablespoons Vegit

Mix ingredients thoroughly.

Variation for salad dressing: Add 2 teaspoons Marakun rice vinegar.

4 2-ounce servings

Nutritional Information (PER SERVING)

Calories	160	Cholesterol mg	20
Carbohydrate g (%)	16 (39)	Sodium mg	280
Fat g (%)	0.4 (2)	Chromium mcg	22
Protein g (%)	24 (59)		

FROZEN SHAKE

4 ounces frozen strawberries

2 ounces frozen blueberries

2 ounces frozen raspberries

2 tablespoons plain nonfat yogurt

½ package Sweet 'n' Low or 1½ teaspoons fructose

1 teaspoon lemon juice

1 teaspoon lime juice

2 egg whites

Combine all the ingredients in the bowl of a food processor or blender. Process until desired consistency is reached (aim for the consistency of a McDonalds's milkshake), about 2 minutes.

2 servings

Nutritional Information (PER SERVING)

Calories	92	Cholesterol mg	1
Carbohydrate g (%)	19 (75)	Sodium mg	51
Fat g (%)	1 (9)	Chromium mcg	9
Protein g (%)	4 (16)		

GRILLED BROCCOLI

2 large heads of broccoli
1 tablespoon extra virgin olive oil
PAM

Preheat broiler to 500°. Wash broccoli. Peel away and discard the tough, outer layer of the stalk leaving the tender, pale interior. Cut the broccoli (florets and stalk) into small (two-bite) portions. Put in a bowl with the olive oil, and gently turn so that the oil coats the broccoli. Spray a large cookie sheet with PAM, spread the broccoli on the sheet, and broil for 8 minutes, or until tips are slightly dark.

4 servings

Nutritional Information (PER SERVING)

Calories	50	Cholesterol mg	0
Carbohydrate g (%)	4 (28)	Sodium mg	21
Fat g (%)	4 (57)	Chromium mcg	15
Protein g (%)	2 (16)		

GRILLED EGGPLANT

3 small, long eggplants, sliced in half lengthwise
1 tablespoon olive oil

Preheat broiler to 500°. Place eggplant face up on broiler pan and brush with oil. With pan about 6 inches below heating element, cook until just fork tender and browned, from 10 to 30 minutes depending on size of eggplant. Baste twice with oil during cooking.

3 servings

Nutritional Information (PER SERVING)

Calories	57	Cholesterol mg	0
Carbohydrate g (%)	4 (28)	Sodium mg	22
Fat g (%)	5 (69)	Chromium mcg	15
Protein g (%)	0.5 (4)		

GRILLED LOBSTER TAIL

½ cup fresh lime juice
¼ cup fresh lemon juice
½ cup shallots, finely chopped
¼ cup olive oil
½ teaspoon paprika
black pepper to taste
5 large, fresh or frozen lobster tails
chopped parsley, radishes, and sliced lemon for garnish

In a large mixing bowl, whisk together lime juice, lemon juice, shallots, olive oil, and spices. Pour mixture over lobster tails and marinate for 2 hours. Preheat broiler to 450°. Arrange on broiler pan, place pan about 8 inches below heating element, and grill for about 7 minutes (watch carefully to avoid charring). Serve surrounded by parsley, whole radishes and large slices of lemon.

5 servings

Nutritional Information (PER SERVING)

Calories	343	Cholesterol mg	156
Carbohydrate g (%)	12 (14)	Sodium mg	828
Fat g (%)	11 (30)	Chromium mcg	30
Protein g (%)	49 (57)		

GRILLED SALMON

½ cup lemon juice
¼ cup scallions
2 tablespoons olive oil
fresh or dried dill to taste
black pepper to taste
4 3½-ounce salmon steaks
chopped parsley, radishes, and large lemon slices for garnish

Whisk together lemon juice, scallions, olive oil, dill, and pepper. Pour over salmon steaks and marinate for 2 hours. Preheat broiler to 450°. Grill for 7 minutes (watch carefully to avoid charring). Serve surrounded by parsley, whole radishes, and large slices of lemon.

4 servings

Nutritional Information (PER SERVING)

Calories	252	Cholesterol mg	49
Carbohydrate g (%)	3 (5)	Sodium mg	59
Fat g (%)	14 (51)	Chromium mcg	6
Protein g (%)	28 (44)		

GRILLED TUNA

½ cup lime juice
¼ cup scallions
¼ cup olive oil
black pepper or pepper flakes to taste
4 3½-ounce tuna steaks
chopped parsley, radishes, and large lemon slices for garnish

Whisk together lime juice, scallions, olive oil, and pepper. Pour over tuna steaks and marinate for 2 hours. Preheat broiler to 450°. Grill for 7 minutes (watch carefully to avoid charring). Serve surrounded by parsley, whole radishes, and large slices of lemon.

4 servings

Nutritional Information (PER SERVING)

Calories	312	Cholesterol mg	49
Carbohydrate g (%)	3 (4)	Sodium mg	51
Fat g (%)	20 (58)	Chromium mcg	4
Protein g (%)	30 (38)		

HALF-THE-FAT HUMMUS

½ package (3 ounces) Casbah instant hummus
4 ounces firm tofu
½ cup water

In a blender, combine the instant hummus with the tofu and water until the mixture is creamy and smooth.

4 2-ounce servings

Nutritional Information (PER SERVING)

Calories	164	Cholesterol mg	0
Carbohydrate g (%)	11 (48)	Sodium mg	71
Fat g (%)	8 (45)	Chromium mcg	10
Protein g (%)	11 (27)		

HASH BROWN POTATOES

2 teaspoons olive oil
6 to 8 boiled potatoes, peeled and diced, to make about 2½ cups
Vegit and black pepper to taste

In a skillet, heat olive oil. Add potatoes, sprinkle with Vegit and pepper, and press them down firmly with a spatula. Cover the pan and allow potatoes to cook over medium-low heat until a golden-brown crust forms on the bottom, about 15 minutes. Turn out of pan upside down on a plate or fold over like an omelette.

4 servings

Nutritional Information (PER SERVING)

Calories	224	Cholesterol mg	0
Carbohydrate g (%)	48 (83)	Sodium mg	13
Fat g (%)	2 (10)	Chromium mcg	37
Protein g (%)	4 (7)		

HIGH-CHROMIUM GINGERS

¼ cup canola oil
¼ cup dark brown sugar
1¼ cup blackstrap molasses
¾ cup cold water
5 cups whole wheat flour
1 cup wheat bran
3 teaspoons cinnamon
3 teaspoons ground ginger
2 teaspoons ground allspice
2 teaspoons ground cloves
4 teaspoons baking powder
1 package rapid-rise yeast
2 tablespoons brewer's yeast
PAM

In a large mixing bowl, combine thoroughly the oil, sugar, and molasses. Stir in cold water. Sift the dry ingredients together, and stir them into the oil-sugar mixture (this will make a very thick dough). Chill in the refrigerator for 40 minutes. Preheat oven to 350°. Spray a baking sheet with PAM. Roll out dough to ½ to ¾ inch thick, and cut into cookies with a 2½- to 3-inch cookie cutter (or use the top of a jar the same size) (thickness and diameter can vary according to taste). Place cookies 1 inch apart on the baking sheet. Bake until no imprint remains when touched with a finger, about 18 minutes.

2½ dozen tempting cookies

Nutritional Information (PER COOKIE)

Calories	71	Cholesterol mg	0
Carbohydrate g (%)	13 (72)	Sodium mg	13
Fat g (%)	2 (23)	Chromium mcg	21
Protein g (%)	1 (5)		

HIGH-CHROMIUM MEAT LOAF

½ pound leanest chuck (95 percent fat-free), ground
4 slices whole grain bread, broken into coarse bread crumbs
½ cup wheat bran
2 tablespoons brewer's yeast
1 whole egg
1 egg white
1 carrot, finely chopped
3 stalks celery, diced
1 small onion, finely chopped
½ cup beer
1 teaspoon dried thyme
1 tablespoon Vegit
black pepper to taste
Worcestershire sauce
PAM

Preheat oven to 350°. Spray a 1-quart casserole dish or 8 × 3 inch loaf pan with PAM. Mix all ingredients in a large bowl. Transfer to prepared pan. Bake uncovered for 45 minutes. Delicious topped with Worcestershire sauce.

4 servings

Nutritional Information (PER SERVING)

Calories	237	Cholesterol mg	94
Carbohydrate g (%)	25 (31)	Sodium mg	281
Fat g (%)	7 (20)	Chromium mcg	36
Protein g (%)	40 (50)		

HIGH-CHROMIUM MUFFINS

1¾ cups wheat bran
¼ cup raw wheat germ
½ cup whole wheat flour
2 teaspoons baking powder
1½ teaspoons baking soda
1 tablespoon brown sugar (optional)
1½ tablespoons brewer's yeast
1 banana
1 apple with skin
¼ cup large prunes, pitted and chopped
¼ cup dates, chopped
1 whole egg
1 egg white

2 teaspoons canola oil
2 tablespoons molasses
2 tablespoons vanilla
1½ to 2 cups water
PAM

Preheat oven to 350°. Spray PAM on a nonstick muffin pan with large or medium-sized muffin cups. In a large bowl, mix all the dry ingredients. In a food processor, separately puree banana, apple, dates, and prunes, and add to dry ingredients. In a small bowl, lightly beat the egg and egg white. Add the eggs and the other wet ingredients, except water, to the dry ingredients. Gradually mix in enough water to make a batter a little thicker than pancake batter. Make sure the dates and prunes are well distributed, but do not overmix. Spoon batter into 6 large or 9 medium-sized muffin cups. Bake for 40 minutes.

6 large or 9 medium muffins

Nutritional Information (PER SERVING)

Calories	171	Cholesterol mg	44
Carbohydrate g (%)	34 (69)	Sodium mg	335
Fat g (%)	4 (17)	Chromium mcg	59
Protein g (%)	7 (14)		

HIGH-CHROMIUM SALAD

¾ cup whole wheat couscous
1½ cups water
1 cup cooked smoked or regular turkey, diced
12 red or dark green lettuce leaves
2 medium scallions, diced
3 tablespoons parsley, minced
1 large fresh tomato, sliced
4 ounces mushrooms, sliced
1 red pepper, sliced
black pepper to taste

YOGURT, MINT, AND GARLIC DRESSING

¾ cup plain nonfat yogurt
1 tablespoon fresh mint, minced
1 small clove garlic, put through a press

Add couscous to 1½ cups boiling water, return to boil, cover, reduce heat to low, and simmer for 35 minutes, or until moisture is absorbed. Add turkey and chill. Place lettuce leaves on a platter and arrange couscous and turkey, scallions, parsley, tomato, mushrooms, and red pepper in a decorative manner. Top with black pepper. Whisk the yogurt, mint, and garlic together and pour on top of salad.

4 servings

Nutritional Information (PER SERVING)

Calories	180	Cholesterol mg	32
Carbohydrate g (%)	32 (58)	Sodium mg	80
Fat g (%)	3 (12)	Chromium mcg	15
Protein g (%)	16 (29)		

HIGH-CHROMIUM SPREAD

4 tablespoons Paul's peanuts, unsalted, or other low-fat peanuts
2 tablespoons brewer's yeast
2 tablespoons Fromage Blanc

In a food processor or blender, combine all ingredients until creamy. Great on sprouted wheat bagels with Sorrell Ridge blueberry conserve. Refrigerate and use by the tablespoon.

6 servings (2 tablespoons each)

Nutritional Information (PER SERVING)

Calories	62	Cholesterol mg	0.4
Carbohydrate g (%)	3 (19)	Sodium mg	81
Fat g (%)	3 (49)	Chromium mcg	34
Protein g (%)	5 (31)		

HIGH-CHROMIUM STUFFING

3 stalks celery, diced
1 large onion, coarsely chopped
1 tablespoon olive oil
½ package frozen corn
6 slices seven-grain, corn bread, or the best whole wheat with bran bread you can find, broken into coarse crumbs
1½ teaspoons dried sage
1 teaspoon dried thyme
Vegit and black pepper to taste

In a medium-sized, cast iron skillet, sauté celery and onion in olive oil. Add corn and ½ cup water. Break up corn with fork, lower the heat, and cook corn for 2 minutes. Add bread crumbs and seasonings, gently turning to mix all ingredients well. Serve with roast chicken or lean pork chops.

4 large or 6 medium servings

Nutritional Information (PER SERVING)

Calories	112	Cholesterol mg	0
Carbohydrate g (%)	19 (64)	Sodium mg	160
Fat g (%)	3 (23)	Chromium mcg	38
Protein g (%)	4 (13)		

HUEVOS RANCHEROS

2 corn tortillas
3 egg whites
½ cup leftover black beans, Little Bear canned refried beans, or Fantastic Foods instant refried beans mix, prepared

according to package directions
½ *ounce (2 tablespoons) low-fat cheese, shredded*
3 *avocado slices (½ avocado, sliced)*
salsa
PAM

Preheat oven to 350°. Bake tortillas for 3 minutes. In a small skillet sprayed with PAM, scramble the egg whites. Top tortillas with eggs, beans, and cheese. Serve with avocado and salsa on the side.

2 servings

Nutritional Information (PER SERVING)

Calories	250	Cholesterol mg	0.25
Carbohydrate g (%)	31 (46)	Sodium mg	249
Fat g (%)	8 (26)	Chromium mcg	19
Protein g (%)	19 (28)		

ISADORE'S BULGUR SALAD (FROM THE MANSION ON TURTLE CREEK, DALLAS, TEXAS)

1 *cup bulgur*
1 *tablespoon lemon juice*
1 *tablespoon lime juice*
2 *tablespoons chopped parsley*
⅓ *cup feta cheese*
½ *cup chopped tomato*
Vegit and black pepper to taste

Soak the bulgur in hot water to cover for 1 hour. Drain well. Combine remaining ingredients and stir in the bulgur.

4 servings

Nutritional Information (PER SERVING)

Calories	165	Cholesterol mg	2
Carbohydrate g (%)	34 (82)	Sodium mg	30
Fat g (%)	1 (5)	Chromium mcg	28
Protein g (%)	5 (12)		

JALAPENO CORN MUFFINS

2 cups corn meal
1 cup whole wheat flour
2 teaspoons baking powder
1 package frozen corn (unsalted), broken up into separate kernels
4 fresh or canned jalapeno peppers, seeded and chopped
3 ounces low-fat cheese, grated
2 tablespoons olive or canola oil
4 egg whites
2 cups nonfat buttermilk (low-sodium)
PAM

Preheat oven to 400°. Spray a nonstick muffin tin with medium-sized muffin cups with PAM. In a bowl, combine corn meal, flour, and baking powder. Stir in corn, peppers, and cheese. In another bowl, mix oil, egg whites, and buttermilk. Add this to corn mixture, stirring just to moisten dry ingredients. Spoon batter into muffin cups and bake for 20 minutes.

9 medium-sized muffins

Nutritional Information (PER SERVING)

Calories	252	Cholesterol mg	2
Carbohydrate g (%)	39 (60)	Sodium mg	256
Fat g (%)	8 (23)	Chromium mcg	13
Protein g (%)	11 (17)		

JOHN'S SCALLOPS

1 clove garlic, minced
¼ teaspoon fresh ginger, grated
1 tablespoon olive oil
¾ cup white wine
10 ounces sea scallops, chopped
4 ounces shiitake mushrooms
1 cup white Chinese cabbage, shredded
½ teaspoon low-sodium tamari

Sauté garlic and ginger in olive oil until golden. Add wine to skillet and let boil down slightly. Add scallops, mushrooms, and cabbage. Simmer until half of the moisture is absorbed. Add the tamari.

4 servings

Nutritional Information (PER SERVING)

Calories	150	Cholesterol mg	38
Carbohydrate g (%)	5 (18)	Sodium mg	269
Fat g (%)	7 (37)	Chromium mcg	18
Protein g (%)	17 (46)		

KETCHUP FROM LAUREL'S KITCHEN*

1 12-ounce can tomato paste (unsalted)
½ cup cider vinegar
½ cup water
1 teaspoon oregano
⅛ teaspoon cumin
⅛ teaspoon nutmeg
⅛ teaspoon pepper
½ teaspoon mustard powder
dash garlic powder

Mix all ingredients.

1¾ cups (serving size—1 tablespoon)

Nutritional Information (PER SERVING)

Calories	6	Cholesterol mg	0
Carbohydrate g (%)	1 (87)	Sodium mg	4
Fat g (%)	0 (0)	Chromium mcg	6
Protein g (%)	0.2 (13)		

*Reprinted from *The New Laurel's Kitchen* © 1976, 1986 by The Blue Mountain Center of Meditation, Inc., with permission by Ten Speed Press, Berkeley, CA.

KILLER CHROMIUM CHILI

- *1 pound light red kidney beans*
- *3 bay leaves*
- *3 teaspoons dried oregano*
- *3 teaspoons black pepper*
- *3 stalks celery, diced*
- *1 large hot chili pepper, seeded and finely chopped*
- *1 large onion, coarsely chopped*
- *2 cloves garlic, minced*
- *1 28-ounce can whole tomatoes*
- *1 28-ounce can crushed tomatoes*
- *1 12-ounce can tomato paste (unsalted)*
- *4 tablespoons chili powder*
- *2 tablespoons ground cumin*
- *Vegit to taste*
- *6 ounces ground chuck (the leanest you can find)*
- *8 ounces beer*
- *¼ cup brewer's yeast*

Rinse and sort through beans. Soak beans overnight or use the quick-soak method (see page 244). Drain beans and cover with 2 inches cold water, bring to a boil with 3 bay leaves, 1 teaspoon oregano, and 1 teaspoon black pepper, and simmer covered for 1½ hours. In a large pot steam celery, chili pepper, onion, and garlic in 1 cup water until softened. Add tomatoes, tomato paste, chili powder, cumin, remaining 2 teaspoons oregano, remaining 2 teaspoons pepper, and Vegit. Remove from heat. In a separate skillet, brown meat and add to the tomatoes. Mash half of the cooked kidney beans and add them and the unmashed beans to the tomato-beef mixture. Stir while bringing to a boil, reduce heat to simmer, and add beer. Adjust seasoning. Let simmer for 15 minutes. Mix in brewer's yeast just before serving.

8 servings (freezes well)

Nutritional Information (PER SERVING)

Calories	345	Cholesterol mg	19
Carbohydrate g (%)	47 (58)	Sodium mg	298
Fat g (%)	5 (15)	Chromium mcg	35
Protein g (%)	22 (26)		

LIMA AND PESTO SAUCE

1 cup dried baby limas, cooked (see pages 244–245)
¼ cup ready-made pesto (remove as much olive oil as possible soon after purchasing)
¼ cup Fromage Blanc

Drain cooked limas and puree in a food processor. Combine lima puree with pesto and Fromage Blanc.

4 servings

Nutritional Information (PER SERVING), sauce alone

Calories	131	Cholesterol mg	0
Carbohydrate g (%)	14 (43)	Sodium mg	171
Fat g (%)	6 (42)	Chromium mcg	20
Protein g (%)	5 (15)		

LIMA CASSEROLE

1 pound large dried lima beans
1 large onion, minced
1 large green pepper, chopped
4 fresh basil leaves, chopped, or 1½ teaspoons dried basil
2 teaspoons olive oil (optional)
Vegit and black pepper to taste

Soak limas overnight or by the quick-soak method (see page 244). Rinse, drain, and cover with 2 inches of water. Bring to a boil, reduce heat, and simmer covered for 1 hour. In a small skillet, steam pepper, onion, and basil in water or sauté in 2 teaspoons olive oil. Add to limas. Continue cooking limas uncovered for about 15 more minutes on low to moderate heat, so the limas form their own creamy consistency. Season to taste with black pepper and Vegit.

6 servings

Nutritional Information (PER SERVING)

Calories	102	Cholesterol mg	0
Carbohydrate g (%)	20 (76)	Sodium mg	13
Fat g (%)	0.4 (3)	Chromium mcg	18
Protein g (%)	5 (21)		

LIMA FRITTATA

- *1 tablespoon olive oil or canola oil*
- *1 small onion, coarsely chopped*
- *1 cup leftover lima casserole or 1 cup cooked large lima beans*
- *2 whole eggs*
- *10 egg whites*
- *2 ounces low-fat Swiss cheese, grated*
- *1 tablespoon Vegit*
- *black pepper to taste*

Preheat broiler to 500°. In a 10-inch skillet, sauté onions in oil until softened. Add limas. In a separate bowl, combine eggs, egg whites, Swiss cheese, Vegit, and pepper, and whisk until yolks are dispersed. Turn up heat and add egg mixture to skillet. Keep heat high for approximately 2 minutes. Lower heat to medium for about 1½ minutes, until the eggs are set on the bottom but still moist on top. Place the skillet under broiler for an additional 4 minutes until the frittata is slightly puffed and golden brown.

4 servings

Nutritional Information (PER SERVING)

Calories	205	Cholesterol mg	138
Carbohydrate g (%)	11 (22)	Sodium mg	235

Fat g (%)	10 (44)	Chromium mcg	19
Protein g (%)	17 (34)		

LIMA PUREE

1 cup dried baby lima beans

Soak limas overnight or by the quick-soak method (see page 244). Drain and cover with 2 inches water. Bring to a boil, reduce heat, and simmer covered for 1½ hours, or until liquid is almost completely absorbed and limas are tender. Drain in a colander. In a food processor, puree limas in batches until they are the consistency of mashed potatoes. Serve hot with any of a variety of toppings, such as pesto, salsa, tomato sauce, or clam sauce.

4 servings

Nutritional Information (PER SERVING)

Calories	189	Cholesterol mg	0
Carbohydrate g (%)	34 (69)	Sodium mg	2
Fat g (%)	1 (5)	Chromium mcg	24
Protein g (%)	13 (26)		

LINN'S COLE SLAW

- *2 tablespoons cider vinegar*
- *⅛ teaspoon fructose or honey*
- *1 tablespoon lemon juice*
- *⅛ teaspoon paprika*
- *½ cup low-fat mayonnaise (see page 275)*
- *Vegit and black pepper to taste*
- *1 medium head red cabbage, shredded*

Mix vinegar, fructose, lemon juice, paprika, Vegit, and pepper with mayonnaise and pour over cabbage.

5 servings

Nutritional Information (PER SERVING)

Calories	60	Cholesterol mg	3
Carbohydrate g (%)	9 (52)	Sodium mg	30
Fat g (%)	2 (31)	Chromium mcg	14
Protein g (%)	3 (17)		

LOW-FAT MAYONNAISE

½ cup nonfat yogurt
2 tablespoons Hellman's light mayonnaise

Mix yogurt and mayonnaise with a fork.

½ cup (1 serving = 2 tablespoons)

Nutritional Information (entire amount)

Calories	143	Cholesterol mg	12
Carbohydrate g (%)	11 (30)	Sodium mg	87
Fat g (%)	8 (52)	Chromium mcg	0
Protein g (%)	7 (18)		

LOW-FAT SOUR CREAM

½ cup ½%-fat Breakstone cottage cheese
¼ cup nonfat buttermilk (low-sodium)
dash lemon juice

In a food processor, electric mixer, or with a wire whisk, beat cottage cheese, buttermilk, and lemon until completely blended and smooth. The low-fat sour cream can be used in place of Fromage Blanc in any recipe except Scallops and Vodka.

2 servings

Nutritional Information (PER SERVING)

Calories	43	Cholesterol mg	3
Carbohydrate g (%)	2 (21)	Sodium mg	37
Fat g (%)	0.4 (9)	Chromium mcg	0
Protein g (%)	7 (70)		

MILK-SOAKED HADDOCK

4 3-ounce haddock fillets
2 cups skim milk
1 cup yellow corn meal
black pepper to taste
PAM or olive oil for coating pan

Soak haddock in milk for 3 hours. Preheat oven to 350°. Remove haddock from milk and roll the fillets in the corn meal and pepper. Place the haddock in a baking pan sprayed with PAM or lightly coated with olive oil. Bake until just done and corn meal is a little crunchy, about 12 minutes. Serve with red clam sauce either homemade (see page 291) or a ready-made brand such as Contadina.

4 servings

Nutritional Information (PER SERVING)

Calories	226	Cholesterol mg	114
Carbohydrate g (%)	29 (49)	Sodium mg	196
Fat g (%)	3 (11)	Chromium mcg	10
Protein g (%)	23 (39)		

MINESTRONE ALLA BURRINI*

4½ cups (3 cans) Health Valley or Pritikin beef broth
1 beef bone, without fat
1 large onion, diced
3 carrots, cut in chunks
3 stalks celery, diced
4–6 fresh basil leaves, chopped
½ head cauliflower, cut into small florets
2 heads broccoli, with stalks peeled and florets and stalks cut in small pieces
4 zucchini, sliced crosswise into ¼-inch pieces

*Reprinted with the permission of Burrini's Prime Meats and Catering, Mendham, NJ.

- ½ *can (1 cup) chick-peas, rinsed thoroughly and drained*
- 3 *28-ounce cans crushed tomatoes*
- 5 *red pepper flakes*
- 1 *teaspoon paprika*
- 1 *tablespoon black pepper*
- 1 *teaspoon rosemary*
- 2 *bay leaves*
- ¾ *pound lean chuck, cut into small cubes*
- 8 *ounces whole wheat spiral pasta*

In a large soup pot, combine beef broth, bone, onion, carrots, and celery. Bring to a boil, reduce heat, and simmer for 10 minutes. Add all the other ingredients except whole wheat spirals and continue simmering for 35 minutes. Skim fat, add pasta and simmer for an additional 12 minutes.

10 servings

Nutritional Information (PER SERVING)

Calories	216	Cholesterol mg	22
Carbohydrate g (%)	28 (50)	Sodium mg	220
Fat g (%)	5 (20)	Chromium mcg	33
Protein g (%)	17 (30)		

MUSHROOM RISOTTO

- 2 *medium cloves garlic, minced*
- 1 *tablespoon olive oil*
- 2 *tablespoons chopped fresh parsley*
- ½ *cup white wine*
- 1 *pound mushrooms, washed and sliced*
- 1½ *cups short grain brown rice*
- 2¾ *cups Health Valley chicken broth*
- 3 *tablespoons grated Parmesan cheese*
- ½ *teaspoon cinnamon*
- *dash nutmeg*
- *black pepper to taste*

In a medium-size saucepan, sauté garlic in olive oil. Add parsley and wine. Add mushrooms and cook over high heat about 3 minutes until all liquid is absorbed. Keeping heat on high, add rice and gently turn to coat with ingredients. Gradually add chicken broth and bring to boil. Cover, reduce heat, and simmer for 40 minutes. Uncover and fluff rice with fork, while mixing in cheese, nutmeg, cinnamon, and pepper.

5 servings

Nutritional Information (PER SERVING)

Calories	215	Cholesterol mg	4
Carbohydrate g (%)	27 (50)	Sodium mg	246
Fat g (%)	8 (32)	Chromium mcg	31
Protein g (%)	10 (18)		

•

NITZA'S TOMATO SAUCE

- *1½ tablespoons olive oil*
- *1 large Spanish onion, coarsely chopped*
- *1 carrot, finely chopped (or shredded)*
- *3 large cloves garlic, minced*
- *1 28-ounce can crushed tomatoes*
- *1 28-ounce can whole tomatoes*
- *¼ cup chopped Italian parsley*
- *5 fresh basil leaves, chopped,* or *2 teaspoons dried basil*
- *2½ teaspoons dried oregano*
- *dash of red pepper flakes*
- *⅓ cup wine (optional)*
- *black pepper to taste*

In a large skillet, heat olive oil. Add onion and sauté until translucent. Add carrot. In a corner of the pan (away from other ingredients), add garlic, sauté until just golden, and quickly stir into carrot-onion mixture. Add both kinds of tomatoes, breaking up the whole tomatoes. Add parsley, basil, oregano, pepper flakes, and pepper. Simmer slowly uncovered for about 30 minutes, tasting periodically and adjusting seasoning. Add wine about 5 minutes before serving. Serve over pasta, chicken, rice, or potatoes.

10 ½-cup servings

Nutritional Information (PER SERVING)

Calories	78	Cholesterol mg	0
Carbohydrate g (%)	6 (48)	Sodium mg	142
Fat g (%)	2 (36)	Chromium mcg	15
Protein g (%)	2 (16)		

NONFAT YOGURT DESSERT

8 ounces plain nonfat yogurt
4 ounces unsweetened applesauce
¼ cup Sorrell Ridge blueberry conserve
2 teaspoons Grape Nuts

In a mixing bowl, combine yogurt, applesauce, and conserve. Divide the mixture between 2 1½-cup bowls and top each with Grape Nuts. Put in the freezer for 15 minutes.

2 servings

Nutritional Information (PER SERVING)

Calories	162	Cholesterol mg	6
Carbohydrate g (%)	42 (80)	Sodium mg	120
Fat g (%)	2 (9)	Chromium mcg	2
Protein g (%)	6 (11)		

GENUINE AUSTIN OMELETTE

1 pound mushrooms, washed and sliced
1 green pepper, coarsely chopped
2 jalapeno peppers, fresh or canned, finely chopped
2 teaspoons canola oil
6 egg whites
2 whole eggs
Vegit and black pepper to taste
1 teaspoon fresh cilantro, finely chopped

2 ounces low-fat Swiss cheese, grated
2 corn tortillas baked at 450° for 3 minutes and broken into pieces

In a 9-inch nonstick skillet, sauté mushrooms and peppers in oil until mushrooms just begin to brown. In a separate bowl, whisk eggs, seasonings, cilantro, and cheese together. Raise heat and pour in eggs. Sprinkle broken tortilla pieces on top of eggs. Lower heat a bit and allow eggs to firm up (about 4 minutes). Gently lift up one side with a spatula and fold in half, pressing the filling down so it cooks as much as possible without burning. Serve immediately.

2 servings

Nutritional Information (PER SERVING)

Calories	310	Cholesterol mg	222
Carbohydrate g (%)	35 (40)	Sodium mg	756
Fat g (%)	12 (31)	Chromium mcg	18
Protein g (%)	25 (29)		

ORANGE PEANUT BREAD

2 cups whole wheat flour
2 teaspoons baking powder
1 teaspoon baking soda
¼ cup crunchy, unhydrogenated peanut butter, with all oil poured off
2 tablespoons honey
2 egg whites
3 heaping tablespoons freshly grated orange peel
½ cup fresh orange juice
¾ cup skim milk
¼ cup Paul's Peanuts (unsalted)

Preheat oven to 350°. Spray a 9 × 5-inch loaf pan with PAM. In a food processor, using short pulses, coarsely chop peanuts (be careful they do not turn into peanut butter) and reserve. In a large bowl, blend flour, baking powder, and baking soda. With a fork, cut in peanut butter and honey until the mixture is the consistency of coarse meal (this takes a little while). In a separate bowl, combine egg whites, orange peel, orange juice, and milk. Add to flour mixture, stirring until well blended. Fold in chopped peanuts. Pour batter into pan. Bake for 45 minutes.

10 servings (10 slices)

Nutritional Information (PER SERVING)

Calories	175	Cholesterol mg	1
Carbohydrate g (%)	25 (55)	Sodium mg	135
Fat g (%)	5 (26)	Chromium mcg	9
Protein g (%)	8 (18)		

PASTA DE MARÉ SAUCE

1 tablespoon olive oil
3 shallots, minced
1 sweet onion, coarsely chopped
1 teaspoon hot red pepper flakes
1 bay leaf
1 32-ounce can crushed tomatoes
2 teaspoons fresh frozen basil
black pepper
8 ounce fresh shrimp, clams, scallops or lobster (optional)

In a large skillet sauté shallots and onion in oil until golden. Add red pepper flakes, bay leaf, tomatoes, pepper, and basil, bringing up heat to boil, and then simmer uncovered for 30 minutes, adding seafood as close to serving as possible so as not to overcook (no more than 3 minutes before serving). Use on pasta, baked potatoes, or high-chromium grain such as cracked wheat.

6 servings for pasta

Nutritional Information (PER SERVING)

Calories	120	Cholesterol mg	20
Carbohydrate g (%)	12 (39)	Sodium mg	300
Fat g (%)	3 (22)	Chromium mcg	22
Protein g (%)	12 (39)		

PRIMAVERA

½ package frozen corn
¼ package frozen green beans
½ package frozen peas
1 cooked sweet potato, cubed
2 zucchini, diced, or ¾ cup any leftover green vegetable
½ cup thinly sliced carrots (optional)
1 recipe cheese sauce (see page 249)
1 pound whole wheat, whole wheat amaranth, or quinoa spaghetti

Start to bring water to boil for pasta. Steam all vegetables (except potato) together for 3 minutes. Add vegetables and potato to cheese sauce. Prepare pasta according to directions on box and drain. Add sauce and vegetables to pasta, toss, and serve hot.

8 servings

Nutritional Information (PER SERVING)

Calories	256	Cholesterol mg	0
Carbohydrate g (%)	52.6 (82)	Sodium mg	35.6
Fat g (%)	1.1 (4)	Chromium mcg	23
Protein g (%)	9.1 (14)		

PASTA WITH BRAISED LENTILS

1 large onion, coarsely chopped
2 cloves garlic, minced
2 medium-sized pickled canned jalapeno peppers, chopped
½ cup sun-dried tomatoes, chopped

1 cup dried lentils
3 cups chicken broth (unsalted) or Gaylord Hauser vegetable broth
½ cup fresh parsley, chopped
2 ounces feta cheese, crumbled
2 ounces Fromage Blanc
6 whole walnuts, chopped (optional)
1 12-ounce whole wheat or quinoa pasta

In a medium saucepan, steam the onion, garlic, and peppers in water, stirring occasionally, until onions are softened. Stir in lentils, broth, and tomatoes, bring to a boil, and simmer covered until tender and most of the liquid is absorbed (1¼ to 1½ hours). Stir in the parsley. Combine feta, Fromage Blanc, and walnuts, and add to the lentils just before serving. Prepare pasta according to directions on package. Drain and serve with lentil mixture as a pasta sauce.

6 servings

Nutritional Information (PER SERVING)

Calories	330	Cholesterol mg	16
Carbohydrate g (%)	49 (61)	Sodium mg	310
Fat g (%)	6 (17)	Chromium mcg	28
Protein g (%)	18 (22)		

PASTA WITH SCALLOPS, PEAS, AND VODKA

1 tablespoon olive oil
3 cloves garlic, minced
1 fresh or canned jalapeno pepper, seeded and chopped
½ cup fresh basil, chopped
5 canned plum tomatoes, diced (1 cup)
¾ pound frozen peas, steamed
juice of ½ lemon
1 pound sea scallops, cut into bite-size chunks
⅓ cup vodka
½ cup Fromage Blanc, after draining overnight (see page 257)

1½ tablespoons grated Parmesan cheese
black pepper to taste
1 pound amaranth pasta

Start to bring water to boil for pasta. In a large saucepan, sauté garlic in olive oil. Add peppers, basil, and tomatoes. Heat over medium-low heat for about 2 minutes. Turn up heat, and add peas, lemon juice, scallops, and vodka (be careful as vodka will bubble and spatter). Boil at high heat to reduce liquid for about 1 minute. Lower heat and fold in the Fromage Blanc. Prepare pasta according to directions on package and spoon scallop mixture over pasta. Top with black pepper and Parmesan and serve immediately.

6 servings

Nutritional Information (PER SERVING)

Calories	460	Cholesterol mg	41
Carbohydrate g (%)	67 (62)	Sodium mg	320
Fat g (%)	7 (13)	Chromium mcg	29
Protein g (%)	31 (27)		

PERFECT POTATO SALAD

3 pounds small red potatoes, scrubbed in skins
½ cup nonfat yogurt
1 tablespoon Hellman's light mayonnaise
1 teaspoon cider vinegar
1½ teaspoons dill (dried) or 1 tablespoon fresh
black pepper to taste
1 medium Vadalia onion or other sweet mild onion, coarsely chopped
6 radicchio leaves

Add the potatoes to a large saucepan of boiling water. When the water returns to a boil, lower heat and cook at a slow boil about 10 minutes, or until potatoes are just done but are still firm. Drain and chill. Mix yogurt, mayonnaise, vinegar, dill, pepper, and onions and add to potatoes when ready to serve. Mix well. Serve on leaves of radicchio.

5 servings

Nutritional Information (PER SERVING)

Calories	269	Cholesterol mg	1
Carbohydrate g (%)	59 (86)	Sodium mg	32
Fat g (%)	1 (4)	Chromium mcg	51
Protein g (%)	7 (10)		

PIZZA CRUST

PIZZA DOUGH

(Adapted with the permission of The Greens restaurant, San Francisco)

3 tablespoons hot water
3 tablespoons skim milk
½ package (about 1¼ teaspoons) active dry yeast
pinch sugar or honey
1 tablespoon olive oil
1 tablespoon rye flour
2 tablespoons whole wheat flour
⅝ cup unbleached white flour

Combine the water and milk (the mixture should be warm, not hot). Add yeast and sugar and stir to dissolve yeast. Mix in the olive oil, rye flour, and whole wheat flour. Gradually add the white flour, stirring to make a soft workable dough. Add only enough flour to keep the dough from sticking—the dough should be a little moist. Turn out onto a lightly floured surface and knead for about 5 minutes. Put the dough in a lightly oiled bowl and turn once to coat the surface with oil. Cover the bowl and let the dough rise in a warm spot about 35 to 40 minutes.

Preheat oven to 500°. To shape the pizza, first form the dough into a ball and then roll it out on a floured surface to flatten it into a disk. Pick up the dough and stretch it gently and evenly. Stretch and roll the dough as necessary to form a 10-inch circle. Transfer to a baking sheet or pizza pan and add chosen topping. Bake at 500° for 13 to 15 minutes in the top third of the oven until the crust is golden brown.

5 servings as an appetizer, 4 as a main dish

Nutritional Information (PER SERVING)

Calories	118	Cholesterol mg	0.1
Carbohydrate g (%)	18 (61)	Sodium mg	6
Fat g (%)	3 (28)	Chromium mcg	5
Protein g (%)	3 (11)		

POLENTA

3 cups cold water
2½ cups coarse yellow corn meal
3 cups boiling water
4.5 ounces shredded low-fat Swiss, skim-milk mozzarella, mild goat cheese or other low-fat cheese or a mixture of cheeses

In a bowl, mix corn meal into the 3 cups of cold water. Slowly add this mixture to a large pot with the boiling water. Reduce heat to medium low. Stir frequently with a wooden paddle for about 45 minutes, or until the mixture is thick, pulls away from the side of the pot, and is beginning to form a crust around the bottom. Add cheeses and mix gently. Serve hot with a sauce. (*Note:* This recipe can be made in 5 minutes using instant polenta.)

To grill polenta, pour into loaf pan and chill thoroughly. Turn out of pan and cut into ½-inch thick slices. Grill under broiler or brown in hot skillet sprayed with PAM.

4 servings

Nutritional Information (PER SERVING)

Calories	384	Cholesterol mg	1.1
Carbohydrate g (%)	57 (59)	Sodium mg	158
Fat g (%)	11 (26)	Chromium mcg	25
Protein g (%)	14.7 (15)		

PORCINI PIZZA SAUCE

1½ ounces dried porcini mushrooms
1 28-ounce can crushed tomatoes
1 teaspoon black pepper and red pepper flakes to taste
1 teaspoon thyme
1 cup cooked rice or other cooked grain, such as kashi pilaf or bulgur
1½ ounces low-fat Swiss cheese or other low-fat cheese
4 tablespoons grated Parmesan cheese

In a mixing bowl, cover mushrooms with 1 cup boiling water and let soak for 20 minutes. While mushrooms are soaking, heat tomatoes and spices in a saucepan. Drain mushrooms and rinse quickly under water to remove any sand. Add mushrooms, cooked rice, and Swiss cheese to tomatoes. Top pizza shell with mixture and sprinkle with Parmesan. Sauce is equally delicious on pasta, potatoes, and vegetables.

Enough sauce for 1 10-inch pizza (4 servings)

Nutritional Information (PER SERVING)

Calories	147	Cholesterol mg	1.6
Carbohydrate g (%)	22.6 (59)	Sodium mg	405
Fat g (%)	4 (23)	Chromium mcg	19
Protein g (%)	6.7 (18)		

POTATO AND BROCCOLI PIZZA

1 tablespoon olive oil
1 small onion, coarsely chopped
½ teaspoon dried thyme
½ teaspoon dried sweet marjoram
2 large baking potatoes, peeled and thinly sliced
½ cup canned crushed tomatoes
1 tablespoon balsamic vinegar
2 broccoli spears, florets and peeled stalks cut into 1-inch pieces
2 ounces Calamata olives, pitted and coarsely chopped (optional)
Vegit and black pepper to taste
2 ounces shredded smoked Gruyere cheese (or whatever cheese on hand)
1 corn meal pizza dough recipe (see page 252) or 1 Grain Dance whole wheat pizza shell

Preheat oven to 500°. In a large, heavy skillet, sauté onions in olive oil over medium heat. Add thyme, marjoram, and potatoes, gently turning to coat potatoes with the mixture. Add tomatoes and vinegar, heat briefly, cover, and reduce heat to simmer for approximately 8 minutes until potatoes are tender. Steam broccoli in a separate saucepan for 3 minutes and add to potatoes along with olives. Add Vegit and pepper. Shape dough according to recipe directions. Spoon topping onto corn meal pizza shell or Grain Dance shell and cover with cheese. Bake in the top third of the oven for about 13 minutes, or until crust is golden and the cheese is melted.

5 servings as an appetizer, 3 as a main dish

Nutritional Information (PER SERVING)

Calories	385	Cholesterol mg	20
Carbohydrate g (%)	60 (61)	Sodium mg	304
Fat g (%)	9 (21)	Chromium mcg	69
Protein g (%)	18 (18)		

POTATO PANCAKES

4 medium baking potatoes, peeled and grated
1 medium onion, diced
2 egg whites, lightly beaten
2 tablespoons whole grain bread crumbs
1 tablespoon brewer's yeast
black pepper to taste
2 teaspoons olive oil

In a large bowl, add onion to grated potatoes. Mix in egg whites, bread crumbs, brewer's yeast, and pepper. Heat olive oil in a nonstick skillet. Cook pancakes, using 1 large serving spoonful per pancake.

4 servings

Nutritional Information (PER SERVING)

Calories	139	Cholesterol mg	0
Carbohydrate g (%)	25 (72)	Sodium mg	41
Fat g (%)	3 (19)	Chromium mcg	35
Protein g (%)	3 (9)		

PRUNE WHIP

1 cup whole, pitted prunes
1 tablespoon grated orange peel
2 teaspoons grated lemon rind
1 teaspoon whole cloves
2 teaspoons cinnamon
2 cups water
½ cup skim-milk ricotta cheese

In a saucepan, combine prunes, orange peel, lemon peel, spices, and water. Bring to a boil and simmer uncovered for 40 minutes, or until most of the moisture is absorbed. Chill. In a food processor or blender, mix prunes with ricotta until thoroughly blended and creamy.

10 servings

Nutritional Information (PER SERVING)

Calories	40	Cholesterol mg	4
Carbohydrate g (%)	7 (63)	Sodium mg	16
Fat g (%)	1 (22)	Chromium mcg	15
Protein g (%)	2 (16)		

QUICK CHROMIUM MUFFINS

1½ cups wheat bran
1 cup whole wheat flour
2 tablespoons baking powder
2 tablespoons brewer's yeast
2 tablespoons canola oil
¼ cup blackstrap molasses
1 egg, lightly beaten
¼ cup prunes, pitted and chopped
1 cup water

Preheat oven to 350°. Spray PAM on a muffin tin with medium-sized cups. In a large mixing bowl, combine dry ingredients. Add oil, molasses, egg, and prunes. Slowly add water, mixing only until dry ingredients are moistened. Spoon batter into 9 muffin cups. Bake for 25 minutes.

9 muffins

Nutritional Information (PER SERVING)

Calories	135	Cholesterol mg	30
Carbohydrate g (%)	23 (63)	Sodium mg	19
Fat g (%)	4 (25)	Chromium mcg	34
Protein g (%)	4 (11)		

QUINOA SPAGHETTI WITH LIMA SAUCE

2 cups dried baby limas
1 tablespoon olive oil
4 large cloves garlic, minced
1 large sweet onion, coarsely chopped
1 16-ounce can tomatoes, chopped

1 *teaspoon dried rosemary* or ½ *teaspoon fresh rosemary, crushed*
¼ *cup fresh parsley, chopped*
black pepper to taste
1 *pound quinoa spaghetti*
grated Parmesan

Soak limas overnight or by the quick-soak method (see page 244). Rinse beans and cover with 2 inches water. Bring to a boil, reduce heat, and simmer uncovered for 1¼ hours, or until beans are soft. Puree cooked limas in a food processor. In a large saucepan, warm olive oil and sauté garlic and onions until golden. Add tomatoes, rosemary, and pureed limas to onions, stirring often over medium heat for 15 minutes. Add parsley and pepper. Prepare pasta according to directions on the package. Toss with sauce and top with Parmesan.

6 servings

Nutritional Information (PER SERVING)

Calories	383	Cholesterol mg	0.8
Carbohydrate g (%)	69 (71)	Sodium mg	162
Fat g (%)	4 (10)	Chromium mcg	29
Protein g (%)	18 (19)		

RED OR WHITE CLAM SAUCE*

3 *tablespoons olive oil*
3 *whole cloves garlic*
1 *cup fresh parsley, chopped*
8 *ounces chowder clams, chopped, with juice (many fish stores will prepare clams)* or 8 *ounces swordfish, cut into small pieces*
½ *cup dry white wine (for white clam sauce only)*
1 *16-ounce can whole tomatoes (for red clam sauce only)*
black pepper to taste

*Reprinted with permission of Ambrosino's Seafood Market, Mendham, NJ.

Sauté garlic in olive oil until golden. Add parsley, clams and juice, and tomatoes or wine. Reduce heat and simmer uncovered for a scant 5 minutes. Add pepper to taste. Serve over pasta.

6 servings

Nutritional Information (PER SERVING)

Calories	103	Cholesterol mg	12
Carbohydrate g (%)	5 (20)	Sodium mg	142
Fat g (%)	7 (59)	Chromium mcg	35
Protein g (%)	5 (21)		

RIBOLLITA

½ loaf excellent whole grain bread, broken into coarse crumbs
3 tablespoons mixed sage, oregano, basil, black pepper, and Vegit
6–7 cups Zuppa di verdure (see page 310) or minestrone alla Burrini (see page 276)
4–5 tablespoons grated Parmesan cheese
⅓ cup olive oil (or less)
balsamic vinegar to taste
PAM

Ribollita means "reboiled" in Italian. It makes use of leftover soups, turning them into a vegetable and bread casserole.

Preheat oven to 350°. Spray a 14-inch casserole dish with PAM. Mix seasonings with bread crumbs in a food processor. Spread a layer of the crumbs on the bottom of the casserole. Add a layer of soup, another layer of crumbs, and another layer of soup. Top with a handful of crumbs mixed with the Parmesan. Sprinkle oil over the top. Bake uncovered for 35 to 40 minutes until the top is well browned and crunchy. Serve with balsamic vinegar.

6 servings

Nutritional Information (PER SERVING)

Calories	316	Cholesterol mg	3
Carbohydrate g (%)	41 (50)	Sodium mg	223
Fat g (%)	14 (38)	Chromium mcg	29
Protein g (%)	9 (12)		

RICE SALAD

2 cups cooked long grain brown rice
4 ounces frozen corn, steamed
1 sweet potato, baked and diced
4 ounces firm tofu, diced
1 apple, cored, peeled, and diced
1 small red onion, cut into slivers
2 stalks celery, diced
1 ounce Paul's peanuts (unsalted), coarsely chopped
1 carrot, diced
¼ avocado, cut into thin slivers
6 ounces mushrooms, sliced
3 tablespoons olive oil
3 tablespoon balsamic vinegar

In a large bowl, combine all ingredients except oil and vinegar. Whisk olive oil and vinegar together and pour over salad just before serving.

6 servings as a main dish

Nutritional Information (PER SERVING)

Calories	238	Cholesterol mg	0
Carbohydrate g (%)	29 (47)	Sodium mg	56
Fat g (%)	11 (41)	Chromium mcg	24
Protein g (%)	7 (12)		

ROASTED SWEET RED PEPPERS

4 sweet red peppers, washed and pricked with a fork

Preheat broiler and grill peppers for 8 to 10 minutes 5 inches from the flame or until the skin is charred in a few places. Allow to cool and remove skin.

2 servings

Nutritional Information (PER SERVING)

Calories	36	Cholesterol mg	0
Carbohydrate g (%)	7.9 (74)	Sodium mg	4
Fat g (%)	0.7 (14)	Chromium mcg	28
Protein g (%)	1.3 (12)		

SEAFOOD SALAD

- *3 cups cooked shrimp, lobster, or crab*
- *½ cup lemon juice*
- *½ avocado, thinly sliced*
- *3 hard-boiled egg whites*
- *3 stalks celery, diced*
- *4 scallions, chopped*
- *1 small cucumber, diced*
- *½ cup low-fat mayonnaise (see page 275) or ⅓ cup vinaigrette dressing (see page 306)*
- *1 bunch watercress, large stems removed and coarsely chopped*

Combine all ingredients except the mayonnaise or vinaigrette and watercress. Stir in the mayonnaise or vinaigrette. Serve on a bed of watercress.

6 servings

Nutritional Information (PER SERVING)

Calories	148	Cholesterol mg	161
Carbohydrate g (%)	6 (17)	Sodium mg	242
Fat g (%)	5 (28)	Chromium mcg	18
Protein g (%)	21 (55)		

SEAFOOD SAUCE

- *1 tablespoon olive oil*
- *3 shallots, minced*
- *1 sweet onion, coarsely chopped*

1 teaspoon red pepper flakes
1 bay leaf
1 32-ounce can crushed tomatoes
2 teaspoons chopped fresh or frozen basil
black pepper to taste
8 ounces fresh shrimp (shelled and deveined), clams (removed from shell and chopped), lobster meat, cut into chunks (optional), or scallops (sliced if large)

In a large skillet, sauté shallots and onion in oil until golden. Add red pepper flakes, bay leaf, tomatoes, basil, and pepper. Bring to boil and then simmer uncovered for 30 minutes. Add seafood no more than 3 minutes before serving so as not to overcook. Use on pasta, baked potatoes, or grain such as bulgur.

6 servings

Nutritional Information with shrimp (PER SERVING)

Calories	120	Cholesterol mg	111
Carbohydrate g (%)	12 (39)	Sodium mg	300
Fat g (%)	3 (22)	Chromium mcg	22
Protein g (%)	12 (39)		

SHRIMP CREOLE

1 teaspoon olive oil
2 cups chopped onion
2 cups diced celery
2 large cloves garlic, minced
2 cups chopped green and red peppers
2 28-ounce cans whole tomatoes with juice
2 bay leaves
1 cup water
¼ teaspoon dried thyme
1 pound fresh or frozen shrimp, shelled and deveined
4 tablespoons chopped fresh parsley
5 drops Tabasco or less to taste
black pepper to taste
2 cups cooked long grain brown rice

In a large skillet, sauté onion, celery, garlic, and peppers in olive oil until softened. Add tomatoes, bay leaves, and thyme, and simmer uncovered for 30 minutes. In a saucepan, drop shrimp into large pot boiling water, return to a boil, and cook for a scant 3 minutes. Drain immediately, run cold water over them, and drain again. Add shrimp, parsley, Tabasco, and black pepper to tomatoes. Serve over rice.

5 servings

Nutritional Information (PER SERVING)

Calories	211	Cholesterol mg	115
Carbohydrate g (%)	28 (52)	Sodium mg	350
Fat g (%)	3 (13)	Chromium mcg	38
Protcin g (%)	19 (35)		

SHRIMP SALAD

- *6 ounces fresh or frozen shrimp, cooked and chopped*
- *1 stalk celery, finely diced*
- *4 small sweet bread and butter pickles, chopped*
- *1 tablespoon pickle juice*
- *1 small white onion, chopped fine*
- *⅓ teaspoon chopped fresh dill* or *1 teaspoon dried dill weed*
- *black pepper to taste*
- *⅓ cup low-fat mayonnaise (see page 275)*

Combine shrimp, celery, pickles, pickle juice, and onion. Season the salad with dill and black pepper. Fold in the mayonnaise. Serve the salad well chilled.

3 servings

Nutritional Information (PER SERVING)

Calories	128	Cholesterol mg	112
Carbohydrate g (%)	12 (39)	Sodium mg	332

Fat g (%)	2 (18)	Chromium mcg	15
Protein g (%)	14 (43)		

SPAGHETTI ALLA PUTTANESCA

- 2 *tablespoons olive oil*
- 2 *cloves garlic, minced*
- 1 *16-ounce can tomatoes, chopped*
- 1 *tablespoon capers*
- 12–16 *Calamata olives, pitted and coarsely chopped*
- 1 *hot chili pepper, with seeds removed and left whole (for milder sauce) or finely chopped (for hot sauce)*
- 2 *teaspoons fresh oregano, finely chopped,* or 1 *teaspoon dried oregano*
- *black pepper to taste*
- 4 *anchovies, chopped*
- 2 *tablespoons chopped fresh parsley*
- 1 *pound whole wheat, amaranth, or quinoa spaghetti*

In a large skillet, sauté garlic in olive oil. Add tomatoes, capers, olives, chili pepper, oregano, and pepper. Cook over a brisk heat for 20 minutes. Add anchovies and parsley, lower heat, and cook gently for 2 minutes. Remove the chili pepper. (If a very hot sauce is desired, use chopped pepper, which will remain in sauce.) Prepare pasta according to package instructions.

4 servings

Nutritional Information (PER SERVING)

Calories	505	Cholesterol mg	0
Carbohydrate g (%)	87 (68)	Sodium mg	375
Fat g (%)	11 (19)	Chromium mcg	31
Protein g (%)	17 (13)		

SPINACH SAUTÉ

1½ pounds chopped spinach
1 tablespoon olive oil
1 teaspoon garlic, minced
1 tablespoon crumbled feta cheese
6 walnuts, broken into pieces

Wash spinach well and drain. In a large skillet, sauté garlic in olive oil over medium high heat. Add spinach with the water that clings to the leaves and cook for 2½ to 3 minutes until wilted. Top with feta and walnuts.

3 servings

Nutritional Information (PER SERVING)

Calories	117	Cholesterol mg	2
Carbohydrate g (%)	9 (26)	Sodium mg	195
Fat g (%)	8 (52)	Chromium mcg	14
Protein g (%)	8 (23)		

SPLIT PEA AND ROSEMARY SOUP

2 teaspoons olive oil
2 bay leaves
1 teaspoon rosemary, coarsely chopped
1 large yellow onion, coarsely chopped
4 stalks celery, diced
2 carrots, chopped
½ cup white wine
2 cups green split peas
8 cups water or vegetable stock
1 tablespoon white miso
1 tablespoon brewer's yeast
grated Parmesan cheese (optional)

In a large pot, gradually warm olive oil with bay leaves and rosemary. Add vegetables and cook for 5 minutes over medium heat, stirring occasionally. Pour in the wine. Add peas and the water or stock. Bring to a boil, simmer covered until the peas are completely soft, about 1½ hours. For a creamier soup, puree in batches, but it's not necessary. Just before serving, stir in miso and brewer's yeast (be careful not to heat yeast for more than 1 minute as it destroys nutrients). Serve with Parmesan, if desired.

6 servings

Nutritional Information (PER SERVING)

Calories	198	Cholesterol mg	0
Carbohydrate g (%)	32 (63)	Sodium mg	87
Fat g (%)	4 (18)	Chromium mcg	25
Protein g (%)	10 (19)		

STIR-FRIED CHICKEN WITH CHROMIUM-RICH VEGETABLES

1 tablespoon canola oil
1 head broccoli, florets and peeled stalk cut into bite-sized pieces
3 ounces frozen peas
3 ounces snow peas
½ red pepper, sliced
½ green pepper, sliced
4 leaves Chinese lettuce
6 ounces chicken cutlet, cooked and cut into 1-inch chunks
6 ounces mushrooms, washed and sliced
1 can whole water chestnuts, drained
5 dashes hot oil
1 tablespoon reduced-sodium tamari

In a large wok, heat canola oil. Add chicken strips and cook quickly, just until no longer pink. Remove from wok with a slotted spoon. Add broccoli, green peas, snow peas, peppers, lettuce, mushrooms, and water chestnuts. Return chicken to wok. Add hot oil and tamari. Heat and serve.

4 servings

Nutritional Information (PER SERVING)

Calories	259	Cholesterol mg	36
Carbohydrate g (%)	30 (45)	Sodium mg	125

Fat g (%)	7 (24)	Chromium mcg	58
Protein g (%)	21 (31)		

SUCCOTASH

3 tablespoons Fromage Blanc
3 tablespoons olive oil
12 ounces frozen corn (unsalted)
12 ounces frozen limas
12 ounces frozen string beans (unsalted)
black pepper

Hang Fromage Blanc in cheesecloth overnight to allow liquid to drip off (see page 257). Add olive oil to fromage blanc and chill. Steam all the frozen vegetables, being careful not to overcook. Set aside and chill. Combine vegetables and chilled Fromage Blanc–olive oil mixture. Top with black pepper.

6 servings

Nutritional Information (PER SERVING)

Calories	227	Cholesterol mg	0.6
Carbohydrate g (%)	38 (61)	Sodium mg	33
Fat g (%)	7 (25)	Chromium mcg	23
Protein g (%)	8 (14)		

SWEET POTATO SAUCE

4 cloves garlic, minced
2 tablespoons olive oil
4 medium sweet potatoes, baked, peeled, and cut in chunks
6 fresh basil leaves, chopped
black pepper to taste
2 tablespoons grated Parmesan cheese

In a heavy skillet, sauté garlic in oil. Add sweet potato and basil and turn gently to distribute garlic and oil.

Serve as a pasta sauce topped with black pepper and Parmesan.

4 servings

Nutritional Information (PER SERVING)

Calories	195	Cholesterol mg	2.5
Carbohydrate g (%)	29 (58)	Sodium mg	71
Fat g (%)	7.5 (35)	Chromium mcg	14
Protein g (%)	3.5 (7)		

TOMATO ZUCCHINI SAUCE

- *2 cloves garlic, minced*
- *¼ cup water*
- *4 zucchini, cubed*
- *3 medium fresh tomatoes, peeled, seeded, and coarsely chopped*
- *1 28-ounce can crushed tomatoes*
- *5 leaves fresh basil, chopped*
- *1 tablespoon vinegar*
- *1 teaspoon fructose red pepper flakes to taste*
- *½ cup red wine*

In a large saucepan, steam the garlic in the water. Add zucchini and cook another 3 minutes. Add the fresh and canned tomatoes, basil, vinegar, fructose, and pepper flakes. Bring to a boil, reduce heat, and simmer about 15 minutes. Add wine and cook another 5 minutes. Serve over pasta. Also delicious with potatoes, grains, and steamed vegetables.

6 servings

Nutritional Information (PER SERVING)

Calories	88	Cholesterol mg	0
Carbohydrate g (%)	17 (85)	Sodium mg	381
Fat g (%)	0 (0)	Chromium mcg	20
Protein g (%)	3 (15)		

QUICKER TOMATO SAUCE

- *1 tablespoon olive oil*
- *2 cloves garlic*
- *½ cup plum tomatoes*
- *¼ cup fresh Italian parsley, diced*

In a medium-sized skillet, sauté garlic in olive oil. Add tomatoes, reduce heat to a simmer, and cook for 10 minutes. Add parsley and serve.

1 serving

Nutritional Information (PER SERVING)

Calories	156	Cholesterol mg	0
Carbohydrate g (%)	8.2 (20)	Sodium mg	203
Fat g (%)	13.9 (76)	Chromium mcg	4
Protein g (%)	1.8 (4)		

TUNA SALAD

- *1 can water-packed white tuna, rinsed in water to remove salt*
- *½ cup plain nonfat yogurt*
- *1 tablespoon Hellman's light mayonnaise*
- *4 small sweet pickles, chopped*
- *2 teaspoons pickle juice*
- *1 small onion, finely chopped*
- *1 stalk celery, coarsely chopped*
- *1 teaspoon chopped fresh dill or ½ teaspoon dried dill weed*
- *black pepper to taste*
- *3 whole wheat pita breads*
- *1 tomato, finely chopped*
- *wheat sprouts to taste*

Flake tuna with a fork. Mix yogurt and mayonnaise in a separate bowl. Add pickles, pickle juice, onion, and celery to tuna. Then add mayonnaise mixture and gently combine. Add dill and pepper and mix again. Stuff into pita pockets and top with tomato and sprouts.

3 servings

Nutritional Information (PER SERVING)

Calories	220	Cholesterol mg	14
Carbohydrate g (%)	34 (62)	Sodium mg	536
Fat g (%)	3 (12)	Chromium mcg	29
Protein g (%)	14 (26)		

TURKEY OR SWORDFISH KABOBS

½ cup olive oil
½ cup red wine for swordfish only
¼ cup cider vinegar
¼ cup lemon juice
¼ cup lime juice
red pepper flakes to taste
black pepper to taste
8 ounces skinned turkey breast, cut into 1½-inch chunks or 8 ounces swordfish
2 red peppers, cut into 1½-inch wedges
2 green peppers, cut into 1½-inch wedges
3 large sweet onions, cut into 1½-inch chunks
1½ pounds fresh mushrooms, washed and stems removed
16 bamboo skewers

In a large shallow bowl, mix oil (and wine for swordfish), vinegar, lemon juice, lime juice, red pepper flakes, and black pepper. Add turkey and vegetables and marinate at least 1 hour. Preheat broiler to 500° or ready your outside grill. Thread on bamboo skewers, in the following order: 1 mushroom, 1 piece red pepper, 1 piece onion, 1 piece turkey, 1 piece green pepper. Repeat until all skewers are filled. Grill under broiler 10 inches from flame for 10 minutes (8 minutes for swordfish) or on outdoor grill for 6 minutes.

4 servings

Nutritional Information for Turkey (PER SERVING)

Calories	302	Cholesterol mg	47
Carbohydrate g (%)	12 (16)	Sodium mg	36

Fat g (%)	20 (60)	Chromium mcg	38
Protein g (%)	21 (24)		

Nutritional Information for Swordfish (PER SERVING)

Calories	331	Cholesterol mg	28.6
Carbohydrate g (%)	17.5	Sodium mg	74
Fat g (%)	22	Chromium mcg	40
Protein g (%)	7.4		

TUSCAN WHITE BEAN SALAD

- ½ *pound dried white haricot or great northern beans*
- 1 *can water-packed white tuna, rinsed in water to remove salt*
- 3 *tablespoons olive oil*
- 3 *tablespoons balsamic vinegar*
- 2 *cloves garlic, thinly sliced*
- 5 *fresh basil leaves, chopped*
- *black pepper to taste*
- 2 *ounces skim-milk mozzarella, shredded (optional)*
- *chopped fresh parsley and lemon slices for garnish*

Soak beans overnight or by the quick-soak method (see page 244). Drain and cover with 2 inches of water. Bring to a boil, reduce heat, and simmer for 1½ hours, or until beans are tender but still firm. Drain and chill. Flake tuna with a fork. Add to the beans with olive oil, vinegar, garlic, and basil. Top with mozzarella (optional) and black pepper and serve surrounded by fresh parsley and lemon.

5 servings

Nutritional Information (PER SERVING)

Calories	235	Cholesterol mg	13
Carbohydrate g (%)	21 (35)	Sodium mg	127
Fat g (%)	11 (41)	Chromium mcg	28
Protein g (%)	15 (24)		

TWINFAST SHAKE

1 scoop (3 tablespoons) Twin Laboratories Twinfast shake, vanilla, chocolate, or strawberry
1¼ cups water
½ cup crushed ice or small cubes

In a food processor or blender, mix all ingredients for 1 minute.

Nutritional Information (PER SERVING)

Calories	80	Cholesterol mg	0
Carbohydrate g (%)	5 (25)	Sodium mg	180
Fat g (%)	0 (0)	Chromium mcg	50
Protein g (%)	15 (75)		

Variations

Strawberry banana: Use strawberry base and add 1 small banana.

Rich banana: Use vanilla base and add 1 large banana and ¼ teaspoon vanilla extract

Cantaloupe: Use vanilla base and add 8 ounces cantaloupe chunks.

Chocolate banana: Use chocolate base and add 1 small banana.

Butterscotch: Use vanilla base and add ⅔ scoop Jello sugar-free butterscotch pudding (can use as a drink or pudding).

Chocolate fudge: Use chocolate base and add ½ scoop Jello sugar-free chocolate pudding (drink or pudding).

Pistachio: Use vanilla base and add ⅔ scoop Jello sugar-free pistachio pudding.

1 serving

VEGETABLE PIZZA

2 cups mixed vegetables (broccoli, tomatoes, mushrooms, eggplant), cubed
1 tablespoon olive oil
1 teaspoon fresh rosemary, chopped
1 Grain Dance whole wheat pizza shell
¼ cup feta cheese, crumbled
PAM

Preheat oven to 450–500°. Arrange vegetables on baking sheet sprayed with PAM. Top vegetables with olive oil and rosemary and grill approximately 8 inches from heat for 15 minutes. Add vegetables to pizza shell, top with feta cheese, and cook in top third of oven for 5 minutes.

4 servings

Nutritional Information (PER SERVING)

Calories	207	Cholesterol mg	13
Carbohydrate g (%)	25 (48)	Sodium mg	319
Fat g (%)	9 (38)	Chromium mcg	25
Protein g (%)	8 (15)		

VINAIGRETTE DRESSING

⅓ cup olive oil
¼ cup balsamic vinegar
2 tablespoons red wine vinegar
2 cloves garlic, minced
black pepper

Allow garlic to steep in oil for 40 minutes or more. Whisk all ingredients together and serve.

4 servings

Nutritional Information (PER SERVING)

Calories	168	Cholesterol mg	0
Carbohydrate g (%)	9 (4)	Sodium mg	1

Fat g (%)	18 (95)	Chromium mcg	2
Protein g (%)	0 (0)		

WHIPPED BUTTERMILK POTATOES

6 baking potatoes, cooked and peeled
1 cup nonfat buttermilk (low-sodium)
1 teaspoon brewer's yeast
1 teaspoon fresh dill
grated Parmesan cheese (optional)

In a large bowl, break up the potatoes into medium-sized chunks. With a hand-held mixer, gradually beat in buttermilk. As the potatoes reach a creamy consistency, add yeast and dill. Top with black pepper and Parmesan (optional).

4 servings

Nutritional Information (PER SERVING)

Calories	250	Cholesterol mg	3
Carbohydrate g (%)	54 (88)	Sodium mg	97
Fat g (%)	1 (1)	Chromium mcg	41
Protein g (%)	7 (11)		

WHOLE WHEAT FETTUCINE WITH ZUCCHINI AND SMOKED SALMON

2 tablespoons olive oil
2 medium cloves garlic, minced
3 medium zucchini, diced
⅓ cup skim-milk ricotta cheese
2 teaspoons fresh tarragon, minced, or ½ teaspoon dried tarragon
1 tablespoon lemon juice
1 teaspoon grated lemon rind
12 ounces whole wheat fettucine or wide noodles
1 tablespoon small capers
4 ounces smoked salmon, thinly sliced and cut into ¼-inch strips
black pepper

Heat oil in a large skillet. Sauté garlic and zucchini over medium high heat for about 2 minutes. Add ricotta and tarragon and simmer until slightly thickened, about 2 more minutes. Stir in lemon juice and rind. Remove sauce from heat and keep covered. Prepare pasta according to directions on box, drain well, and toss with sauce. Turn pasta onto serving plate, arrange salmon and capers on top, and sprinkle with black pepper.

4 servings

Nutritional Information (PER SERVING)

Calories	431	Cholesterol mg	13
Carbohydrate g (%)	64 (59)	Sodium mg	249
Fat g (%)	11 (23)	Chromium mcg	23
Protein g (%)	18 (17)		

WHOLE WHEAT NOODLES WITH PEANUT SAUCE

1 pound whole wheat, amaranth, or quinoa pasta
1 small sweet onion, diced
½ cup water
1 tablespoon sesame butter (oil removed)
3 tablespoons crunchy, unsalted, unhydrogenated peanut butter (oil removed)
2 tablespoons tahini (oil removed)
2 teaspoons low-sodium tamari
5 drops hot sesame oil
1 teaspoon cider vinegar
1 tablespoon dark brown sugar

Prepare pasta as directed on the package. Drain and chill. In a 2-quart saucepan over medium low heat, steam the onion in water until softened. Add the remaining ingredients, mashing with the back of a spoon until slightly creamy. Add a little bit of water at a time until consistency resembles creamy peanut butter. Remove from heat. Add 1 tablespoon of sauce per serving of pasta.

6 servings

Nutritional Information (PER SERVING)

Calories	325	Cholesterol mg	0
Carbohydrate g (%)	57 (71)	Sodium mg	184
Fat g (%)	4 (11)	Chromium mcg	20
Protein g (%)	14 (18)		

WINTER WHEAT, CORN, AND CHEESE CASSEROLE

1¼ cups winter wheat berries
1 10-ounce package frozen corn
1 onion, coarsely chopped
4 ounces low-fat cheese, grated
1½ cups skim milk
2 canned jalapeno or other hot chili peppers, seeded and chopped
1 teaspoon chili powder
black pepper
paprika
PAM

In a 4-quart pot, bring wheat berries and 2 quarts water to a boil. Cook partially covered at rapid simmer for 1½ hour or longer, until berries are tender. Preheat oven to 350°. Drain wheat berries and combine with the remaining ingredients, except paprika and PAM. Pour into a 2-quart casserole sprayed with PAM, sprinkle with paprika, and bake for 40 to 45 minutes.

6 servings

Nutritional Information (PER SERVING)

Calories	244	Cholesterol mg	7
Carbohydrate g (%)	38 (60)	Sodium mg	168

Fat g (%)	6 (20)	Chromium mcg	23
Protein g (%)	13 (20)		

WINTER WHEAT SHRIMP SALAD

1¼ cups winter wheat berries
1 red onion, cut in 1-inch slices
2 heads broccoli, florets and peeled stems cut into bite-sized pieces
2 carrots, scraped and diced
1 pound cooked fresh or frozen shrimp
½ cup vinaigrette dressing (see page 306)

In a 4-quart pot, bring wheat berries and 2 quarts water to a boil. Cook partially covered at rapid simmer for 1½ hours. Steam broccoli until just tender but still crisp. Combine all the ingredients except vinaigrette and chill. Toss with vinaigrette before serving.

4 servings

Nutritional Information (PER SERVING)

Calories	234	Cholesterol mg	220
Carbohydrate g (%)	29 (45)	Sodium mg	284
Fat g (%)	2 (7)	Chromium mcg	30
Protein g (%)	31 (48)		

ZUPPA DI VERDURE

2 cups white beans (great northern, white haricot, fagioli)
10 cups water
3½ tablespoons Gaylord Hauser's vegetable broth
1 pound carrots, scraped and cut into big chunks
6 stalks celery, diced
3 small cloves garlic, minced
1 white turnip, diced
3 ripe tomatoes, chopped
3 small onions, cut into rings
black pepper (lots)
Vegit to taste

1 10-ounce package frozen peas
5 white boiling potatoes, peeled and cut into chunks
1 pound fresh or frozen green beans, rinsed and cut in thirds
grated Parmesan cheese

Soak the beans by the overnight or quick-soak method (see page 244). Drain and put in a large soup pot with 10 cups of water. Add the broth, carrots, celery, garlic, turnip, tomatoes, onions, pepper, and Vegit, and bring to a boil. Reduce heat and simmer covered for 1½ hours. Add potatoes, peas, and green beans. Raise heat slightly and cook uncovered for an additional 20 to 30 minutes. If necessary, thin with additional water, but soup should be thick. Serve with grated Parmesan.

14 1¾-cup servings

Nutritional Information (PER SERVING)

Calories	175	Cholesterol mg	0
Carbohydrate g (%)	37 (81)	Sodium mg	82
Fat g (%)	0.7 (3)	Chromium mcg	15
Protein g (%)	7 (16)		

NINE

THE CHROMIUM PROGRAM EXERCISE PLAN: PUTTING CHROMIUM TO WORK

The Chromium Program exercise plan is a six-week upper body, lower body, and abdominal strengthening program. Specific instructions are given for males and females in groups I and II. The muscles worked, equipment, starting position, and action are described for each exercise. Specific weights, repetitions, sets, and holds are given in a progression table. Several advanced exercises are provided for those who wish to continue beyond the level they will attain in six weeks. Group III members should continue the strengthening program they already practice and should refer to Appendix D, the weight training regimen followed by the athletes in Dr. Gary Evans's research. The purpose of the Chromium Program for groups I and II is to firm, tone, and define muscles and to increase strength and stamina, not to bulk up. There is no heavy weight lifting in the exercise plan. The exercises require no weights at all or no more than 20 pounds.

EQUIPMENT

For lower body exercises, women in group I need a 5-pound set of adjustable ankle weights with velcro attachments. These sets have pockets that allow you to change the sandbag weights to create any total weight from 1 to 5 pounds. Group II women need a 10-pound set and an extra 1-pound weight. Men in both group I and Group II need a 20-pound set of adjustable ankle weights. These can be purchased in many sporting goods stores and are also available through surgical supply houses.

For the upper body exercises, group I women need a 3-pound set of dumbbells and an adjustable 20-pound set. Group II women and both group I and group II men need an adjustable 45-pound set of dumbbells. These weights are sold in sporting goods stores and in some department stores and health clubs. Shiny, chrome-plated dumbbells are attractive, but more expensive and no better than durable cast iron ones. Some of the exercises also use items that are found in the home, such as broomsticks, chairs, and books.

If you have any difficulty in locating the dumbbells, ankle weights, or any other equipment you might want to use in addition to that required by this program, Country Technology, P.O. Box 87, Gays Mills, WI, (608) 735-4718, FAX (608) 735-4859, has a wide variety of fitness material at reasonable prices.

Although it is strongly recommended that you use the equipment described in the exercises, there may be times when you need alternatives, such as when you travel. You can use jugs of water, large tomato paste cans, or even heavy telephone books as substitutes for dumbbells.

HOW OFTEN AND HOW RAPIDLY TO WORK OUT

Abdominal muscles should be worked every day, but upper and lower body exercises should be performed on alternate days. Each time you work these muscles properly, you actually create microscopic tears in the fibers. With a day's rest, the fibers heal stronger and larger than before, but they need that rest.

It is recommended that group I men and women do

the entire lower and upper body workout 3 times a week, with at least 1 day rest in between workouts. Each workout will take 30 to 40 minutes. Group II members will be performing a more extensive upper and lower body program. Although you also may do the entire workout 3 times a week, it will take almost an hour, and it is recommended that instead you work out for 20 to 30 minutes 6 days a week, alternating lower and upper body exercises.

In general, rest 15 to 20 seconds between sets of an exercise and about 1 minute between exercises. However, if as you advance in your program, you find this rest period isn't long enough, you can extend it slightly.

LOWER BODY STRENGTHENING PROGRAM

1. STRAIGHT LEG RAISES

MUSCLES WORKED Strengthen and tone front of thighs (quadriceps).

EQUIPMENT

Group I
Females: adjustable ankle weights, 2 to 5 pounds
Males: adjustable ankle weights, 3 to 8 pounds

Group II
Females: adjustable ankle weights, 2 to 6 pounds
Males: adjustable ankle weights, 5 to 10 pounds

STARTING POSITION Attach ankle weight (see progression table) to your right ankle. Lie flat on your back on the floor. Straighten your right leg and bend your left knee. Rest your arms either behind your head or at your sides. Press the small of your back into the floor.

ACTION Slowly raise your right leg to the height of your bent left knee. Hold the required number of seconds (see progression table). Slowly lower to starting position. Exhale as you lift your leg; inhale as you lower it. Perform the required number of repetitions and sets (see progression table). Switch ankle weight to left leg and repeat the entire exercise.

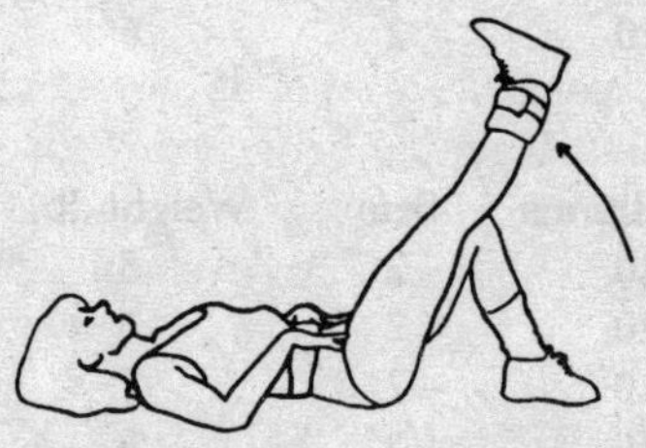

Straight leg raises

PROGRESSION

Group I

FEMALES

Week	Repetitions	Sets	Weight (lb)	Hold (sec)
1	10	2	0	2
2	10	2	2	2
3	10	2	3	2
4	10	2	3	2
5	10	2	4	2
6	10	2	5	2

MALES

Week	Repetitions	Sets	Weight (lb)	Hold (sec)
1	10	2	3	2
2	10	2	4	2
3	10	2	5	2
4	10	2	6	2
5	10	2	7	2
6	10	2	8	2

Group II

FEMALES

Week	Repetitions	Sets	Weight (lb)	Hold (sec)
1	10	2	2	0
2	10	2	2	2
3	10	2	3	2
4	10	2	4	2
5	10	2	5	2
6	10	2	6	2

MALES

Week	Repetitions	Sets	Weight (lb)	Hold (sec)
1	10	2	5	2
2	10	2	6	2
3	10	2	7	2
4	10	2	8	2
5	10	2	9	2
6	10	2	10	2

2. SIDE LEG RAISES (TOP LEG)

MUSCLES WORKED Strengthen and tone outside of thigh (quadriceps). Especially good for women.

EQUIPMENT

Group I
Females: adjustable ankle weights, 2 to 5 pounds
Males: omit exercise

Group II
Females: adjustable ankle weights, 2 to 6 pounds
Males: omit exercise

STARTING POSITION Attach ankle weight to right ankle. Lie on the floor on your left side. Bend your left elbow and rest your head in your left hand. Place your right hand on the floor in front of your chest for support.

Bend your left (bottom) knee to a 90° angle. Straighten your right (top) leg.

ACTION Slowly lift right leg off the floor to the height of your head. Hold required number of seconds. Slowly lower to starting position. Exhale as you lift your leg; inhale as you lower it. Perform the required number of repetitions and sets. Switch ankle weight to left leg and repeat the entire exercise.

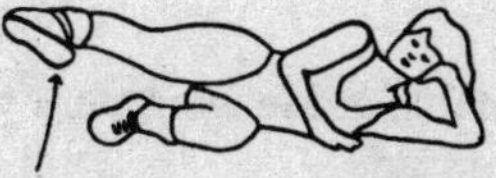

Side leg raises (top leg)

PROGRESSION

Group I

FEMALES

Week	Repetitions	Sets	Weight (lb)	Hold (sec)
1	10	2	0	2
2	10	2	2	2
3	10	2	3	2
4	10	2	3	2
5	10	2	4	2
6	10	2	5	2

MALES: OMIT

Group II

FEMALES

Week	Repetitions	Sets	Weight (lb)	Hold (sec)
1	10	2	2	0
2	10	2	2	2
3	10	2	3	2
4	10	2	4	2
5	10	2	5	2
6	10	2	6	2

MALES: OMIT

3. SIDE LEG RAISES (BOTTOM LEG)

MUSCLES WORKED Strengthen and tone inside of thigh (quadriceps). Especially good for women.

EQUIPMENT

Group I
Females: adjustable ankle weights, 1 to 5 pounds
Males: omit exercise

Group II
Females: adjustable ankle weights, 1 to 5 pounds
Males: omit exercise

STARTING POSITION Attach ankle weight to right ankle. Lie on the floor on your right side. Bend your right elbow and support your head with your right hand. Place your left hand on the floor in front of your chest for support. Straighten your right (bottom) leg. Bend your left (top) knee to about a 45° angle and rest your left foot on the floor.

ACTION Slowly lift your right (bottom) leg up 6 inches. Hold required number of seconds. Slowly lower to starting position. Exhale as you lift your leg; inhale as you lower it. Perform the required number of repetitions and sets. Switch ankle weight to left ankle and repeat the entire exercise.

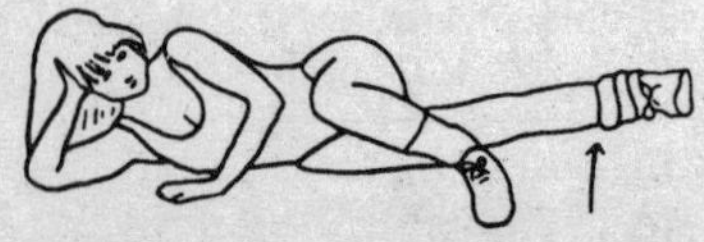

Side leg raises (bottom leg)

PROGRESSION

Group I

FEMALES

Week	Repetitions	Sets	Weight (lb)	Hold (sec)
1	10	2	0	2
2	10	2	1	2
3	10	2	2	2
4	10	2	3	2
5	10	2	4	2
6	10	2	5	2

MALES: OMIT

Group II

FEMALES

Week	Repetitions	Sets	Weight (lb)	Hold (sec)
1	10	2	0	2
2	10	2	1	2
3	10	2	2	2
4	10	2	3	2
5	10	2	4	2
6	10	2	5	2

MALES: OMIT

4. HIP EXTENSIONS

MUSCLES WORKED Strengthen and tone back of thigh (hamstrings).

EQUIPMENT

Group I

Females: adjustable ankle weights, 2 to 5 pounds
Males: adjustable ankle weights, 3 to 8 pounds

Group II

Females: adjustable ankle weights, 2 to 7 pounds
Males: adjustable ankle weights, 5 to 10 pounds

STARTING POSITION Attach weight to right ankle. Lie on the floor on your abdomen with a pillow under your waist. Rest your arms at your sides. Straighten both legs.

ACTION Keeping leg and foot straight, lift right leg off the floor 6 inches. Hold required number of seconds. Slowly lower to starting position. Exhale as you lift your leg; inhale as you lower it. Perform required number of repetitions and sets. Switch ankle weight to left ankle and repeat the entire exercise.

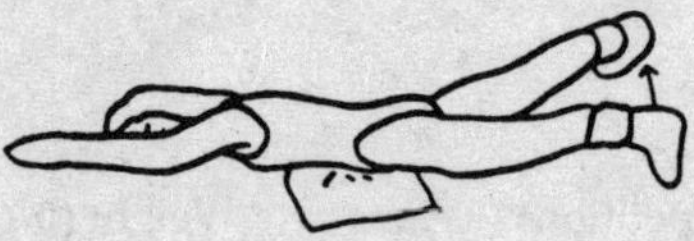

Hip extensions

PROGRESSION

Group I

FEMALES

Week	Repetitions	Sets	Weight (lb)	Hold (sec)
1	10	2	0	2
2	10	2	2	2
3	10	2	3	2
4	10	2	3	2
5	10	2	4	2
6	10	2	5	2

MALES

Week	Repetitions	Sets	Weight (lb)	Hold (sec)
1	10	2	3	2
2	10	2	4	2
3	10	2	5	2
4	10	2	6	2
5	10	2	7	2
6	10	2	8	2

Group II

FEMALES

Week	Repetitions	Sets	Weight (lb)	Hold (sec)
1	10	2	2	2
2	10	2	3	2
3	10	2	4	2
4	10	2	5	2
5	10	2	6	2
6	10	2	7	2

MALES

Week	Repetitions	Sets	Weight (lb)	Hold (sec)
1	10	2	5	2
2	10	2	6	2
3	10	2	7	2
4	10	2	8	2
5	10	2	9	2
6	10	2	10	2

5. SQUATS

MUSCLES WORKED Strengthen and tone buttocks, hips, and thighs (gluteus maximus, quadriceps, hamstrings) and the upper back. Especially good for women.

EQUIPMENT

Group I

Females: 5-pound ankle weight

Males: adjustable ankle weights, 5 to 15 pounds

Group II

Females: adjustable ankle weights, 5 to 10 pounds

Males: adjustable ankle weights, 5 to 20 pounds

STARTING POSITION Place a straight-backed chair behind you for a height mark. Wrap ankle weight firmly around the center of a broomstick handle (if possible, use a broom that has a detachable head). Place the broomstick behind your head, resting the weight against the base of your neck. Grasp the broomstick with both hands about 1 foot on either side of your head. Stand erect with knees straight and feet pointing forward and spread apart slightly more than shoulder width.

ACTION Keeping your back straight, slowly lower yourself to the edge of the chair seat, as if you were going to sit down. Make certain that your knees do not go farther forward than your toes as you lower yourself. Hold required number of seconds. Slowly return to starting position, pushing off from your heels as you rise. Inhale as you lower yourself; exhale as you rise. Perform required number of repetitions and sets.

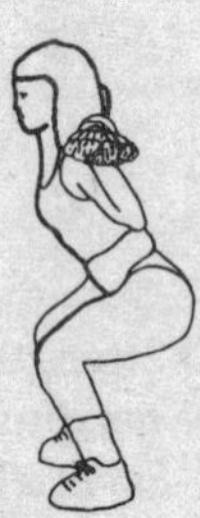

Squats

PROGRESSION

Group I

FEMALES

Week	Repetitions	Sets	Weight (lb)	Hold (sec)
1				
2				
3				
4	5	3	0	0
5	8	3	0	2
6	8	3	5	2

MALES

Week	Repetitions	Sets	Weight (lb)	Hold (sec)
1	10	3	0	2
2	10	3	5	2
3	10	3	7	2
4	10	3	10	2
5	10	3	12	2
6	10	3	15	2

Group II

FEMALES

Week	Repetitions	Sets	Weight (lb)	Hold (sec)
1				
2				
3	8	3	0	2
4	8	3	5	2
5	8	3	7	2
6	8	4	10	2

MALES

Week	Repetitions	Sets	Weight (lb)	Hold (sec)
1	10	3	5	2
2	10	3	7	2
3	10	3	10	2
4	10	3	12	2
5	10	3	15	2
6	10	3	20	2

6. TOE RAISES

MUSCLES WORKED Strengthen and tone shin muscles (tibialis anterior). Especially good for runners.

EQUIPMENT

Group I

Females: omit exercise

Males: omit exercise

Group II
Females: no equipment needed
Males: no equipment needed

STARTING POSITION Stand facing a wall, feet shoulder width apart and 3 feet from the wall. Place your hands against the wall for support.

ACTION Raise toes on both feet 3 inches off the floor. Hold required number of seconds. Return to starting position. Perform required number of repetitions and sets.

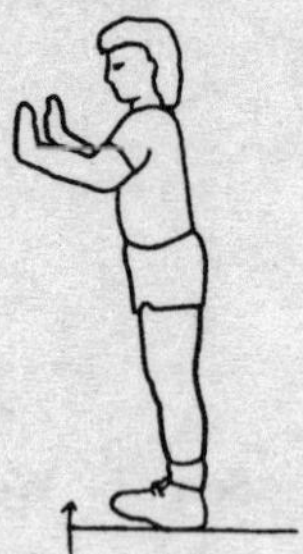

Toe raises

PROGRESSION

Group I
FEMALES: OMIT
MALES: OMIT

Group II
FEMALES

Week	Repetitions	Sets	Weight (lb)	Hold (sec)
1	10	2	0	0
2	10	2	0	1
3	10	3	0	2
4	10	3	0	3
5	10	3	0	4
6	10	3	0	5

MALES

Week	Repetitions	Sets	Weight (lb)	Hold (sec)
1	10	3	0	0
2	10	3	0	2
3	15	3	0	3
4	15	3	0	4
5	20	3	0	4
6	20	3	0	5

7. CALF RAISES

MUSCLES WORKED Strengthen and tone the calf (gastrocnemius). Especially good for runners.

EQUIPMENT

Group I
Females: omit exercise
Males: omit exercise

Group II
Females: no equipment needed
Males: no equipment needed

STARTING POSITION Stand erect on the edge of a step with the back half of your feet off the step. Place your hands against a wall or hold on to a sturdy bannister or door frame for support.

ACTION Rise up on the balls of your feet. Hold required number of seconds. Slowly lower to starting position. Perform required number of repetitions and sets.

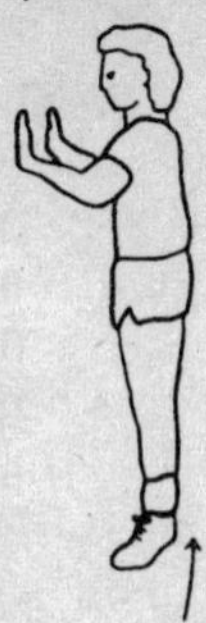

Calf raises

PROGRESSION

Group I

FEMALES: OMIT

MALES: OMIT

Group II

FEMALES

Week	Repetitions	Sets	Weight (lb)	Hold (sec)
1	10	2	0	0
2	10	2	0	1
3	10	3	0	2
4	10	3	0	3
5	10	3	0	4
6	10	3	0	5

MALES

Week	Repetitions	Sets	Weight (lb)	Hold (sec)
1	10	3	0	0
2	10	3	0	2
3	15	3	0	3
4	15	3	0	4
5	20	3	0	4
6	20	3	0	5

8. SIDE LUNGES

MUSCLES WORKED Strengthen and tone front and back of thigh (quadriceps and hamstrings).

EQUIPMENT

Group I

Females: omit exercise

Males: adjustable ankle weights, 5 to 15 pounds

Group II

Females: omit exercise

Males: adjustable ankle weights, 5 to 20 pounds

STARTING POSITION Wrap ankle weight firmly around the center of a broomstick handle (if possible, use a broom that has a detachable head). Place the broomstick behind your head, resting the weight against the base of your neck. Grasp the broomstick with both hands about 1 foot on either side of your head. Stand erect with legs about 4 feet apart.

ACTION Slowly step to the right as far as possible, keeping the toe pointing forward and bending the leg at a 45° angle as far as possible (lunge). Hold required number of seconds. Return to starting position. Exhale as you lunge; inhale as you return to starting position. Repeat to the left. A lunge to the right and one to the left constitute one repetition. Perform required number of repetitions and sets.

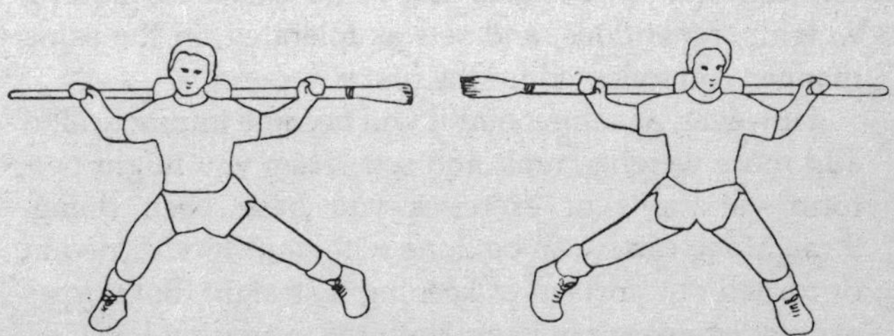

Side lunges

PROGRESSION

Group I

FEMALES: OMIT

MALES

Week	Repetitions	Sets	Weight (lb)	Hold (sec)
1				
2				
3	10	3	5	0
4	10	3	10	1
5	10	3	12	2
6	10	3	15	2

Group II

FEMALES: OMIT

MALES

Week	Repetitions	Sets	Weight (lb)	Hold (sec)
1	10	3	5	1
2	10	3	7	2
3	10	3	10	2
4	10	3	12	2
5	10	3	15	2
6	10	3	20	2

ADVANCED LOWER BODY EXERCISES

Once you have finished the six-week lower body exercise plan for your group, you have several options. You can continue to perform the same exercises, adding weights, repetitions, and sets as tolerated, in the same manner you followed for the first six weeks.

However, at some point it will become impractical to add more weights, reps, and sets. Then you might perform variations of exercises you have been doing. Straight leg raises can be done with your foot turned in or turned out, instead of keeping it straight. Both types of side leg raises can begin with the exercising leg at either a 45° or 90° angle instead of straight. This uses different, but related muscles.

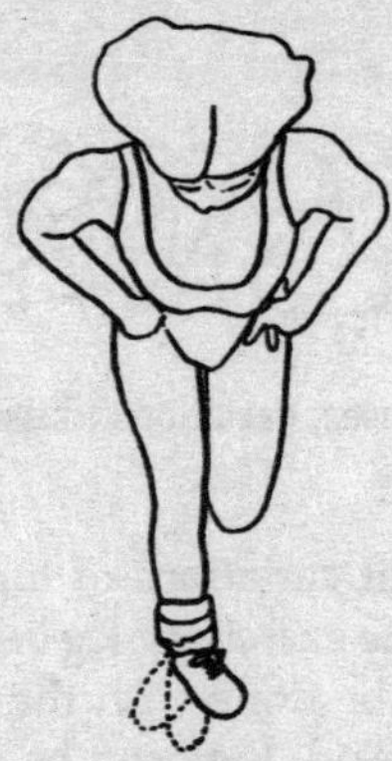

Straight leg raises, variation: foot can be turned in, which exercises the outside of the thigh, or foot can be turned out, which exercises the inside of the thigh.

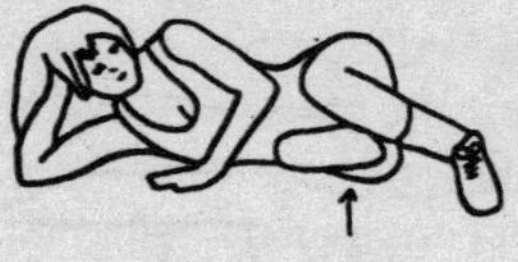

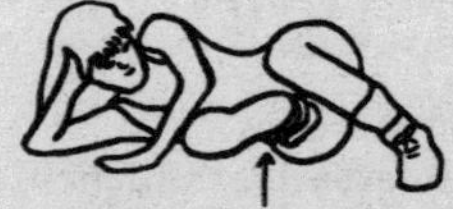

Side leg raises, variation (inside of thigh)

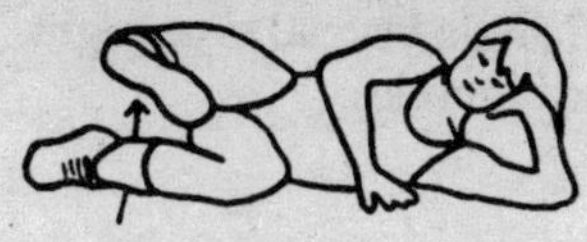

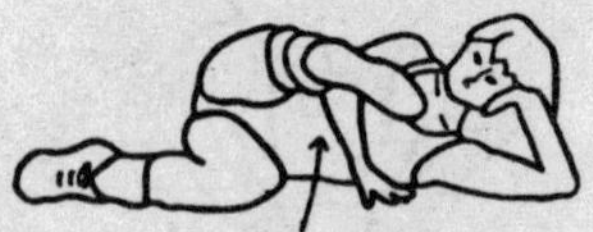

Straight leg raises, variations (outside of thighs)

There are several variations of hip extensions. They can be done with the exercising leg bent to 90° instead of straight. They can be done with the legs separated instead of together. And, they can be done both legs to-

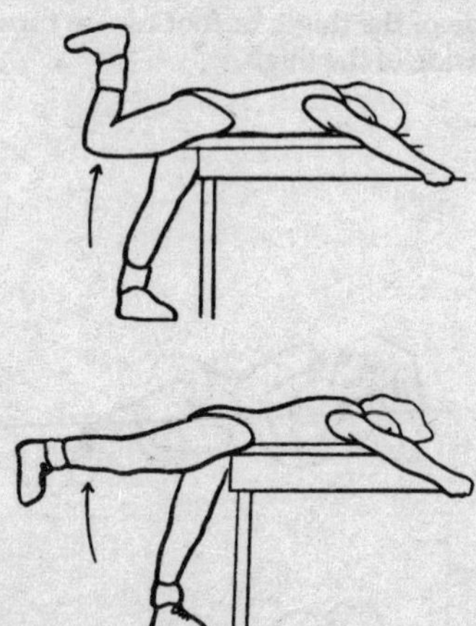

Sample Hip Extension Exercises

Upper exercise: hip extension variation, lying on table, extending one hip (right), knee bent

Lower exercise: hip extension variation, lying on table, extending one hip (right), knee straight

gether. The starting position can be changed from lying on the floor to placing the body on an elevated surface, such as a table, with the legs at floor level. These variations can be combined in different ways to give several more variations.

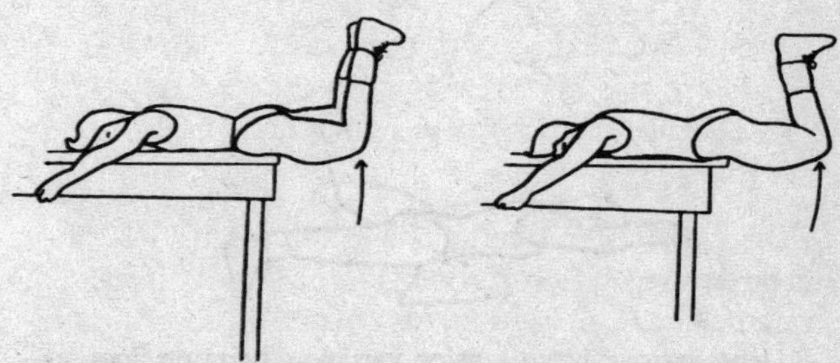

Left exercise: hip extension variation, lying on table, extending both hips, knees bent, legs apart

Right exercise: hip extension variation, lying on table, extending both hips, knees bent, legs together

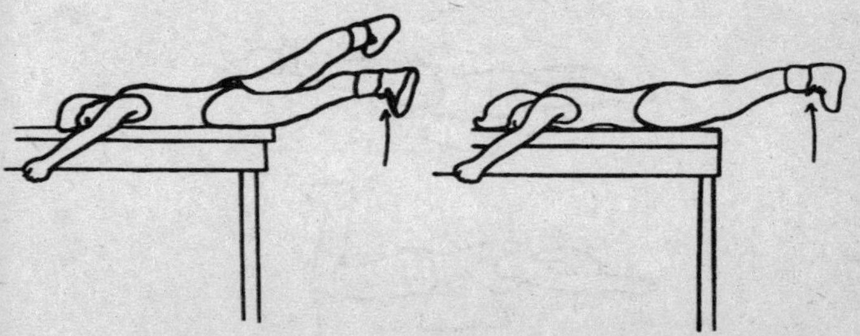

Left exercise: hip extension variation, lying on table, extending both hips, knees straight, legs apart

Right exercise: hip extension variation, lying on table, extending both hips, knees straight, legs together

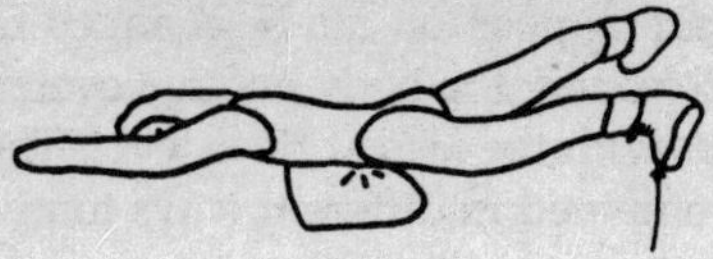

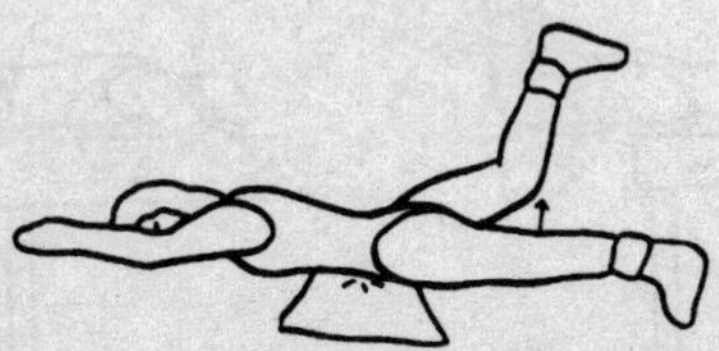

Upper exercise: hip extension variation, lying on floor, extending both hips, knees straight, legs apart

Lower exercise: hip extension variation, lying on floor, extending one hip, knee bent, legs apart

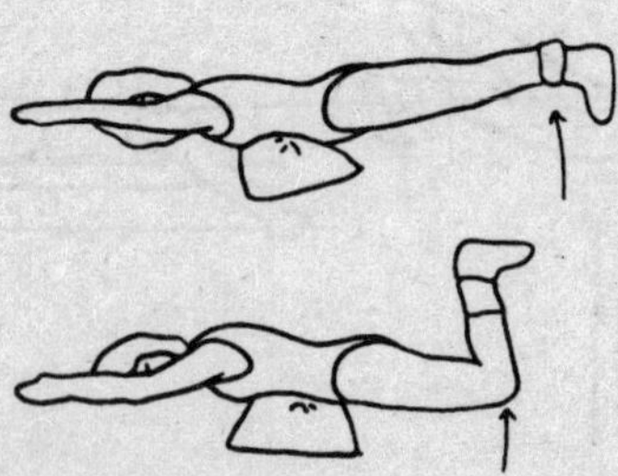

Upper exercise: hip extension variation, lying on floor, extending both hips, knees straight, legs together

Lower exercise: hip extension variation, lying on floor, extending both hips, knees bent, legs together

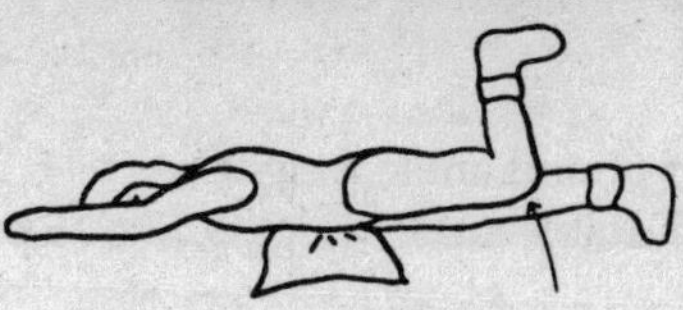

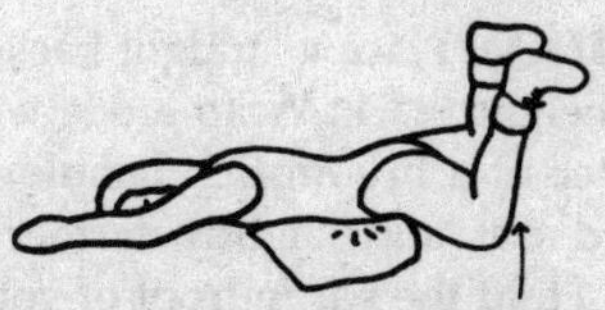

Upper exercise: hip extension variation, lying on floor, extending one hip, knee bent, legs together

Lower exercise: hip extension variation, lying on floor, extending both hips, knees bent, legs apart

You can also begin exercises that were not in first six-week plan for your group, but were being done by another group. For example, group I women could add side lunges, toe raises, and calf raises, and groups I and II men could add side leg raises.

Finally, you can add new exercises. As with any of the other options, you can add the new exercises to your present plan or replace others with them. Substitution may be more practical, so you don't end up with too many exercises, but remember always replace an an exercise with one that works the same muscles. For the lower body, there are two new exercises in the advanced category.

9. DEAD LIFTS

MUSCLES WORKED Strengthen and tone buttocks, hips, thighs (gluteus maximus, quadriceps, hamstrings), and the upper back. Especially good for women.

EQUIPMENT

Group I

Females: 5-pound ankle weight
Males: adjustable ankle weights, 5 to 15 pounds

Group II

Females: adjustable ankle weights, 5 to 10 pounds
Males: adjustable ankle weights, 5 to 20 pounds

STARTING POSITION Place a straight backed chair behind you for a height mark. Wrap ankle weight firmly around the center of a broomstick handle. Stand erect with feet turned out and slightly farther apart than shoulder width. Hold the bar in front of your hips with one hand on either side of the weight.

ACTION Slowly lower yourself to the edge of the chair seat, as if you were going to sit down. Keep your knees over your turned out feet. Hold required number of seconds. Slowly return to starting position, pushing off from your heels as you rise. Inhale as you lower yourself; exhale as you rise. Perform required number of repetitions and sets.

PROGRESSION Same as pp. 322–323.

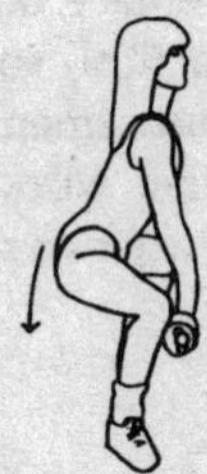

Dead lifts

10. FRONT LUNGES

MUSCLES WORKED Strengthen and tone front and back of thigh (quadriceps, hamstrings).

EQUIPMENT

Group I

Females: omit exercise

Males: adjustable ankle weights, 5 to 15 pounds

Group II

Females: omit exercise

Males: adjustable ankle weights, 5 to 20 pounds

STARTING POSITION Wrap ankle weights firmly around the center of a broomstick handle. Place the broomstick behind your head, resting the weight against the base of your neck. Grasp the broomstick with both hands 1 foot on either side of your head. Stand erect with legs about 4 feet apart.

ACTION Step forward and kneel on right knee. Hold required number of seconds. Return to starting position. Exhale as you lunge; inhale as you return to starting position. Repeat, kneeling on left knee. A lunge onto the right knee and one onto the left knee constitute one repetition. Perform required number of repetitions and sets.

PROGRESSION See pp. 328.

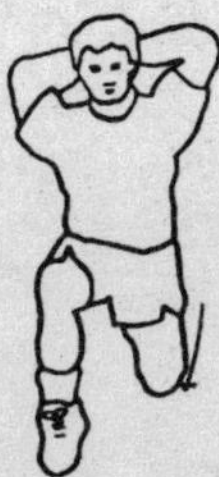

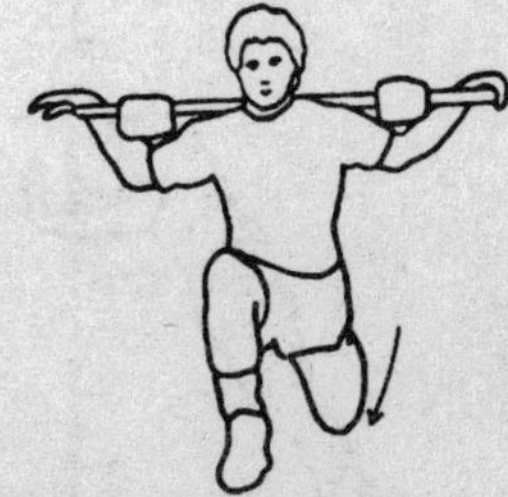

Front lunges

UPPER BODY STRENGTHENING PROGRAM

1. WALL PUSHUPS

MUSCLES WORKED Strengthen and tone chest and back of upper arm (pectoralis major and minor, triceps).

EQUIPMENT

Group I
Females: no equipment needed
Males: no equipment needed

Group II
Females: no equipment needed
Males: omit exercise

STARTING POSITION Stand erect about 3 feet from a wall. Lean forward and place your hands on the wall at shoulder height.

ACTION Bend your elbows, drawing your head and chest to the wall. Allow your heels to rise off the ground until your forehead gently touches the wall. Hold required number of seconds. Return to starting position. Exhale as you lean toward the wall; inhale as you return to starting position. Perform required number of repetitions and sets.

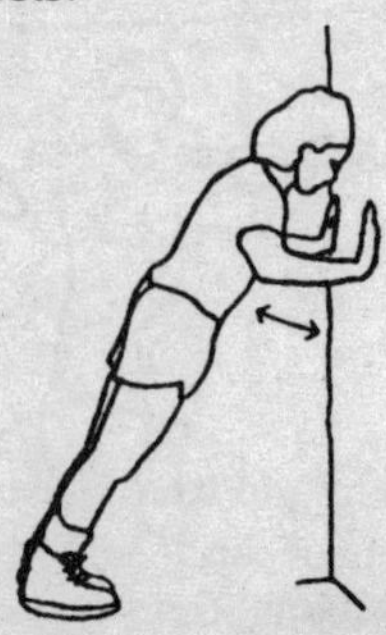

Wall pushups

PROGRESSION

Group I

FEMALES

Week	Repetitions	Sets	Weight (lb)	Hold (sec)
1	10	3	0	2
2	10	3	0	4
3	progress to bent knee pushups			
4				
5				
6				

MALES

Week	Repetitions	Sets	Weight (lb)	Hold (sec)
1	10	3	0	0
2	progress to bent knee pushups			
3				
4				
5				
6				

Group II

FEMALES

Week	Repetitions	Sets	Weight (lb)	Hold (sec)
1	10	3	0	2
2	progress to bent knee pushups			
3				
4				
5				
6				

MALES: OMIT

2. BENT KNEE PUSHUPS

MUSCLES WORKED Strengthen and tone chest and back of upper arm (pectoralis major and minor, triceps). Works muscles more than wall pushups.

EQUIPMENT

Group I
Females: no equipment needed
Males: no equipment needed

Group II
Females: no equipment needed
Males: omit exercise

STARTING POSITION Lie on the floor on your abdomen with your arms bent and your hands at shoulder height slightly farther apart than shoulder width. Bend your knees. Straighten your arms, keeping your back straight, to lift your body off the floor.

ACTION Slowly lower your body by bending only your arms, keeping your back straight, until your chin just touches the floor. Hold required number of seconds. Return to starting position. Exhale as you lower your body; inhale as you return to starting position. Perform required number of repetitions and sets.

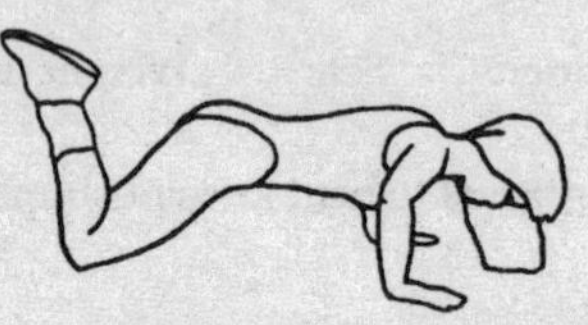

Bent knee pushups

PROGRESSION

Group I

FEMALES

Week	Repetitions	Sets	Weight (lb)	Hold (sec)
1	wall pushups			
2	wall pushups			
3	10	2	0	0
4	10	3	0	0

5	10	3	0	2
6	10	3	0	3

MALES

Week	Repetitions	Sets	Weight (lb)	Hold (sec)
1	wall pushups			
2	10	3	0	4
3	progress to straight pushups			
4				
5				
6				

Group II

FEMALES

Week	Repetitions	Sets	Weight (lb)	Hold (sec)
1	wall pushups			
2	10	3	0	0
3	10	3	0	2
4	10	3	0	3
5	10	3	0	5
6	progress to straight pushups			

MALES: OMIT

3. STRAIGHT PUSHUPS

MUSCLES WORKED Strengthen and tone chest and back of upper arm (pectoralis major and minor, triceps). Works muscles more than wall and bent knee pushups.

EQUIPMENT

Group I

Females: omit exercise

Males: no equipment needed

Group II

Females: no equipment needed

Males: no equipment needed

STARTING POSITION Lie on the floor on your abdomen with your arms bent, your hands at shoulder height slightly farther apart than shoulder width, and your legs straight. Raise your body off the floor by straightening your arms and balancing on your toes.

ACTION Slowly lower your body by bending only your arms, keeping your back straight, until your chest lightly touches the floor. Hold required number of seconds. Return to starting position. Exhale as you lower your body; inhale as you return to starting position. Perform required number of repetitions and sets.

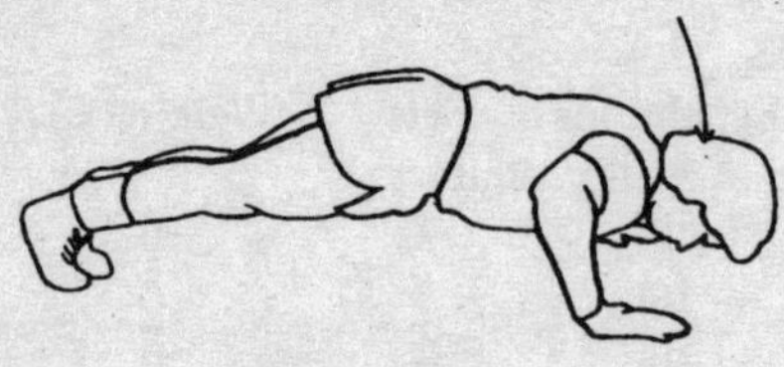

Straight pushups

PROGRESSION

Group I

FEMALES: OMIT

MALES

Week	Repetitions	Sets	Weight (lb)	Hold (sec)
1	bent knee pushups			
2	bent knee pushups			
3	10	3	0	0
4	10	3	0	1
5	10	3	0	2
6	10	3	0	3

Group II

FEMALES

Week	Repetitions	Sets	Weight (lb)	Hold (sec)
1	wall pushups			
2	bent knee pushups			

3	bent knee pushups			
4	bent knee pushups			
5	bent knee pushups			
6	5	2	0	0

MALES

Week	Repetitions	Sets	Weight (lb)	Hold (sec)
1	10	3	0	0
2	10	3	0	1
3	10	3	0	3
4	10	3	0	4
5	10	3	0	5
6	15	3	0	5

4. FLIES

MUSCLES WORKED Strengthen and tone chest and front of upper arm (pectoralis major and minor, biceps).

EQUIPMENT

Group I

Females: 3-pound dumbbells; adjustable dumbbells, 5 to 7½ pounds

Males: adjustable dumbbells, 5 to 10 pounds

Group II

Females: 3-pound dumbbells; adjustable dumbbells, 5 to 10 pounds

Males: adjustable dumbbells, 5 to 17½ pounds

STARTING POSITION Hold a dumbbell in each hand. Lie on the floor on your back with your knees bent and your arms stretched to the side at shoulder level.

ACTION Slowly raise arms as if you were hugging a large object. Hold required number of seconds. Return to starting position. Exhale as you raise you arms; inhale as you return to starting position. Perform required number of repetitions and sets.

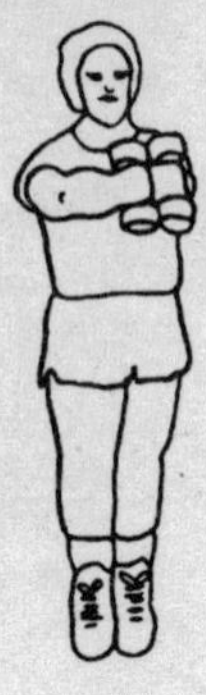

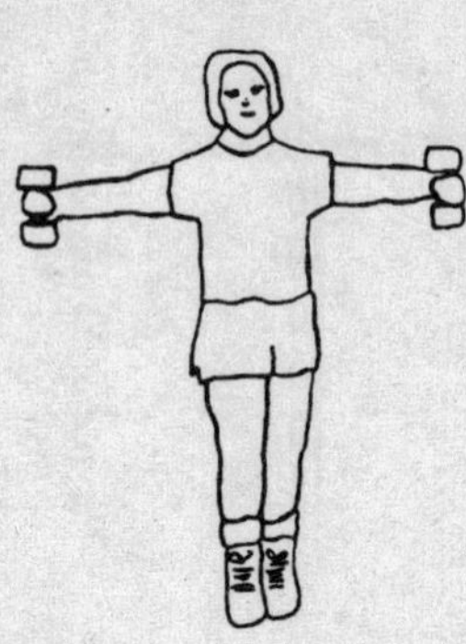

Flies

PROGRESSION

Group I

FEMALES

Week	Repetitions	Sets	Weight (lb)	Hold (sec)
1	10	2	3	0
2	10	3	3	0
3	10	2	5	0
4	10	3	5	0
5	10	3	5	0
6	10	3	7½	0

MALES

Week	Repetitions	Sets	Weight (lb)	Hold (sec)
1	10	2	5	0
2	10	3	5	0
3	10	2	7½	0
4	10	3	7½	0
5	10	2	10	0
6	10	3	10	0

Group II

FEMALES

Week	Repetitions	Sets	Weight (lb)	Hold (sec)
1	10	3	3	0
2	10	2	5	0
3	10	3	5	0
4	10	2	7½	0
5	10	3	7½	0
6	10	2	10	0

MALES

Week	Repetitions	Sets	Weight (lb)	Hold (sec)
1	10	3	5	0
2	10	3	7½	0
3	10	3	10	0
4	10	3	12½	0
5	10	3	15	0
6	10	3	17½	0

5. DOUBLE ARM PULLOVERS

MUSCLES WORKED Strengthen and tone back of upper arm and large muscle in the back (triceps, latissimus dorsi).

EQUIPMENT

Group I

Females: 3-pound dumbbells; adjustable dumbbells, 5 to 7½ pounds

Males: adjustable dumbbells, 5 to 12½ pounds

Group II

Females: 3-pound dumbbells; adjustable dumbbells, 5 to 10 pounds

Males: adjustable dumbbells, 7½ to 15 pounds

STARTING POSITION Hold one dumbbell with both hands. Lie flat on your back on the floor. Bend your knees. Place your arms on the floor with your hands above your head and your elbows slightly bent.

ACTION Slowly raise your arms until they are perpendicular to your body. Hold required number of seconds. Slowly return to starting position. Exhale as you raise your arms; inhale as you lower them. Perform required number of repetitions and sets.

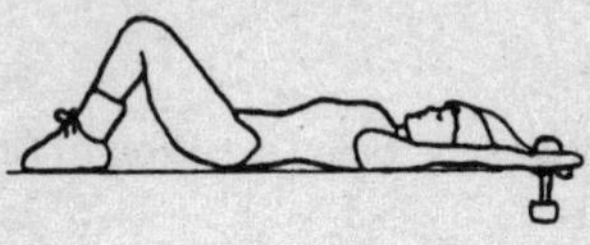

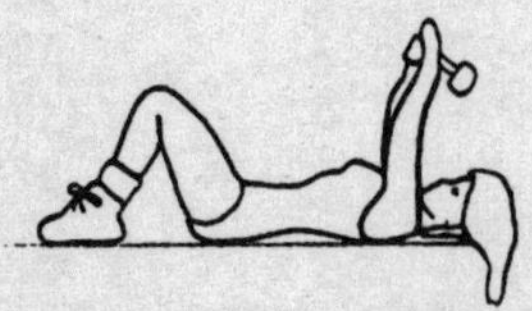

Double arm pullovers

PROGRESSION

Group I

FEMALES

Week	Repetitions	Sets	Weight (lb)	Hold (sec)
1	10	3	3	0
2	10	3	3	2
3	10	3	5	0
4	10	3	5	2
5	10	3	7½	0
6	10	3	7½	2

MALES

Week	Repetitions	Sets	Weight (lb)	Hold (sec)
1	10	2	5	0
2	10	3	7½	0

3	10	3	7½	2
4	10	3	10	0
5	10	3	10	2
6	10	3	12½	2

Group II

FEMALES

Week	Repetitions	Sets	Weight (lb)	Hold (sec)
1	10	3	3	2
2	10	3	5	0
3	10	3	5	2
4	10	3	7½	0
5	10	3	7½	2
6	10	3	10	2

MALES

Week	Repetitions	Sets	Weight (lb)	Hold (sec)
1	10	3	7½	0
2	10	3	7½	2
3	10	3	10	0
4	10	3	10	2
5	10	3	12½	2
6	10	3	15	2

6. SHOULDER PRESSES

MUSCLES WORKED Strengthen and tone shoulder and back of upper arm (deltoid, triceps).

EQUIPMENT

Group I

Females: omit exercise

Males: adjustable dumbbells, 5 to 12½ pounds

Group II

Females: 3-pound dumbbells; adjustable dumbbells, 5 to 10 pounds

Males: adjustable dumbbells, 7½ to 20 pounds

STARTING POSITION Hold a dumbbell in each hand. Sit erect in a chair with your arms positioned at shoulder height.

ACTION Push right arm straight up parallel with your body. Hold required number of seconds. Return to starting position. Exhale as you raise your arm; inhale as you lower it. Repeat with left arm. One action with right arm and one with the left constitute one repetition. Perform the required number of repetitions and sets.

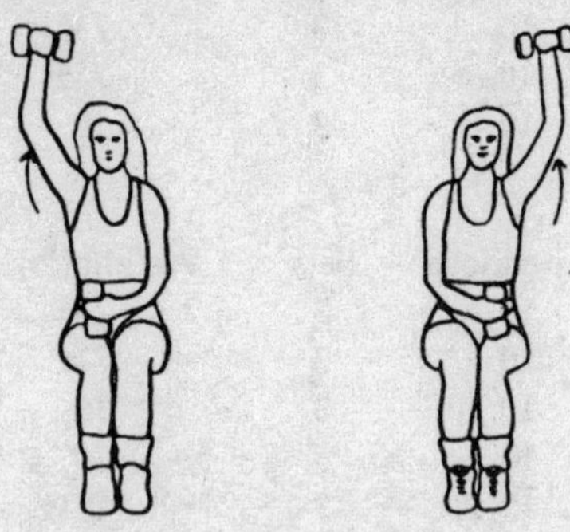

Shoulder press

PROGRESSION

Group I

FEMALES: OMIT EXERCISE

MALES

Week	Repetitions	Sets	Weight (lb)	Hold (sec)
1				
2				
3	10	2	5	2
4	10	3	7½	2
5	10	3	10	2
6	10	3	12½	2

Group II

FEMALES

Week	Repetitions	Sets	Weight (lb)	Hold (sec)
1	10	3	3	0
2	10	3	5	0
3	10	3	5	2
4	10	3	7½	0
5	10	3	7½	2
6	10	3	10	2

MALES

Week	Repetitions	Sets	Weight (lb)	Hold (sec)
1	10	3	7½	2
2	10	3	10	2
3	10	3	12½	2
4	10	3	15	2
5	10	3	17½	2
6	10	3	20	2

7. LATERAL RAISES

MUSCLES WORKED Strengthen and tone the muscles that stabilize the shoulder joint—the rotator cuff.

EQUIPMENT

Group I
Females: omit exercise
Males: omit exercise

Group II
Females: omit exercise
Males: adjustable dumbbells, 5 to 10 pounds

STARTING POSITION Hold a dumbbell in each hand. Stand erect with your arms straight and at your sides and palms facing your body.

ACTION Slowly raise arms sideways to shoulder height with palms facing down. Hold required number of seconds. Slowly lower arms to starting position. Exhale as you raise your arms; inhale as you lower them. Perform required number of repetitions and sets.

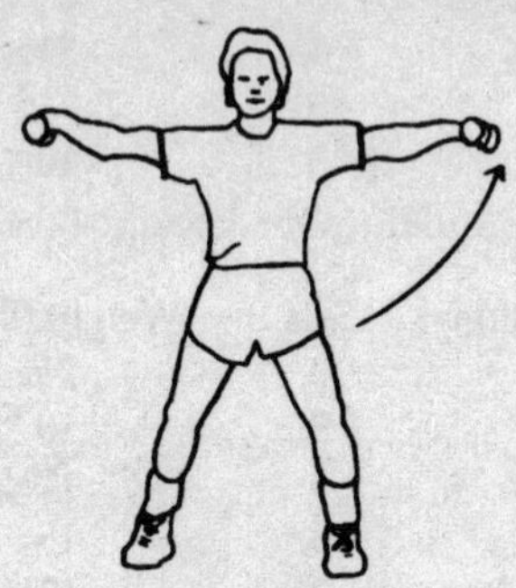

Lateral raises

PROGRESSION

Group I

FEMALES: OMIT EXERCISE

MALES: OMIT EXERCISE

Group II

FEMALES: OMIT EXERCISE

MALES

Week	Repetitions	Sets	Weight (lb)	Hold (sec)
1	10	3	5	0
2	10	3	5	2
3	10	3	7½	0
4	10	3	7½	2
5	10	3	10	0
6	10	3	10	2

8. UPRIGHT ROWS

MUSCLES WORKED Strengthen and tone shoulder, upper arm, and upper back (deltoid, biceps, rhomboideus major and minor)

EQUIPMENT

Group I

Females: 3-pound dumbbells; adjustable dumbbells, 5 to 10 pounds

Males: adjustable dumbbells, 5 to 15 pounds

Group II

Females: adjustable dumbbells, 5 to 12½ pounds

Males: adjustable dumbbells, 10 to 20 pounds

STARTING POSITION Hold a dumbbell in each hand. Stand erect with your arms straight and in front of you, palms facing toward your body. Bend your knees slightly.

ACTION Bend your elbows keeping palms toward your body, slowly raising your arms until your hands reach

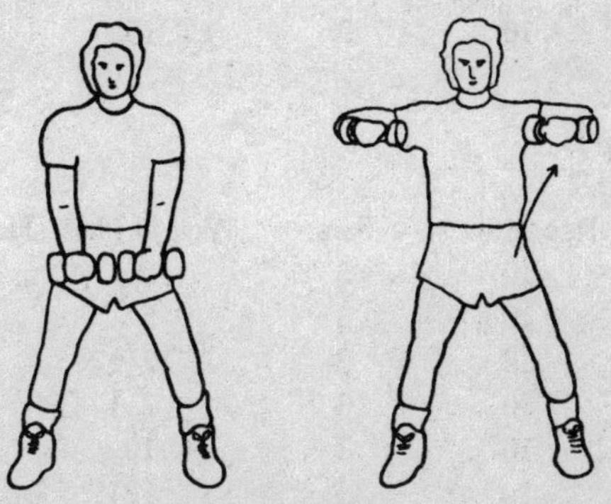

Upright rows

shoulder height. Hold the required number of seconds. Slowly return to starting position. Exhale as you raise your arms; inhale as you lower them. Perform required number of repetitions and sets.

PROGRESSION

Group I

FEMALES

Week	Repetitions	Sets	Weight (lb)	Hold (sec)
1	10	3	3	2
2	10	3	5	2
3	10	3	7½	0
4	10	3	7½	2
5	10	3	10	0
6	10	3	10	2

MALES

Week	Repetitions	Sets	Weight (lb)	Hold (sec)
1	10	3	5	2
2	10	3	7½	2
3	10	3	10	0
4	10	3	10	2
5	10	3	12½	2
6	10	3	15	2

Group II

FEMALES

Week	Repetitions	Sets	Weight (lb)	Hold (sec)
1	10	3	5	0
2	10	3	5	2
3	10	3	7½	0
4	10	3	7½	2
5	10	3	10	2
6	10	3	12½	2

MALES

Week	Repetitions	Sets	Weight (lb)	Hold (sec)
1	10	3	10	0
2	10	3	10	2
3	10	3	12½	2
4	10	3	15	2
5	10	3	17½	2
6	10	3	20	2

9. BICEPS CURLS

MUSCLES WORKED Strengthen and tone front of upper arm (biceps).

EQUIPMENT

Group I
Females: 3-pound dumbbells; adjustable dumbbells, 5 to 10 pounds
Males: adjustable dumbbells, 5 to 15 pounds
Group II
Females: adjustable dumbbells, 5 to 12½ pounds
Males: adjustable dumbbells, 7½ to 20 pounds

STARTING POSITION Hold a dumbbell in your right hand. Sit erect in a chair with your arms at your sides. Keeping your elbow at your side lift your forearm with your palm facing upward and turn arm out about 45° to the side. Support your elbow with your left hand.

ACTION Slowly raise your forearm until it reaches shoulder height. Slowly return to starting position. Exhale as you raise your arm; inhale as you lower it. Perform required number of repetitions and sets. Transfer dumbbell to left hand and repeat entire exercise.

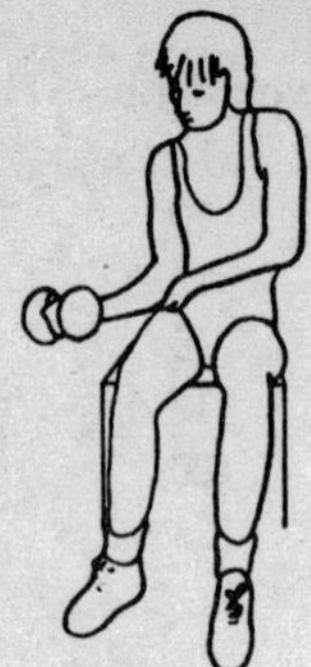
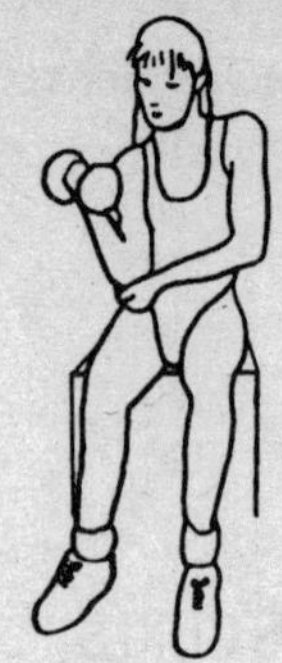

Biceps curls

PROGRESSION

Group I

FEMALES

Week	Repetitions	Sets	Weight (lb)	Hold (sec)
1	10	3	3	0
2	10	2	5	0
3	10	3	5	0
4	10	2	7½	0
5	10	3	7½	0
6	10	3	10	0

MALES

Week	Repetitions	Sets	Weight (lb)	Hold (sec)
1	10	3	5	0
2	10	2	7½	0
3	10	3	7½	0
4	10	3	10	0
5	10	3	12½	0
6	10	3	15	0

Group II
FEMALES

Week	Repetitions	Sets	Weight (lb)	Hold (sec)
1	10	3	5	0
2	10	3	5	0
3	10	3	7½	0
4	10	3	7½	0
5	10	3	10	0
6	10	3	12½	0

MALES

Week	Repetitions	Sets	Weight (lb)	Hold (sec)
1	10	3	7½	0
2	10	3	10	0
3	10	3	12½	0
4	10	3	15	0
5	10	3	17½	0
6	10	3	20	0

10. WRIST CURLS

MUSCLES WORKED Strengthen and tone forearm (flexors, extensors).

EQUIPMENT
Group I
Females: omit exercise
Males: omit exercise
Group II
Females: omit exercise
Males: adjustable dumbbells, 5 to 10 pounds

STARTING POSITION Hold a dumbbell in your right hand. Sit in a chair. Support your forearm on your right leg your wrist extending beyond your knee and your palm facing upward.

ACTION Slowly roll your right hand toward your chest (flex your wrist) until it is as high up as it will go. Slowly return to starting position. Exhale as you roll your hand up; inhale as you lower it. Perform required number of repetitions and sets. Transfer dumbbell to left hand and repeat entire exercise.

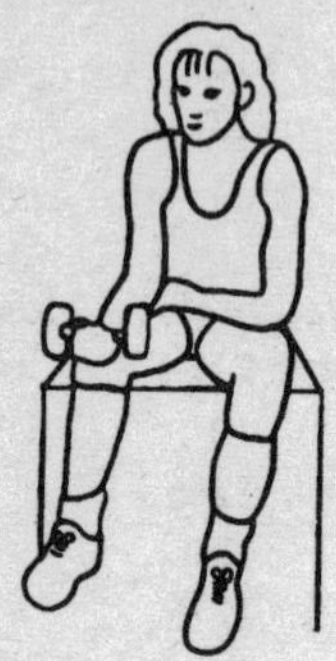
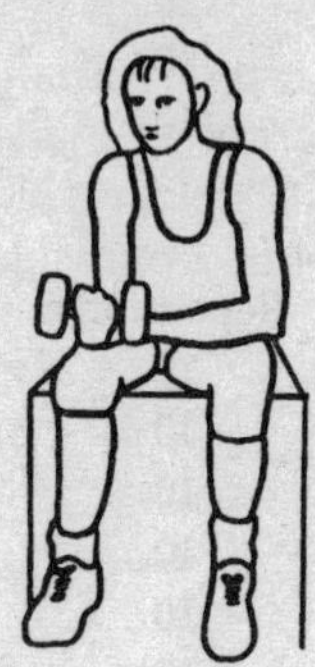

Wrist curls

PROGRESSION

Group I

FEMALES: OMIT

MALES: OMIT

Group II

FEMALES: OMIT

MALES

Week	Repetitions	Sets	Weight (lb)	Hold (sec)
1	10	3	5	0
2	10	3	5	0
3	10	3	7½	0
4	10	3	7½	0
5	10	3	10	0
6	10	3	10	0

ADVANCED UPPER BODY EXERCISES

As with the lower body exercises, you can proceed in several ways once you have completed the six-week plan. You can do the same exercises, adding more weights, repetitions, and sets, until it becomes impractical.

You can do variations of some of the exercises. The pushups can be made more difficult by elevating your arms on books or blocks, by elevating your feet on a bench or bed, or by elevating both your arms and feet.

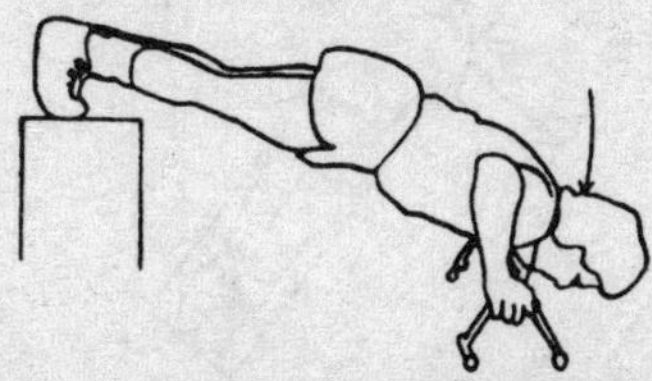

Pushups, variation

You can vary the flies by lying on an inclined bench with your head higher than your feet (incline fly) or with your feet higher than your head (decline fly). In lateral raises you can grip the dumbbells with your palms facing up to work slightly different rotator cuff muscles. By performing biceps curls with your arm turned in instead of out, you work the biceps in a slightly different way.

You can incorporate some exercises from other groups. For example, group I females can add shoulder presses, and group I males and group II females can add wrist curls.

And there are some new exercises that you can add to or substitute for those you've been doing.

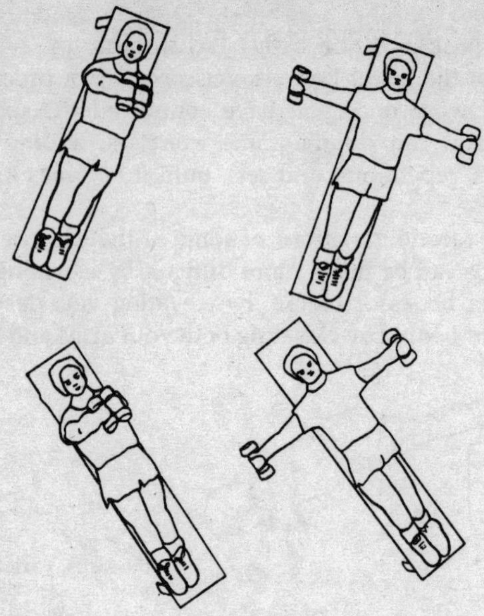

Flies, variations

11. HANDSTAND PUSHUPS

MUSCLES WORKED Strengthen and tone chest and back of upper arm (pectoralis major and minor, triceps). Works muscles more than straight pushups.

EQUIPMENT

All groups: 2 pillows

STARTING POSITION Place the pillows on the floor against a wall shoulder width apart. Place your body in a handstand position, with your hands on the pillows.

ACTION Keeping your body straight, slowly lower yourself until your shoulders touch the pillows. Return to starting position. *This is a very difficult and advanced exercise and should only be attempted after all the other pushup variations have been mastered.*

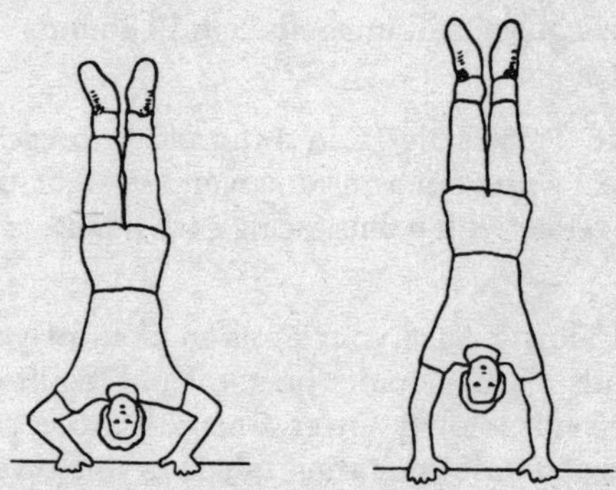

Handstand pushups

PROGRESSION (recommended only for group II males, although if you have mastered all the straight pushup variations, you can try it)

Week	Repetitions	Sets	Weight (lb)	Hold (sec)
1	10	3	0	0
2	10	3	0	1
3	10	3	0	2
4	10	3	0	3
5	10	3	0	4
6	10	3	0	5

12. FORWARD RAISES

MUSCLES WORKED Strengthen and tone the muscles that stabilize the shoulder joint—the rotator cuff.

EQUIPMENT

Group I
Females: omit exercise
Males: omit exercise

Group II
Females: omit exercise
Males: adjustable dumbbells, 5 to 10 pounds

STARTING POSITION Hold a dumbbell in each hand. Stand erect with your arms down and straight and your hands together with palms facing each other.

ACTION Slowly raise your arms in front of you until your hands reach shoulder height. Hold required number of seconds. Slowly lower arms to starting position. Exhale as you raise your arms; inhale as you lower them. Perform required number of repetitions and sets.

This exercise can be varied by beginning with palms facing the body and held facing down as the arm is raised.

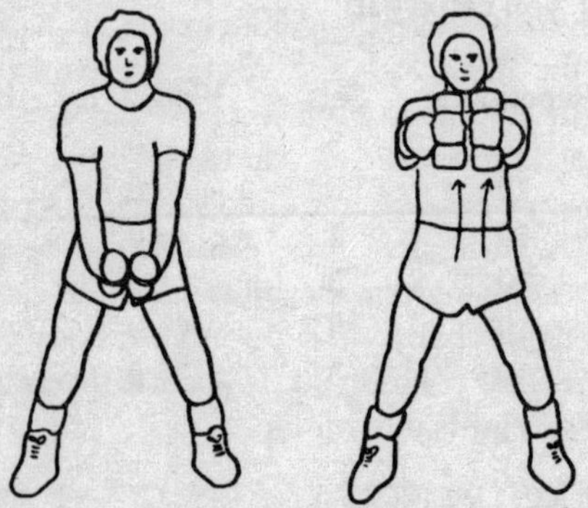

Forward raises

PROGRESSION See pp. 348.

13. DIPS

MUSCLES WORKED Strengthen and tone back of upper arm and large muscle in the back (triceps, latissimus dorsi). Works muscles more than double arm pullovers.

EQUIPMENT

Group I

Females: No weight needed

Males: adjustable ankle weights (to rest in lap) 2 to 4 lbs

Group II

Females: adjustable ankle weights, 2 to 3 lbs

Males: adjustable ankle weights, 2 to 6 lbs

STARTING POSITION Place a sturdy chair against a wall and sit on the floor with your back resting against the front edge of the chair. Place your feet about shoulder width, bend your knees, and draw them to your chest. Bend your elbows and grab the chair behind you.

ACTION Slowly straighten your arms and raise your body off the floor, keeping your feet firmly planted. Hold required numbers of seconds. Slowly return to starting position. Exhale as you raise your body; inhale as you lower it. Perform required number of repetitions and sets. The difficulty of this exercise can be increased by changing the starting position. Use two chairs. Rest your feet on one chair, and support your body with your arms on the chair behind you. To further increase the difficulty, rest weights in your lap.

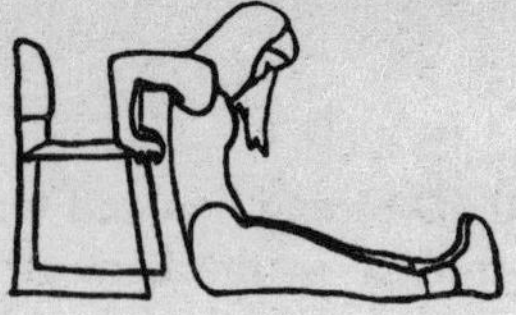

Dips

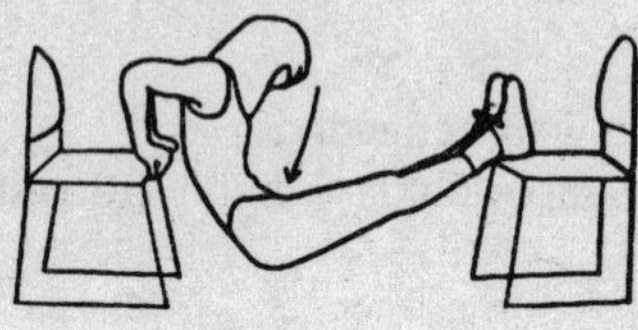

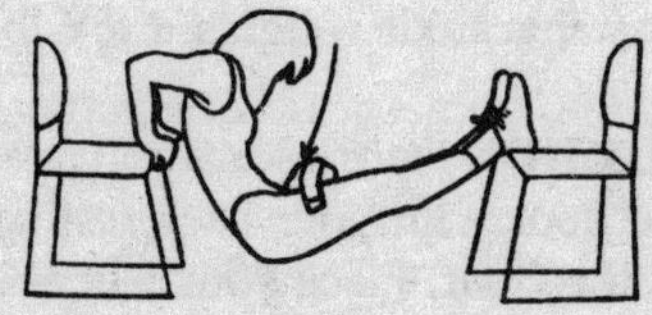

Dips, variation

PROGRESSION

Group I

FEMALES

Week	Repetitions	Sets	Weight (lb)	Hold (sec)
1	10	2	0	0
2	10	3	0	0
3	10	3	0	1
4	10	3	0	2
5	10	3	0	3
6	10	3	0	4

MALES

Week	Repetitions	Sets	Weight (lb)	Hold (sec)
1	10	3	0	0
2	10	3	0	1

3	10	3	0	2
4	10	3	2	3
5	10	3	3	4
6	10	3	4	5

Group II

FEMALES

Week	Repetitions	Sets	Weight (lb)	Hold (sec)
1	10	2	0	0
2	10	3	0	1
3	10	3	0	2
4	10	3	0	3
5	10	3	2	4
6	10	3	3	5

MALES

Week	Repetitions	Sets	Weight (lb)	Hold (sec)
1	10	3	0	1
2	10	3	2	1
3	10	3	3	2
4	10	3	4	3
5	10	3	5	4
6	10	3	6	5

14. PULLUPS

MUSCLES WORKED Depending on the position of the hands and arms, strengthen and tone forearms, upper arms, shoulders, and upper back (flexors and extensors, biceps and triceps, deltoids, trapezius).

EQUIPMENT

All groups: pullup bar

STARTING POSITION Hold onto bar with your arms in front of you, shoulder width apart, palms toward you. Allow your legs to hang down.

ACTION Slowly pull yourself up until your head is above the bar, exhaling as you pull up. Slowly return to starting position; inhale as you lower yourself. Perform required number of repetitions and sets. Holding the bar with your palms facing away from you increases the difficulty of the exercise and involves the forearm more. Holding the bar behind your head strengthens the back much more than the other variations.

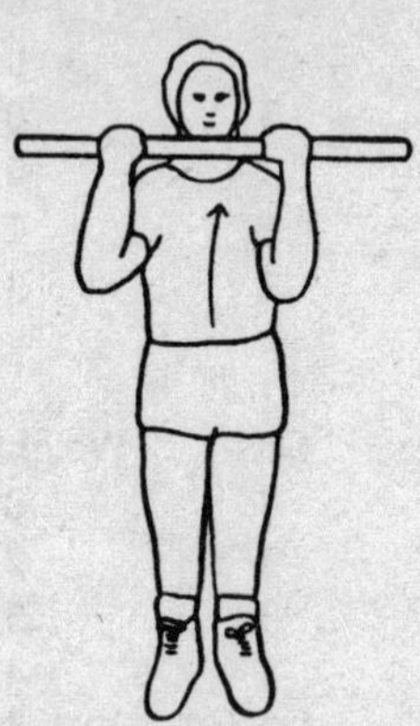

Pullups

PROGRESSION

Group I

FEMALES: OMIT

MALES

Week	Repetitions	Sets
1	10	1
2	12	1
3	15	1
4	10	2
5	12	2
6	10	3

Group II

FEMALES

Week	Repetitions	Sets
1	5	1
2	5	2
3	10	1
4	12	1
5	15	1
6	10	2

MALES

Week	Repetitions	Sets
1	10	1
2	15	1
3	10	2
4	15	2
5	10	3
6	15	3

ABDOMEN STRENGTHENING PROGRAM

1. ABDOMINAL CURLS

MUSCLES WORKED Strengthen and tone upper abdomen (rectus abdominis).

EQUIPMENT

Groups I and II: no equipment needed

STARTING POSITION Lie on the floor on your back. Bend your knees and keep your feet flat on the floor. Interlock your hands behind your head. Press the small of your back into the floor. Tuck your chin to avoid excessive head movement.

ACTION Slowly raise your upper back and shoulder blades off the floor. Hold required number of seconds. Slowly return to starting position. Exhale as you raise shoulders off the floor; inhale as you lower them. Perform required number of repetitions and sets.

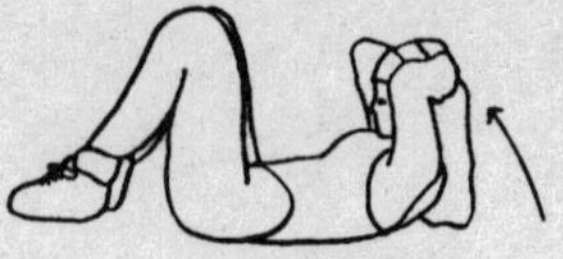

Abdominal curls

PROGRESSION

Group I

FEMALES

Week	Repetitions	Sets	Weight (lb)	Hold (sec)
1	10	2	0	0
2	10	3	0	0
3	10	3	0	0
4	15	3	0	0
5	15	3	0	0
6	15	4	0	0

MALES

Week	Repetitions	Sets	Weight (lb)	Hold (sec)
1	10	3	0	0
2	10	3	0	1
3	10	3	0	2
4	15	3	0	1
5	15	3	0	2
6	15	4	0	1

Group II

FEMALES

Week	Repetitions	Sets	Weight (lb)	Hold (sec)
1	10	2	0	0
2	10	2	0	1

3	10	3	0	2
4	15	2	0	1
5	15	2	0	2
6	15	3	0	2

MALES

Week	Repetitions	Sets	Weight (lb)	Hold (sec)
1	10	3	0	1
2	10	3	0	2
3	15	3	0	1
4	15	3	0	2
5	15	4	0	1
6	15	4	0	2

2. ABDOMINAL CRUNCHES

MUSCLES WORKED Strengthen and tone upper abdomen (rectus abdominis).

EQUIPMENT

Groups I and II: no equipment needed

STARTING POSITION Lie on the floor on your back with your buttocks about 18 inches from a wall. Bend your knees and place your feet against the wall. Interlock your hands behind your head. Press the small of your back into the floor. Tuck your chin to avoid excessive head movement.

ACTION Slowly raise your back and shoulder blades off the floor. Hold required number of seconds. Return to starting position. Exhale as you raise your shoulders; inhale as you lower them. Perform required number of repetitions and sets.

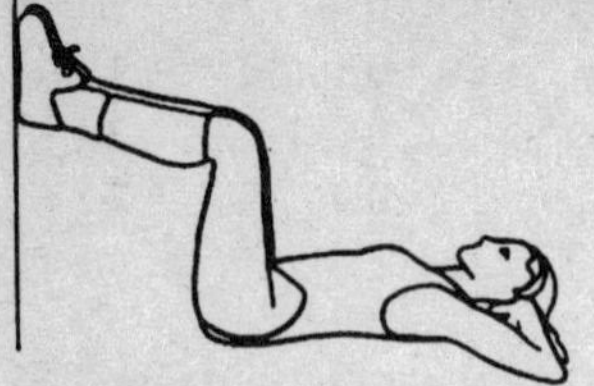
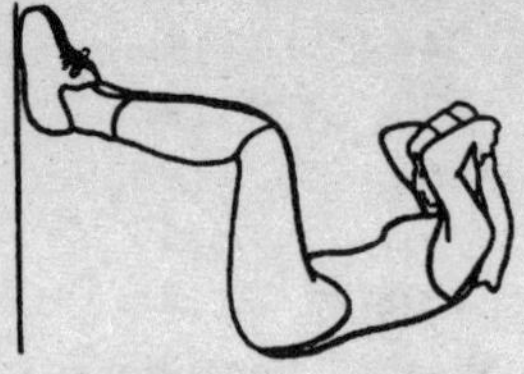

Abdominal crunches

PROGRESSION

Group I

FEMALES

Week	Repetitions	Sets	Weight (lb)	Hold (sec)
1	10	2	0	0
2	10	2	0	0
3	10	3	0	0
4	10	3	0	0
5	15	3	0	0
6	15	3	0	0

MALES

Week	Repetitions	Sets	Weight (lb)	Hold (sec)
1	10	3	0	0
2	10	3	0	1
3	10	3	0	2
4	15	3	0	1
5	15	3	0	2
6	15	4	0	2

Group II

FEMALES

Week	Repetitions	Sets	Weight (lb)	Hold (sec)
1	10	2	0	0
2	10	2	0	1
3	10	3	0	1
4	10	3	0	2
5	15	3	0	1
6	15	3	0	2

MALES

Week	Repetitions	Sets	Weight (lb)	Hold (sec)
1	10	3	0	1
2	10	3	0	2
3	15	3	0	1
4	15	3	0	2
5	15	4	0	1
6	15	4	0	2

3. DOUBLE LEG ABDOMINAL CURLS

MUSCLES WORKED Strengthen and tone upper abdomen (rectus abdominis).

EQUIPMENT

Groups I and II

Females: no equipment needed

Males: omit exercise

STARTING POSITION Lie on the floor on your back with your buttocks close to a wall. Raise your legs straight up and place your feet against the wall. Extend your arms at your sides. Press the small of your back into the floor. Tuck your chin to avoid excessive head movement.

ACTION Slowly raise your back and your shoulder blades off the floor and reach with your hands and arms toward your feet. Hold required number of seconds. Return to starting position. Exhale as you reach up; inhale as you lower your arms and shoulders. Perform required number of repetitions and sets.

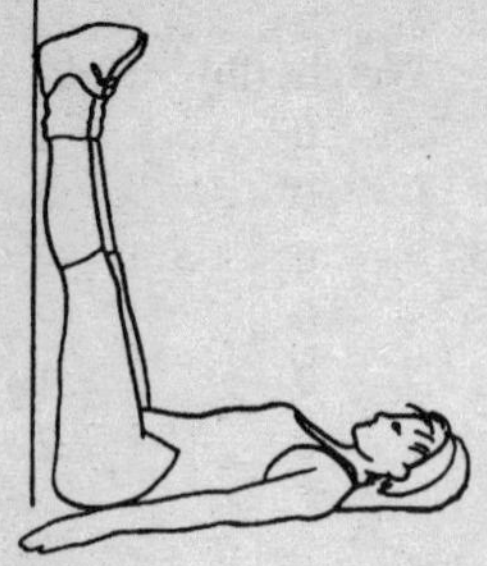
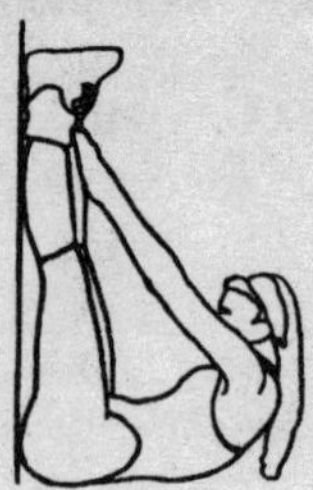

Double leg abdominal curls

PROGRESSION

Group I

FEMALES

Week	Repetitions	Sets	Weight (lb)	Hold (sec)
1				
2				
3				
4	10	2	0	0
5	10	3	0	1
6	10	3	0	2

MALES: OMIT

Group II

FEMALES

Week	Repetitions	Sets	Weight (lb)	Hold (sec)
1				
2				
3				
4	15	3	0	0
5	15	3	0	1
6	15	3	0	2

MALES: OMIT

4. U-POSITION SITUPS

MUSCLES WORKED Strengthen and tone upper and lower abdomen (rectus abdominis, transversus abdominis).

EQUIPMENT

Groups I and II: no equipment needed

STARTING POSITION Lie on the floor on your back. Bend your knees and put your feet flat on the floor. Interlock your hands behind your head. Press the small of your back into the floor. Tuck your chin to avoid excessive head movement.

ACTION Slowly raise your upper back and shoulder blades and at the same time bring your knees toward your chest. Keep your elbows back. Hold the required number of seconds. Return to starting position. Exhale as you bring your body together; inhale as you return to starting position. Perform required number of repetitions and sets.

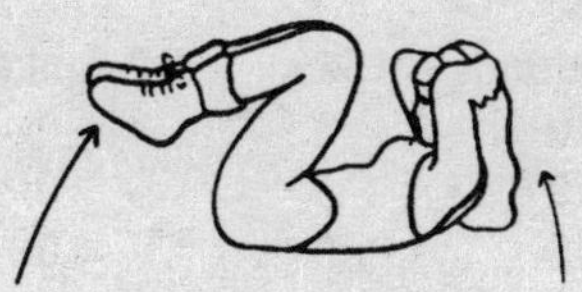

U-position situps

PROGRESSION

Group I

FEMALES

Week	Repetitions	Sets	Weight (lb)	Hold (sec)
1	10	2	0	0
2	10	3	0	0

3	10	3	0	1
4				
5				
6				

MALES

Week	Repetitions	Sets	Weight (lb)	Hold (sec)
1	10	3	0	0
2	10	3	0	1
3	10	3	0	2
4	15	3	0	1
5	15	3	0	2
6	15	4	0	2

Group II

FEMALES

Week	Repetitions	Sets	Weight (lb)	Hold (sec)
1	10	2	0	0
2	10	3	0	1
3	10	3	0	2
4				
5				
6				

MALES

Week	Repetitions	Sets	Weight (lb)	Hold (sec)
1	10	3	0	1
2	10	3	0	2
3	15	3	0	1
4	15	3	0	2
5	15	4	0	1
6	15	4	0	2

5. REVERSE CURLS

MUSCLES WORKED Strengthen and tone lower abdomen (transversus abdominis).

EQUIPMENT

Groups I and II

Females: no equipment needed

Males: omit exercise

STARTING POSITION Lie on the floor on your back. Bend your knees and put your feet flat on the floor. Interlock your hands behind your head. Press the small of your back into the floor.

ACTION Slowly draw your knees toward your chest, lifting your pelvis off the floor. Keep your feet below your knees. Hold required number of seconds. Return to starting position. Exhale as you lift your pelvis; inhale as you lower it. Perform required number of repetitions and sets.

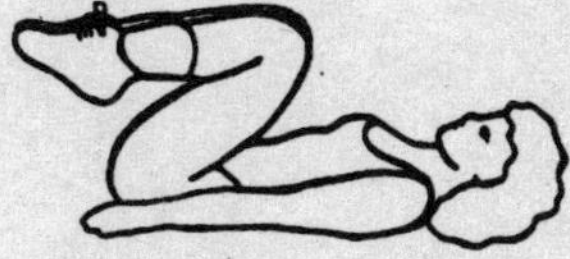

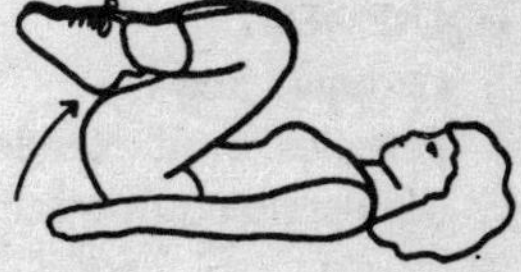

Reverse curls

PROGRESSION

Group I

FEMALES

Week	Repetitions	Sets	Weight (lb)	Hold (sec)
1				
2	10	2	0	0
3	10	2	0	1
4	10	3	0	0
5	10	3	0	1
6	10	3	0	2

MALES: OMIT

Group II

FEMALES

Week	Repetitions	Sets	Weight (lb)	Hold (sec)
1				
2	10	2	0	1
3	10	3	0	1
4	10	3	0	2
5	15	3	0	1
6	15	3	0	2

MALES: OMIT

6. BENT KNEE ROTATIONS

MUSCLES WORKED Strengthen and tone side (internal oblique, external oblique). Especially good for men.

EQUIPMENT

Groups I and II

Females: omit exercise

Males: no equipment needed

STARTING POSITION Lie on the floor on your back. Bend your knees and draw them toward your chest at a 90° angle. Interlock your hands behind your head.

ACTION Rotate your legs to the right. Lower them to the floor and pause. Return to starting position. Repeat on left side. Exhale as you lower your knees; inhale as you raise them. One rotation to the right and one to the left constitute one repetition. Perform required number of repetitions and sets.

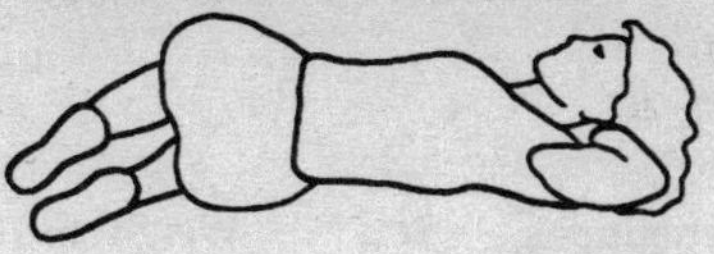

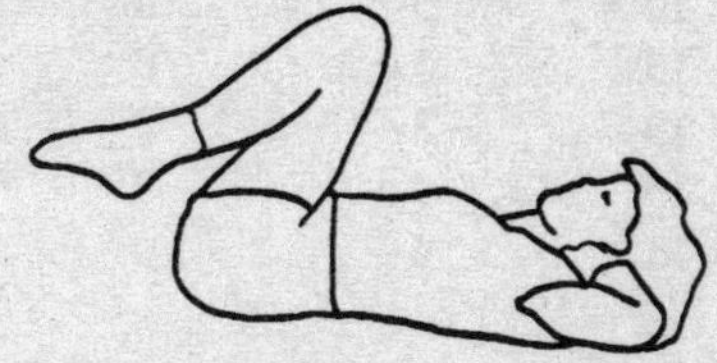

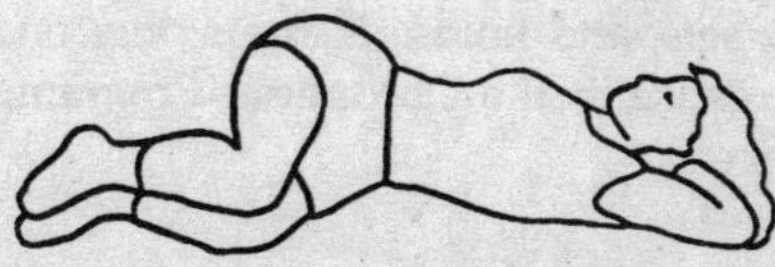

Bent knee rotations

PROGRESSION

Group I

FEMALES: OMIT

MALES

Week	Repetitions	Sets	Weight (lb)	Hold (sec)
1				
2	10	2	0	0
3	10	3	0	0
4	10	4	0	0
5	15	3	0	0
6	15	4	0	0

Group II
FEMALES: OMIT
MALES

Week	Repetitions	Sets	Weight (lb)	Hold (sec)
1	10	2	0	0
2	10	3	0	0
3	15	3	0	0
4	15	3	0	0
5	15	4	0	0
6	15	4	0	0

ADVANCED ABDOMINAL EXERCISES

For further training you may increase the number of repetitions, sets, and holds. There is only one new abdominal exercise in the Chromium Program, and it is very advanced.

7. PULLUP BAR EXERCISES

MUSCLES WORKED Strengthen and tone upper and lower abdomen (rectus abdominis, transversus abdominis).

EQUIPMENT
Groups I and II: pullup bar

STARTING POSITION Grab the pullup bar with both hands, palms facing toward you. Hang from the bar by your arms.

ACTION Raise your knees to your chest. Hold required seconds. Slowly lower knees. Perform required repetitions and sets. As a variation, instead of raising your knees to your chest, raise your legs straight in front of you so your body forms a 90° angle.

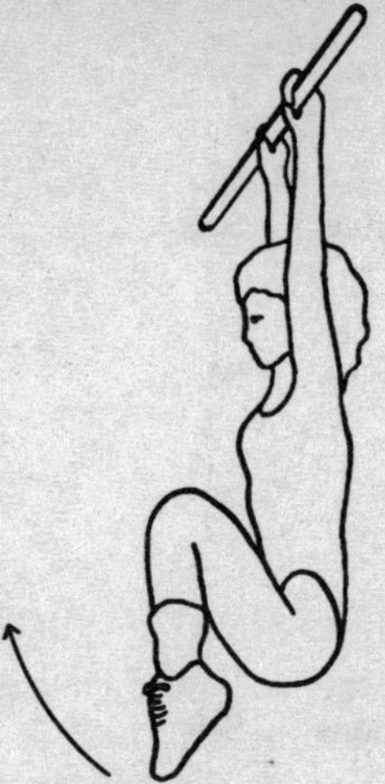

Pullup bar exercises

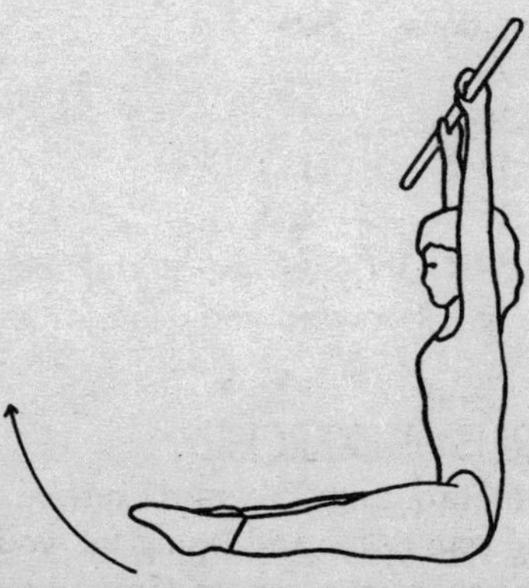

Pullup bar exercises, variation

PROGRESSION

Group I

FEMALES: OMIT

MALES

Week	Repetitions	Sets
1	5	1
2	7	1
3	10	1
4	12	1
5	15	1
6	10	2

Group II

FEMALES

Week	Repetitions	Sets
1	5	1
2	5	1
3	7	1
4	10	1
5	12	1
6	15	1

MALES

Week	Repetitions	Sets
1	7	1
2	10	1
3	12	1
4	15	1
5	10	2
6	15	2

OTHER FORMS OF EXERCISE

Although the Chromium Program exercise plan focuses on increasing lean tissue and losing fat, you should not neglect other beneficial exercises. Group I members who already engage in some sort of regular aerobic activity should continue it. Those who don't should begin. Group III members should be sure to include some sort of aerobics in their overall program. Group II members, of course, already are active in this area and should not alter their regimen.

All groups should also stretch every day in conjunction with aerobic exercise or the exercises of the Chromium Program. Be certain to warm up before you stretch, in order to reduce risk of injury. Maintaining flexibility as you increase strength is crucial.

MEASURING YOUR PROGRESS

By the end of six weeks, if you have adhered to both the diet and exercise plans, you will notice some remarkable changes. You should be at or close to your goal body fat percent, which you can check by the method we used in Chapter 7. You will also notice an increase in strength and stamina, as well as an enhanced appearance, which will undoubtedly bring you compliments from others. It's not necessary, but if you are interested in more objective and sophisticated ways of assessing your progress, Appendix C describes other means of measuring body fat and strength.

APPENDIX A

THE CHROMIUM PROGRAM FOODS RESOURCE LIST

Here is a list of the specific brand names mentioned in the menus and recipes. It tells the type of store in which they are generally available (supermarket or specialty store such as health food store), and gives the companies or distributors from whom they can be ordered, either by you or by a store where you shop, if you cannot obtain them in the stores. The list also includes some general food products, with brand name suggestions, with which you might not be familiar or which may be difficult to find (for example, Fromage Blanc, brewer's yeast, and wheatgrass).

In case any brand is unavailable, or you don't like it for some reason, we list acceptable alternatives. If we don't feel there are suitable alternatives, we suggest some substitution for the food or, if necessary, eliminating it. Try to use the suggested brands. Many available brands are not as rich in chromium or some other supportive nutrients, and our recommendations were made on the basis of taste (admittedly subjective) as well as nutrient values.

Alpine Lace fat-free, low-sodium cheese Distributed by First World Cheese, Inc., Maplewood, NJ 07040. Available nationwide.

Alternative: Any other fat-free cheese (see Dorman's).

Alvarado Street Bakery sprouted wheat bagels Alvarado Street Bakery, (707)-585-9853. Available nationwide in health food stores, and in many supermarkets.

Alternative: Sprouted wheat bread, other whole grain bagels, Pritikin English muffins, whole grain bread (sprouted wheat has higher concentration of chromium, so none of the alternatives is as good).

Altadena nonfat yogurts Altadena Dairy, 17637 E. Valley Blvd., City of Industry, CA 91747, (818)-964-6401. Available nationwide in health food stores.

Alternative: Dannon and Columbo make a nonfat variety, but it contains sugar. If Altadena is unavailable, it is better to get Dannon/Columbo plain nonfat and add unsweetened conserve, preserve, or fresh fruit.

Amaranth pasta See Health Valley.

American Glacé Nonfat frozen dessert available in soft ice cream machines in supermarkets and malls.

Alternative: Other soft frozen desserts (for example, Gisé or Taste D-Lite), nonfat frozen yogurt (such as Élan).

American Grain rice snacks American Grains, Inc., Emeryville, CA 94608. Available nationwide in health food stores.

Alternative: No acceptable alternative. Substitute other foods used as snacks in menus, for example, air-popped popcorn, fruit, whole wheat pretzels, toasted whole wheat pita chips.

American Marketplace Foods 359 McLean Blvd., Paterson, NJ 07513. Makers of Muffin-A-Day, a delicious high-fiber, fat-free muffin that is rich in high-chromium wheat bran. Call 1-800-Muffin-4U.

Arrowhead Mills ready-made corn flakes, raw rye flakes (prepared as a hot cereal) and whole millet (for millet

porridge) Arrowhead Mills, Box 2059, Hereford, TX 79045. Available nationwide in health food stores.

Alternative: Grainfield's oven-toasted corn flakes (see Grainfield's), Health Valley blue corn flakes (see Health Valley), or any other unsweetened corn flakes. Rye flakes and millet can be bought in bulk in many health food stores.

Brewer's yeast Lewis Laboratories International, Ltd., P.O. Box 373, Southport, CT 06490, $7.00 for 16 oz. (postage included), will send free taste sample. Also available in health food stores and some pharmacies. Best-tasting of available brands.

Alternative: Other brewer's yeast or nutritional yeast, but not torula yeast, which is deficient in chromium.

Casbah hummus, Nutted Pilaf, tabouly, soups, breakfast cup Sahara Products, Inc., Berkeley, CA 94710, (415)-548-1868. Available nationwide in health food stores and some supermarkets.

Alternative: Fantastic Foods products; Golden Couscous soups; Health Valley soups.

Chico San popcorn cakes H. J. Heinz Co., Pittsburgh, PA. Available nationwide in supermarkets.

Alternative: Substitute rice cakes (not as good because rice has little chromium).

Christopher's Chewies A satisfying, light, puffed brown rice and tahini chewy snack. Home Again Foods, Inc., Orangeburg, NY 10962, (914)-359-6356. Available nationwide in health food stores.

Alternative: Substitute other food used as snacks in menus, for example, fruit or air-popped popcorn.

Crispini A whole wheat, no-fat flatbread-type cracker with sesame seeds. Rickburn Enterprises, Paterson, NJ. Available nationwide in supermarkets.

Alternative: Substitute whole wheat pita bread toasted to chips. Rye-Krisps and Norwegian flatbread are similar but some people don't like the taste or texture.

Diet Fuel (see Twinlab) No acceptable alternative.

Dorman's Light Slim Jack fat-free cheese and Lo-Chol low-cholesterol cheese Light Skim Jack packed by N. Dorman, Inc., Syosset, NY 11791; Lo-Chol distributed by Dorman-Roth Foods, Inc., Moonachie, NJ 07074.

Alternative: Any other part skim or low-cholesterol cheese.

Dutchie unsalted whole wheat pretzels Parent company, Wege Pretzel Co., P.O. Box 154, Blettner Ave., Hanover, PA 17331, (800)-727-7322. Available nationwide under brand names Wege or Dutchie.

Alternative: Any whole wheat pretzels.

Élan frozen dessert Élan Foods, Buffalo, NY 14202. Available nationwide in supermarkets.

Alternative: Other nonfat frozen yogurts or see recipe for nonfat yogurt dessert.

Fantastic Foods products Fantastic Foods, 106 Galli Drive, Novato, CA 94949, (415)-883-7718, FAX (415)-883-5129. Available nationwide in health food stores. Instant refried beans (just add water), nature's burgers (all vegetable and grain mix), Shells 'N' Curry (curried pasta shell mix to be added to tofu), tofu scrambler (spice mixture to be added to tofu and scrambled as an egg substitute), Quick Pilaf, brown rice with miso mix.

Alternative: For Shells 'n' Curry, substitute another Fantastic Foods mix such as vegetarian chili. For quick pilaf substitute another brand such as Casbah. For nature's burger, substitute Original Near East Falafel Vegetable Burger Mix (Near East Food Products, Inc., Leominster, MA 01453), available in health food stores, following package directions but adding ¼ cup wheat bran per serving. Most other brands of vegetable burgers are high in fat. You might also use texturized vegetable protein (TVP), adding ¼ cup wheat germ or wheat bran per 2 burgers, Worcestershire sauce, and seasoning to taste and cooked as you would nature's burgers.

Fiber One cereal General Mills. Available nationwide in supermarkets.

Alternative: All-Bran, Nabisco 100% Bran (both have sugar, which depletes chromium).

Food for Life seven-grain sprouted cinnamon raisin bread Food for Life, 3580 Pasadena Ave., Los Angeles, CA 90031. Available nationwide in health food stores.

Alternative: Essene bread (available in health food stores), a sprouted bread that is high in calories so only half as much should be used; any other sprouted wheat bread; if no sprouted bread available, find a good whole grain bread.

Fromage Blanc Vermont Butter and Cheese Company, Websterville, VT 05678. $12.20 for three 8-ounce containers. Also available in specialty cheese and gourmet stores, primarily on the East coast. *Note:* Do not buy after the expiration date, as it makes a noticeable difference in taste.

Alternative: See low-fat sour cream recipe (page 275), but try to order this excellent product.

Gaylord Hauser vegetable broth mix, Vegit, and Spike seasoning Modern Products, Inc., Milwaukee, WI, 53209. Available nationwide in health food stores.

Alternative: Any other all vegetable-based broth and salt replacements.

Golden Couscous soups Nile Spice Foods, Box 20581, Seattle, WA 98102. Available nationwide in health food stores.

Alternative: Casbah soups in a cup; Health Valley soups.

Grain Dance whole wheat pizza shells Amberwave Foods, T.F.P., Oakmont, PA 15139, (412)-828-3152. Available in many health food stores.

Alternative: Creative Fun Foods, (603)-464-3400. See recipes for whole wheat and corn meal pizza doughs (pages 285 and 252).

Grainfield's oven toasted corn flakes The Weetabix Co., Inc., 20 Cameron St., Clinton, MA 01510.

Alternative: See Health Valley or Arrowhead Mills.

Green Mountain salsa Hume Specialities, Inc., RD 2, Box 190, Chester, VT 05143. Order directly.

Alternative: Hot Cha Cha! or other ready-made low-sodium, low-fat salsa.

Health Valley amaranth pasta Health Valley Foods, 16100 Foothill Blvd., Irwindale, CA 91706, (818)-334-3241. Available nationwide in health food stores.

Alternative: Other whole grain pastas available in supermarkets and health food stores (but most are not as high in protein).

Health Valley beef and chicken broth and canned soups Health Valley Foods, 16100 Foothill Blvd., Irwindale, CA 91706, (818)-334-3241. Available nationwide in health food stores and many supermarkets. *Note:* We like only the black bean soup a great deal.

Hodgson Mill buttermilk pancake mix and cracked wheat cereal Hodgson Mill Enterprises, Inc., Gainesville, MO 65655. Available nationwide in many supermarkets and health food stores.

Alternative: Arrowhead Mills mixes and cereals (Hereford, TX), available in most health food stores; other whole grain pancake mix; if no acceptable alternative, substitute another breakfast from the menu plan.

Holland's Pride mussels K. J. International Trading Co., Inc., Forked River, NJ 08731. Available in many supermarkets.

Alternative: Other brands of mussels.

Hot Cha Cha! salsa Hot Cha Cha! Division of Allied Old English, 100 Markley St., Port Redding, NJ 07064, (201)-636-2060. Available nationwide in supermarkets.

Alternative: Green Mountain salsa or other ready-made low-sodium, low-fat salsa.

House of Herbs unsulphured blackstrap molasses House of Herbs, Passaic, NJ. Available nationwide in health food stores and many supermarkets. (*Unsulphured* means without the use of sulfur dioxide, a preservative. Preferable but not crucial.)

Alternative: Plantation (see Plantation) or any other blackstrap molasses.

IBC Root Beer St. Louis, MO, (314)-731-7767. Available in supermarkets nationwide.

Alternative: Other sugar-free root beers (but the flavor of others is not as good). (Root beer contains some chromium, but other flavor sodas do not, so the other flavors are not an equivalent substitute.)

Jaclyn's soups, bread crumbs, and breaded mushrooms/cauliflower Jaclyn's Food Products, P.O. Box 1314, Cherry Hill, NJ 05034, (609)-983-2560. Available nationwide in health food stores.

Alternative: Similar Health Valley products.

Kashi pilaf Kashi Company, P.O. Box 8557, La Jolla, CA 92038-8557. A blend of whole oats, brown rice, rye, hard red winter wheat, triticale, raw buckwheat, barley, and sesame seeds. Available nationwide in health food stores and some supermarkets. This is called the breakfast pilaf.

Alternative: Long grain or short grain brown rice.

Little Bear canned refried beans Little Bear Organic Foods, 15200 Sunset Blvd., #202, Pacific Palisades, CA 90277. Ready-to-eat canned refried beans, available nationwide in health food stores.

Alternative: Fantastic Foods instant refried beans (see Fantastic Foods).

Marukan rice vinegar Marukan Vinegar, Inc., Paramount, CA 90723. Available nationwide in specialty stores.

Alternative: Other rice vinegars from specialty stores.

Millet porridge See Arrowhead Mills.

Molasses See House of Herbs and Plantation.

Mueslix Kellogg. Available nationwide in supermarkets.

Alternative: A few chopped dates. *Note:* Mueslix is high in calories and used only as recommended (i.e., no more than ¼ cup).

Newman's Own Old Fashioned Roadside Virgin Lemonade Newman's Own, Westport, CT 06880. Available in supermarkets nationwide. Sweetened with fructose and a good substitute for non-beer drinkers.

Alternative: Homemade lemonade or other unsweetened fruit juices.

New Morning honey graham crackers New Morning, Leominster, MA, 01453. Available nationwide in health food stores.

Alternative: Omit unless another low-sodium, low-fat brand can be found.

Oil Olive oil is richest in the very healthful monounsaturated fats. We've selected extra virgin, because the deeper taste requires less oil. Any brand is acceptable. Because olive oil is unacceptable for most baking, we recommend Puritan oil (canola oil), also high in monounsaturated fats. If you prefer a lighter salad dressing, you may substitute "lite" olive oil or Puritan oil for the more full-bodied extra virgin.

Panda licorice Finn Foods Division of Leaf, Inc., Bannockburn, IL 60015. Available nationwide in health food stores.

Alternative: Other licorice; if none available, substitute a few dates.

Paul's peanuts, unsalted Paul's Peanuts, Inc., P.O. Box 2061, Great Neck, NY 11022. Available in most supermarkets.

Alternative: Weight Watcher's peanuts (not as good because have added dextrose); any other dry roasted, low-fat peanuts.

Perfect Foods frozen wheatgrass juice Perfect Foods, Brooklyn, NY. Available nationwide in health food stores.

Alternative: If no other brand of fresh or frozen concentrate is available, omit.

Pizsoy pizza Tree Tavern Products, 3 Crosby Place, Paterson, NJ 07501, (201)-279-1616. Available nationwide in health food stores.

Alternative: Grain Dance soy cheese pizza.

Polenta Fattorie and Pandea Instant Polenta. Imported by Liberty Imports, Inc., Carlstadt, NJ 07072; distributed by Haddon House Distributors, (609)-654-7901. Available in specialty shops.

Alternative: any other precooked maize flour (polenta), ready in 5 minutes.

Pritikin English muffins and broths Interstate Brands Corp., Kansas City, MO 64111. Available in health food stores nationwide and in some supermarkets (mostly in California).

Alternative: Other whole wheat English muffins (for example, Thomas).

Quinoa and quinoa pasta Available nationwide in health food stores.

Alternative: Other grains and pastas made from them, such as amaranth and amaranth pasta, but quinoa is higher in protein than any other grain.

Ryeflakes See Arrowhead Mills.

Richard Bourclon traditional sourdough bread Berkshire Mountain Bakery, Inc., Housatonic, MA 01236-0785. Available in many health food stores.

Alternative: Crispini crackers, Rye Krisp crackers.

Salsa See Hot Cha Cha!

Shredded Wheat 'N Bran Nabisco, East Hanover, NJ 07936. Available nationwide.

Sorrell Ridge conserves and marmalade and fruit spread Sorrell Ridge Farm, 100 Markley St., Port Redding, NJ 07064. Available nationwide in supermarkets.

Alternative: No-sugar, all-fruit Polaner preserves and conserves, Smucker's Simply Fruit, spreadable fruit.

Twinlab Diet Fuel Twinfast Twin Laboratories, Ronkonkoma, NY 11779. Available nationwide in health food stores and some pharmacies.

Alternative: Other low-fat, liquid meal supplement such as SlimFast (Thompson Medical Inc., 919 Third Ave., 26th floor, New York, NY 10022).

Vegit Modern Products, Inc., Dept. 1, P.O. Box 09398, Milwaukee, WI 53209. Available nationwide in health food stores.

Alternative: Other all-vegetable salt-replacement seasoning.

Vieux Carré's Original New Orleans Seafood Sauce Vieux Carré Foods, Inc., New Orleans, LA 70119, 1-(800)-992-9699. Available nationwide in supermarkets and specialty stores.

Alternative: Other cocktail sauce or salsa, homemade ketchup.

Wheatgrass, wheatgrass juice see Perfect Foods, or available fresh-squeezed in many health food stores.

APPENDIX B

CHROMIUM CONTENT OF FOODS

The following list gives the chromium content of more than a hundred foods known to have a significant amount of chromium. The foods are arranged alphabetically rather than by food group to make it easier for you to find a particular ingredient when you are preparing meals or developing your own high-chromium recipes.

Of course, not all foods are listed. A food that is not on the list may be a healthful food, but one that is low in chromium, for example, rice. Obviously, this does not mean it should not be part of your diet, but it does mean it will not contribute to your chromium requirements.

Another reason for omission of a food is incomplete data. This table is a compilation of results from several analyses of chromium content of foods, but not all ingredients have been studied. For example, although several research papers state that fermented foods, such as sauerkraut, miso, and pickles, are good sources of chromium, no study has adequately analyzed these foods for exact content. Fermented foods are included in the menus, but since their exact chromium content is not known, they were not used in calculating the daily intake of chromium. (The actual chromium intake on those days may be slightly underestimated.) The same is true of root beer; it has been mentioned as a good source of chromium, but no reliable analysis has been performed. As a practical matter, this presents no problem, since the amount of chromium added by inclusion of these ingredients would probably not be more than 10 to 15 micrograms. As nutritional chromium has such low toxicity, there is no risk of getting too much from any food sources.

Remember, also, that this compilation lists only chromium concentration of these foods, not biologically available amounts. The only extensive study on availability was done almost twenty years ago, when analytical techniques were not nearly as sophisticated as they are today, so the values obtained then may not be totally accurate and are certainly not complete. Most people have the ability to convert inactive chromium into the active form, so chromium content can be taken as a fairly reliable guide to how much chromium is able to be used in the body. (For a review of the situations calling for biologically active supplements and a summary of the foods highest in biologically active chromium, see Chapter 6.)

FOOD	CONCENTRATION (MCG/100G)	PORTION SIZE	AMOUNT OF PORTION (G)	AMOUNT OF CHROMIUM (MCG/PORTION)
American cheese	56	1 slice	25	14
Apple	24	1 medium	150	36
Applesauce	8	½ cup	100	8
Asparagus	11	1 cup	100	11
Baked beans	24	1 cup	100	24
Banana	11	1 medium	150	16
Barley	17	¼ cup	50	8.5
Beef (round)	44	3½ ounces	100	44
Beer (average)	30	12 ounces	180	34
Beets	5	1 cup	140	7
Black pepper	370	dash	1	3.7
Blackstrap molasses	115	1 tablespoon	15	17
Blueberries	5	1 cup	140	7
Brewer's yeast	600	1 ounce	28	168
Broccoli	19	1 head	180	34
Brown rice	9	¼ cup	50	4.5

(Continued)

FOOD	CONCENTRATION (MCG/100G)	PORTION SIZE	AMOUNT OF PORTION (G)	AMOUNT OF CHROMIUM (MCG/PORTION)
Brussels sprouts	14	4 small	140	20
Buckwheat	38	⅓ cup	33	13
Butter	15	1 tablespoon	15	2.25
Cabbage	15	1 cup	90	13
Carrots	8	1 medium	80	6.4
Cauliflower	3	1 cup	100	3
Celeriac	4	¼ root	100	4
Celery	18	1 cup	120	21
Chard	6	1 cup raw	115	8
Cheddar cheese	29	1″ cube	30	9
Chicken	14	3½ ounces	100	14
Chick-peas	10	¼ cup	50	5
Chili powder	86	1 teaspoon	5	4.2
Clams	44	6	105	46
Cloves	150	¼ teaspoon	1.25	1.9
Cod	30	3.5 ounces	100	30
Corn	37	1 ear	140	52
Corn flakes	14	1 cup	80	11
Corn meal	11	1 cup	100	11
Corn oil	23	1 tablespoon	15	3.45
Crab	13	3½ ounces	100	13
Cracked wheat (dry)	60	⅓ cup	50	30
Cucumber	17	1 small	180	30
Dates	19	5	40	7.6
Dried liver	170	1 tablespoon	15	25
Eggplant	2	1 cup	200	4
Egg	52	1 medium	50	26
Feta cheese	36	1″ cube	17	6.1
Figs	25	1	40	10
Fortified wine	40	2 ounces	30	12
Garbanzo beans	10	½ cup raw	100	10
Garlic	4	1 clove	3	0.12
Green beans	4	1 cup	100	4
Green pepper	19	1 cup	100	19
Halibut	18	3½ ounces	100	18
Kale	4	¼ pound	115	4.6
Lamb chops	12	3½ ounces	100	12
Leeks	8	3 to 4	100	8

(Continued)

FOOD	CONCENTRATION (MCG/100G)	PORTION SIZE	AMOUNT OF PORTION (G)	AMOUNT OF CHROMIUM (MCG/PORTION)
Lentils	11	½ cup	100	11
Lettuce (iceberg)	17	2 cups	90	15
Lettuce (romaine)	20	2 cup	110	22
Licorice	30	1 stick	32	9.6
Lima beans	10	½ cup	100	10
Liver (calf)	50	3½ ounces	100	50
Lobster	33	1 cup	145	48
Melon	13	¼	100	13
Millet	8	¼ cup raw	25	2
Molasses (blackstrap)	33	1 Tbsp	15	5
Mozzarella cheese	36	1″ cube	30	11
Mushrooms	47	1 cup raw	70	33
Mussels	22	6	150	33
Onions	19	1 cup chopped	160	30
Orange	5	1 medium	180	9
Orange (mandarin)	10	1 medium	100	10
Orange juice	12	1 cup	80	9.6
Oysters	20	6 medium	100	20
Parsley	4	1 tablespoon	4	0.16
Parsnips	13	1 cup	100	13
Peach	8	1 medium	100	8
Peanuts	90	1 tablespoon	9	8
Peanut butter	30	1 Tbsp	15	5
Pear	44	1 small	75	33
Peas	38	1 cup	100	38
Pinto beans	17	½ cup, cooked	100	17
Plum	10	2 medium	100	10
Popcorn	9	3 cups	42	3.8
Pork	10	3½ ounces	100	10
Potato	21	1 medium	250	42
Prunes	100	5	50	25
Radish	3	5 small	5	1.5
Raisins	6	2 tablespoons	18	1.1
Red pepper (sweet)	10	1 cup	100	10
Red wine	10	4 ounces	60	6
Rhubarb	66	½ cup	50	33
Rolled oats	9	1 cup	80	7.2

(*Continued*)

FOOD	CONCENTRATION (MCG/100G)	PORTION SIZE	AMOUNT OF PORTION (G)	AMOUNT OF CHROMIUM (MCG/PORTION)
Rye bread	30	2 slices	50	15
Sardines	20	3½ ounces	100	20
Scallops (sea)	60	6	150	90
Shrimp	30	6	100	30
Sole	40	3½ ounces	100	40
Soybeans	10	¼ cup raw	50	5
Spinach	20	1 cup (raw)	55	11
Split peas	18	½ cup raw	100	18
Squash (winter)	18	¾ cup	100	18
Strawberries	3	1 cup	150	4.5
Sunflower seeds	34	1 tablespoon	18	3
Sweet potatoes/ yams	20	1 medium	180	36
Swiss cheese	36	1″ cube	30	11
Thyme	1,000	¼ teaspoon	1.25	12.5
Tomato	24	1 medium	100	24
Turkey (white meat)	11	3½ ounces	100	11
Turnip greens	5	¼ pound	115	5.6
Walnuts	48	1 tablespoon	8	4
Water chestnuts	4	4	25	1
Watercress	16	1 cup	120	19
Wheat bran	38	¼ cup	25	9.5
Wheat germ	25	¼ cup	25	6
White wine	12	4 ounces	60	7.2
Whole wheat (berries)	29	1 cup cooked	125	36
Zucchini	3	1 cup	205	6

APPENDIX C

ADDITIONAL WAYS OF MEASURING YOUR PROGRESS IN THE CHROMIUM PROGRAM

STRENGTH

In order to measure how much stronger you're becoming, you must have a baseline measurement. Have your strength measured when you begin the program and then at regular intervals. Most physical therapy or sports medicine centers have the necessary equipment.

Although the *Cybex machine* is used primarily for measuring the effects of rehabilitation following injury, it can also be used to gauge your strength. The Cybex employs isokinetic resistance in which the harder you work, the more the resistance increases.

Another, more conventional means of gauging muscular strength is determining your *repetition maximum (RM).* This is the maximum weight that can be lifted a specified number of times, usually 10. *Don't attempt to determine your RM unsupervised.*

BODY FAT

There are several methods of determining body fat (see the table on p. 395). Most of these methods are extremely expensive and are appropriate and available only as research tools. Except for the Wilmore tape and scale method we described earlier (see page 82), the only other one you can employ without having to go to a physician or a sports medicine facility is *skinfold thickness,* an

METHODS OF ESTIMATING BODY FAT AND ITS DISTRIBUTION

METHOD	COST	EASE OF USE	ACCURACY	MEASURES REGIONAL FAT
Height and weight	$	Easy	High	No
Skin folds	$	Easy	Low	Yes
Circumferences	$	Easy	Moderate	Yes
Density				
Immersion	$$	Moderate	High	No
Plethysmograph	$$$	Difficult	High	No
Heavy water				
Tritiated	$$	Moderate	High	No
Deuterium oxide or heavy oxygen	$$	Moderate	High	No
Potassium isotope (^{40}K)	$$$	Difficult	High	No
Conductivity, total body electrical	$$$	Moderate	High	No
Bioelectric impedance	$$	Easy	High	No
Fat-soluble gas	$$	Difficult	High	No
Computed tomography	$$$$	Difficult	High	Yes
Ultrasonography	$$$	Moderate	Moderate	Yes
Neutron activation	$$$$	Difficult	High	No
Magnetic resonance	$$$$	Difficult	High	Yes

$= low cost, $$ = moderate cost, $$$ = high cost, $$$$ = very high cost

Source: G. A. Bray and D. S. Gray, Obesity: part I–pathogenesis, Western Journal of Medicine, *149:429–441, 1988.*

indication of the amount of underlying fat. (Even with this technique, although it is easily mastered, you may not feel competent enough to administer it yourself.) Skinfold calipers vary considerably in price, but acceptable ones are available for around $25. (Country Technology, P.O. Box 87, Gays Mills, WI, (608)-735-4718, has a wide range of skinfold calipers, including computerized models for $450.)

Skinfold testing can become quite detailed if you

measure the thickness of the skin at several body sites (some sources recommend up to seven) and plug the results into an equation. However, since the test isn't extremely accurate to begin with, it's acceptable to use just three sites and estimate body fat from the chart in Figure A1. It takes a little practice to make accurate measurements, so do a few trial runs before using the chart. It's easier to have someone else do the measuring for you. As instructed in the figure, add up your results, draw a line on the chart between your measurements sum and your age, and find where the line intersects the body fat scale for your sex. This technique is accurate to within about 3 to 4 percent.

The three sites to measure for males are chest, abdo-

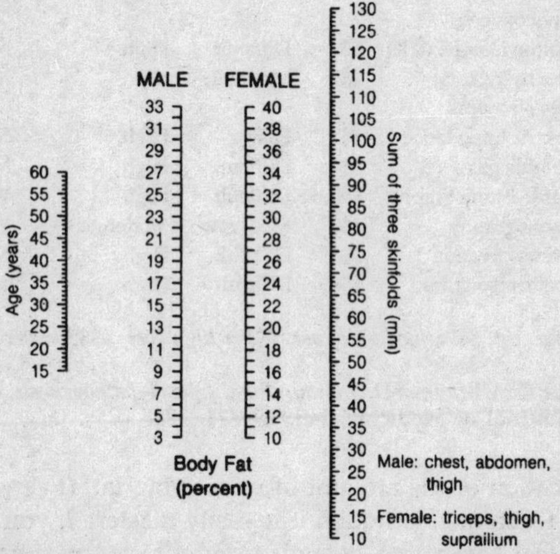

Figure A1. Nomogram for determination of percentage body fat using age and three designated skinfold measurements. To estimate body fat, take three measurements of skinfold thickness (as indicated in the text) and total them. Using a straight edge, draw a line between this sum on the millimeter scale and your age on the years scale. The point where this line intersects the percent scale (for male or female) is your body fat percent.

men, and thigh; for females, triceps, thigh, and suprailium. In each case, grasp a fold of skin, measure the thickness with calipers, and record the result. At the *chest,* take a diagonal fold midway between the right nipple and the front border of the armpit. At the *abdomen,* take a vertical fold about an inch to the right of the belly button. At the *thigh,* take a vertical fold on the front midway between the knee and hip joint when seated with leg flexed. At the *triceps,* take a vertical fold (at the back of the right arm) midway between the shoulder and elbow joints with the arm hanging naturally at the side in a relaxed position. At the *suprailium* just above the crest of the ilium, the bony protuberance of the hip bone), take a vertical fold.

Other more technical methods that are available at some sports medicine centers, health clubs, university medical centers, and doctors' offices are underwater weighing, bioelectrical impedance, and near-infrared interactance.

Underwater weighing measures body density, from which your body fat can be determined. You sit on a large scale, expel the air from your lungs, and get "dunked" under water. The difference between your underwater weight and your weight out of the water is your body density. Since fat is lighter than water, it tends to float; the more fat in a body, the lighter its weight in water. This method is more accurate than skinfold thickness and costs about $50.

The procedure for measuring *bioelectric impedance* is similar to electrocardiography. Electrodes are attached to you and current is pulsed through your body. Since lean tissue conducts better than fat (a good insulator), the greater the resistance, or impedance, to the current flow, the greater the percent fat. Many physicians now have this equipment in their offices, and the test can range from $20 to $50. It is a relatively new technique and some physiologists are still skeptical about its accuracy.

The *near infrared interactance* method is the newest and least proven. The mechanism generates and senses near-infrared light at a wavelength that is absorbed by fat, but not by lean tissue. By measuring absorption at the biceps, a computer estimates the amount of fat in the arm and also calculates an estimate of the amount in the entire body. The test is quick and simple and costs about $25, but because it measures only at one site, its accuracy is questionable.

APPENDIX D

WEIGHT TRAINING PROGRAM USED BY DR. GARY EVANS

The following is the weight training regimen used by the athletes at Bemidji State University (Minnesota) in whom Dr. Gary Evans demonstrated the anabolic effect of chromium. As this is an advanced program, it should be attempted only by experienced weight lifters. It is assumed that anyone who might participate in this program would already be familiar with the exercises, so they are not described.

The program involves four workouts a week for eight weeks. The exercises are divided into two groups, one group performed on Monday and Thursday and the other on Tuesday and Friday. The amount of weight lifted is based on a percentage of the repetition maximum (RM), that is, the maximum amount of weight that can be properly lifted for the given repetitions (reps). Rest periods between sets of an exercise are specified, and a rest of 4 to 5 minutes is taken between exercises.

The workout is designed to work the larger muscle groups first. Failing to follow the prescribed order of the exercises may impede development of the larger muscles. The order of the exercises is:

MONDAY AND THURSDAY

1. Bench press
2. Incline press

3. Close grip bench
4. Squat or leg press
5. Leg extension
6. Leg curl
7. Situp

TUESDAY AND FRIDAY

1. Power clean
2. Behind the neck press
3. Upright row
4. Lat pull
5. Shrug
6. Tricep extension
7. Dip or close grip pushup
8. Bicep curl
9. Hyper extension

DAY	INTENSITY	REST (MIN)	EXERCISE	SETS/REPS	% OF RM
Mon	Low	1–2	Bench	3 × 12	60–65
	Low	1–2	Squat	3 × 12	60–65
	Low	1–2	Others*	3 × 12	70–75 (12 RM)
Tues	Low	1–2	Clean	3 × 12	60–65
	Low	1–2	Press	3 × 12	60–65
	Low	1–2	Others	3 × 12	70–75
Thurs	Low	1–2	Bench	3 × 12	60–65
	Low	1–2	Squat	3 × 12	60–65
	Low	1–2	Others	3 × 12	70–75
Fri	Low	1–2	Clean	3 × 12	60–65
	Low	1–2	Press	3 × 12	60–65
	Low	1–2	Others	3 × 12	70–75
Mon	Low	1–2	Bench	12/10/8†	60/65/70
	Low	1–2	Squat	12/10/8	60/65/70
	Low	1–2	Others	4×10	70–75 (10 RM)

(Continued)

DAY	INTENSITY	REST (MIN)	EXERCISE	SETS/REPS	% OF RM
Tues	Low	1–2	Clean	12/10/8	60/65/70
	Low	1–2	Press	12/10/8	60/65/70
	Low	1–2	Others	4×10	70–75 (10 RM)
Thurs.	Low	1–2	Bench		
	Low	1–2	Squat		
	Low	1–2	Others	4 × 10	70–75
Fri	Low	1–2	Clean		
	Low	1–2	Press		
	Low	1–2	Others	4 × 10	70–75
Mon	Low-mod	2	Bench	4 × 10	50/60/65/70
	Low-mod	2	Squat	4 × 10	50/60/65/70
	Low-mod	2	Others	10/8/6	65/75/80
Tues	Low-mod	2	Clean	4 × 10	50/60/65/70
	Low-mod	2	Press	4 × 10	50/60/65/70
	Low-mod	2	Others	10/8/6/4	65/75/80
Thur	Mod-high	2	Bench	10/8 × 4	50/65/70/75/80
	Mod-high	2	Squat	10/8 × 4	50/65/70/75/80
	Mod-high	2	Others	10/8/6/4	65/75/80/80
Fri	Mod-high	2	Clean	10/8 × 4	50/65/70/75/80
	Mod-high	2	Press	10/8 × 4	50/65/70/75/80
	Mod-high	2	Others	10/8/6/4	65/70/80/80
Mon	Mod-high	2	Bench	10/8/6 × 4	50/65/70/75/80/82
	Mod-high	2	Squat	10/8/6 × 4	50/65/70/75/80/82
	Mod-high	2	Others	8/6/6	70/75/80
Tues	High	2	Clean	10/8/6 × 4	50/65/70/75/80/82
	High	2	Squat	10/8/5 × 4	50/65/70/75/80/85
	High	2	Others	8/6/6	75/80/85
Thur	High	2	Bench	10/8/5 × 4	50/65/70/75/80/85
	High	2	Squat	10/8/5 × 4	50/65/70/75/80/85
	High	2	Others	8/6/6	70/80/85

(Continued)

DAY	INTENSITY	REST (MIN)	EXERCISE	SETS/REPS	% OF RM
Fri	High	2	Clean	10/8/5 × 4	50/65/70/75/80/85
	High	2	Press	10/8/5 × 4	50/65/70/75/80/85
	High	2	Other	8/6/6	70/80/85
Mon	High	2–3	Bench	10/8/6/4/3/2	50/65/70/80/85/90
	High	2–3	Squat	10/8/6/4/3/2	50/65/70/80/85/90
	High	2–3	Others	4 × 5	90–95
Tues	High	2–3	Clean	10/8/6/4/3/2	50/65/70/80/85/90
	High	2–3	Press	10/8/6/4/3/2	50/65/70/80/85/90
	High	2–3	Others	4×5	90–95
Thur	High	2–3	Bench	10/8/5/4/3/2	50/65/70/80/85/90
	High	2–3	Squat	10/8/5/4/3/2	50/65/70/80/85/90
	High	2–3	Others	4 × 5	90–95
Fri	High	2–3	Clean	10/8/5/4/3/2	50/65/75/80/85/90
	High	2–3	Press	10/8/5/4/3/2	50/65/70/80/85/90
	High	2–3	Others	4 × 5	90–95
Mon	High	2–3	Bench	10/5/3/1 × 3	50/65/75/85/95/105
	High	2–3	Squat	10/5/3/1 × 3	50/65/75/85/95/105
	High	2–3	Others	3 × 10	85–90
Tues	High	2–3	Clean	10/5/3/1 × 3	50/65/75/85/95/105
	High	2–3	Press	10/5/3/1 × 3	50/65/75/85/95/105
	High	2–3	Others	3 × 10	85–90
Thur	Low	1–2	Bench	3 × 12	60
	Low	1–2	Squat	3 × 12	60
	Low	1–2	Others	3 × 12	75–80
Fri	Low	1–2	Clean	3 × 12	60
	Low	1–2	Press	3 × 12	60
	Low	1–2	Others	3 × 12	60

(Continued)

DAY	INTENSITY	REST (MIN)	EXERCISE	SETS/REPS	% OF RM
Mon	Mod	2	Bench	4 × 10	50/60/65/70
	Mod	2	Squat	4 × 10	50/60/65/70
	Mod	2	Others	10/8/6	65/75/80
Tues	Mod	2	Clean	4 × 10	50/60/65/70
	Mod	2	Press	4 × 10	50/60/65/70
	Mod	2	Others	10/8/6	65/75/80
Thur	Mod	2	Bench	10/8 × 4	50/65/70/75/80
	Mod	2	Squat	10/8 × 4	50/65/70/75/80
	Mod	2	Others	10/8/6/4	65/70/80/80
Fri	High	2	Clean	10/8 × 4	50/65/70/75/80
	High	2	Press	10/8 × 4	50/65/70/75/80
	High	2	Others	10/8/6/4	65/70/80/80
Mon	High	2	Bench	10/8/6 × 4	50/65/70/75/80/82
	High	2	Squat	10/8/6 × 4	50/65/70/75/80/82
	High	2	Others	8/6/6	70/75/80
Tues	High	2	Clean	10/8/6 × 4	50/65/70/75/80/82
	High	2	Press	10/8/6 × 4	50/65/70/75/80/82
	High	2	Others	8/6/6	70/75/80
Thur	High	2	Bench	10/8/5 × 4	50/65/70/75/80/85
	High	2	Squat	10/8/5 × 4	50/65/70/75/80/85
	High	2	Others	8/6/6	70/75/80
Fri	High	2	Clean	10/8/5 × 4	50/65/70/75/80/85
	High	2	Press	10/8/5 × 4	50/65/70/75/80/85
	High	2	Others	8/6/6	70/75/80

**All other exercises in the group to be done on that day.*
†3 sets with 12 repetitions in the first set, 10 in the second, and 8 in the third, the first set at 60% RM, the second at 65% RM, and the third at 70% RM. Numbers for all exercises work this way.

REFERENCES

CHAPTER 2

Buckley, W. E., C. E. Yesalis III, K. E. Friedl, W. A. Anderson, A. L. Streit, and J. E. Wright. Estimated prevalence of anabolic steroid use among male high school seniors. *Journal of the American Medical Association, 260* (23): 3441–3445, 1988.

Carrasco, D., M. Prieto, L. Pallardo, J. L. Mole, J. M. Cruz, C. Munoz, and J. Berenguer. Multiple hepatic adenomas after long-term therapy with testosterone enanthate. *Journal of Hepatology, 1*:573–578, 1985.

Clarkson, P. M., R. Hintermister, M. Fillyaw, and L. Stylos. High density lipoprotein cholesterol in young adult weight lifters, runners and untrained subjects. *Human Biology, 53*(2):251–257, 1981.

Goldberg, L., D. L. Elliot, R. W. Schultz, and F. E. Kloster. Changes in lipid and lipoprotein levels after weight training. *Journal of the American Medical Association, 252*(4):504–506, 1984.

Hagberg, J. M., A. A. Ehsani, D. Goldring, A. Hernandez, D. R. Sinacore, and J. O. Holloszy. Effect of weight training on blood pressure and hemodynamics in hypertensive adolescents. *Journal of Pediatrics, 104*:147–151, 1984.

Hallagan, J. B., L. F. Hallagan, and M. B. Snyder. Anabolic-androgenic steroid use by athletes. *New England Journal of Medicine, 321*(15):1042–1045, 1989.

Hurley, B. F., J. M. Hagberg, A. P. Goldberg, D. R. Seals, A.

A. Eshani, R. E. Brennan, and J. O. Holloszy. Resistive training can reduce coronary risk factors without altering VO_{2max} or percent body fat. *Medicine and Science in Sports and Exercise, 20*(2):150–154, 1988.

Hurley, B. F., D. R. Seals, A. A. Ehsani, L. J. Cartier, G. P. Dalsky, J. M. Hagberg, and J. O. Holloszy. Effects of high-intensity strength training on cardiovascular function. *Medicine and Science in Sports and Exercise, 16*(5):483–488, 1984.

Hurley, B. F., D. R. Seals, J. M. Hagberg, A. C. Goldberg, S. M. Ostrove, J. O. Holloszy, W. G. Wiest, and A. P. Goldberg. High-density-lipoprotein cholesterol in bodybuilders v. powerlifters. *Journal of the American Medical Association, 252*(4):507–513, 1984.

Johnson, M. D., S. Jay, B. Shoup, and V. I. Rickert. Anabolic steroid use by male adolescents. *Pediatrics, 83*(6):921–924, 1989.

Lamb, D. R. Anabolic steroids in athletics: how well do they work and how dangerous are they? *American Journal of Sports Medicine, 12*(1):31–38, 1984.

McKillop, G. and D. Ballantyne. Lipoprotein analysis in bodybuilders. *International Journal of Cardiology, 17*:281–286, 1987.

Miller, W. J., W. M. Sherman, and J. L. Ivy. Effect of strength training on glucose tolerance and post-glucose insulin response. *Medicine and Science in Sports and Exercise, 16*(6):539–543, 1984.

Overly, W. L., J. A. Dankoff, B. K. Wang, and U. D. Singh. Androgens and hepatocellular carcinoma in an athlete. *Annals of Internal Medicine, 100*(1):158–159, 1984.

Scott, M. J., and M. J. Scott, Jr. HIV infection associated with injections of anabolic steroids. *Journal of the American Medical Association, 262*(2):207–208, 1989.

Seals, D. R., B. F. Hurley, J. M. Hagberg, J. Schultz, B. J. Linder, L. Natter, and A. A. Ehsani. Effects of training on systolic time intervals at rest and during isometric exercise in men and women 61 to 64 years old. *American Journal of Cardiology, 55*:797–800, 1985.

Wadler, G. I., and B. Hainline. *Drugs and the Athlete.* (Philadelphia: Davis, 1989), pp. 55–69.

Webb, O. L., P. M. Laskarzewski, C. J. Glueck. Severe depression of high-density lipoprotein cholesterol levels in weight lifters and body builders by self-administered exogenous testosterone and anabolic-androgenic steroids. *Metabolism,* 33(11):971–975, 1984.

Windsor, R. E., and D. Dumitru. Anabolic steroid use by athletes. *Postgraduate Medicine, 84*(4):37–48, 1988.

Windsor, R. E., and D. Dumitru. Prevalence of anabolic steroid use by male and female adolescents. *Medicine and Science in Sports and Exercise, 21*(5):494–497, 1989.

CHAPTER 3

Evans, G. W. The role of picolinic acid in mineral metabolism. *Life Chemistry Reports, 1*:57–67, 1982.

Evans, G. W., E. E. Roginski, and W. Mertz. Interaction of the glucose tolerance factor (GTF) with insulin. *Biochemical and Biophysical Research Communications, 50*:718–722, 1973.

Gilman, M. B., G. Otte, and G. W. Evans. The effect of chromium picolinate on lean body mass and body fat in exercising males. *Medicine and Science in Sports and Exercise,* in press.

Hasten, D. L., E. P. Rome, B. D. Franks, and M. Hegsted. Effects of chromium picolinate on beginning weight training students. *International Journal of Sports Nutrition, 2*:343–350, 1992.

Kaats, G. R., J. A. Fisher, and K. Blum. The effects of chromium picolinate supplementation on body composition in different age groups. *Age, 14*:138, 1991.

Krieger, I., R. Cash, and G. W. Evans. Picolinic acid in acrodermatitis enteropathica: Evidence for a disorder of tryptophan metabolism. *Journal of Pediatric Gastroenterology and Nutrition, 3*:62–68, 1984.

Lindemann, M. D., C. M. Wood, A. F. Harper, and E. T. Kornegay. Chromium picolinate additions to diets of growing-finishing pigs. *Journal of Animal Science, 71(Supplement 1)*:14, 1993.

Page, T. G., L. L. Southern, T. L. Ward, and D. L. Thompson, Jr. Effect of chromium picolinate on growth and serum carcass traits of growing finishing pigs. *Journal of Animal Science, 71*:656–662, 1993.

CHAPTER 4

Abraham, A. S., M. Sonnenblick, M. Eini, O. Shemesh, and A. P. Batt. The effect of chromium on established atherosclerotic plaques in rabbits. *American Journal of Clinical Nutrition, 33*:2294–2298, 1980.

Anderson, R. A. Chromium metabolism and its role in disease process in man. *Clinical Physiology and Biochemistry, 4*:31–41, 1986.

Anderson, R. A. Nutritional role of chromium. *The Science of the Total Environment, 17*:13–29, 1981.

Anderson, R. A., M. M. Polansky, N. A. Bryden, S. J. Bhathena, and J. J. Canary. Effects of supplemental chromium on patients with symptoms of reactive hypoglycemia. *Metabolism, 36(4)*:351–355, 1987.

Brown, R. O., S. Forloines-Lynn, R. E. Cross, and W. D. Heizer. Chromium deficiency after long-term total parenteral nutrition. *Digestive Diseases Science, 31*:661–664, 1986.

Committee on Dietary Allowances, Food and Nutrition Board, National Research Council Recommended Dietary Allowances, 9th ed., National Academy of Sciences, Washington, D.C., 1980.

Committee on Dietary Allowances, Food and Nutrition Board, National Research Council Recommended Dietary Allowances, 10th ed., National Academy of Sciences, Washington, D.C., 1990.

Evans, G. W. The effect of chromium picolinate on insulin controlled parameters in humans. *International Journal of Biosocial Research;* 1(2), 1990.

Felig P. Amino acid metabolism in man. *Annual Review of Biochemistry,* 44:933–955, 1975.

Freund, H., S. Atamian, and J. E. Fischer. Chromium deficiency during total parenteral nutrition. *Journal of the American Medical Association, 241:*496–498, 1979.

Hambidge, K. M. Chromium nutrition in man. *American Journal of Clinical Nutrition, 27:*505–514, 1974.

Hollenbeck, C., and G. M. Reaven. Variations in insulin-stimulated glucose uptake in healthy individuals with normal glucose tolerance. *Journal of Clinical Endocrinology and Metabolism, 64:*1169–1173, 1987.

Ishiguro, T., Y. Sato, Y. Oshida, K. Yamanouchi, M. Okuyama, and N. Sakamoto. The relationship between insulin sensitivity and weight reduction in simple obese and obese diabetic patients. *Nagoya Journal of Medical Science, 49:*61–69, 1987.

Jeejeebhoy, K. N., R. C. Chu, E. B. Marliss, R. Greenberg, and A. S. Bruce-Robertson. Chromium deficiency, glucose intolerance and neuropathy reversed by chromium supplementation in a patient receiving long-term total parenteral nutrition. *American Journal of Clinical Nutrition, 30:*531–538, 1977.

Jenkins, D. J. A., T. M. S. Wolever, V. Vuksan, and others. Nibbling versus gorging: metabolic advantages of increased meal frequency. *New England Journal of Medicine, 321:*929–934, 1989.

Joven, J., E. Vilella, B. Costa, P. R. Turner, C. Richart, and L. Masana. Concentrations of lipids and apolipoproteins in patients with clinically well-controlled insulin-dependent and non-insulin dependent diabetes. *Clinical Chemistry, 35*(5):813–816, 1989.

Kaplan, N. M. The deadly quartet: upper body obesity, glucose intolerance, hypertriglyceridemia and hypertension. *Archives of Internal Medicine, 149:*1514–1520, 1989.

Laws, A., M. L. Stefanick, and G. M. Reaven. Insulin resistance and hypertriglyceridemia in nondiabetic relatives of patients with non-insulin dependent diabetes mellitus. *Journal of Clinical Endocrinology and Metabolism, 69:*343–347, 1989.

Lee, N. A. and C. A. Reasner. Beneficial effect of chromium supplementation on serum triglyceride levels in NIDDM. *Diabetes Care, 17(12):*1449–1452, 1994.

Lillioja, S., D. M. Mott, B. V. Howard, and others. Impaired glucose tolerance as a disorder of insulin action—longitudinal and cross-sectional studies in Pima Indians. *New England Journal of Medicine, 318:*1217–1225, 1988.

Mertz, W. Chromium occurrence and function in biological systems. *Physiological Reviews, 49:*163–239, 1969.

Mertz, W. Trace minerals and atherosclerosis. *Federation Proceedings, 41:*2807–2812, 1982.

Mertz, W., and E. E. Roginsky. Biological activity and fate of chromium (III) in the rat. *American Journal of Physiology, 209:*489–494, 1965.

Moden, M., H. Halkin, S. Almog, A. Lusky, A. Eshkol, M. Shefi, A. Shitrit, and Z. Fuchs. Hyperinsulinemia: A link between hypertension, obesity and glucose intolerance. *Journal of Clinical Investigation, 75:*809–817, 1985.

Newman, H. A. I., R. F. Leighton, R. R. Lanese, and N. A. Freedland. Serum chromium and angiographically determined coronary artery disease. *Clinical Chemistry, 24:*541–544, 1978.

Offenbacher, E. G., and F. X. Pi-Sunyer. Beneficial effect of chromium-rich yeast on glucose tolerance and blood lipids in elderly subjects. *Diabetes, 29:*919–925, 1980.

Offenbacher, E. G., and F. X. Pi-Sunyer. Chromium in human nutrition. *Annual Review of Nutrition, 8:*543–563, 1988.

Potter, J. F., P. Levin, R. A. Anderson, J. M. Freiberg, R. Andres, and D. Elahi. Glucose metabolism in glucose-intolerant older people during chromium supplementation. *Metabolism, 34*(5):199–214, 1985.

Press, R. I., J. Geller, and G. W. Evans. The effect of chromium picolinate on serum cholesterol and apolipoprotein fractions in human subjects. *Western Journal of Medicine, 152*(1)41–45, 1990.428

Press, R. I., J. Geller, and G. W. Evans. The effect of chromium picolinate on serum glucose, glycosylated hemoglobin and cholesterol of adult onset diabetics. *Metabolism,* in press.

Rabinowitz, M. B., S. R. Levin, and H. C. Gonick. Comparisons of chromium status in diabetic and normal men. *Metabolism, 29*(4):355–364, 1980.

Reaven, G. M. Role of insulin resistance in human disease (Banting Lecture 1988). *Diabetes, 37:*1595–1607, 1988.

Riales, R. R., and M. J. Albrink. Effect of chromium chloride supplementation on glucose tolerance and serum lipids including high-density lipoprotein of adult men. *American Journal of Clinical Nutrition, 34:*2670–2678, 1981.

Schroeder, H. A. The role of chromium in mammalian nutrition. *American Journal of Clinical Nutrition, 21*(3):230–244, 1968.

Schroeder, H. A., A. P. Nason, and I. H. Tipton. Chromium deficiency as a factor in atherosclerosis. *Journal of Chronic Diseases, 23:*123–142, 1969.

Schwartz, K., and W. Mertz. Chromium (III) and the glucose tolerance factor. *Archives of Biochemistry and Biophysics, 85:*292–295, 1959.

Schwartz, K., and W. Mertz. A glucose tolerance factor and its differentiation from factor 3. *Archives of Biochemistry and Biophysics, 72:*515–518, 1957.

Simonoff, M., Y. Llabador, C. Hamon, A. M. Peers, and G. N. Simonoff. Low plasma chromium in patients with coronary artery and heart diseases. *Biological Trace Element Research, 6:*431–439, 1984.

Stout, R. W. Overview of the association between insulin

and atherosclerosis. *Metabolism, 34*(12), suppl. 1:7–12, 1985.

Toepfer, E. W., W. Mertz, M. M. Polansky, E. E. Roginski, and W. R. Wolf. Preparation of chromium-containing material of glucose tolerance factor activity from Brewer's yeast extracts and by synthesis. *Journal of Agricultural Food Chemistry, 25*(1):182–186, 1977.

Zavaroni, I., E. Bonora, M. Pagliara, and others. Risk factors for coronary artery disease in healthy persons with hyperinsulinemia and normal glucose tolerance. *New England Journal of Medicine, 320:*702–706, 1989.

Wing, R. R., C. H. Bunker, L. H. Kuller, and K. A. Matthews. Insulin, body mass index, and cardiovascular risk factors in premenopausal women. *Arteriosclerosis, 9:*479–484, 1989.

CHAPTER 5

Albrecht, M., J. Bianocozy, and G. Tamias. Dental and oral symptoms of diabetes mellitus. *Community Dental and Oral Epidemiology, 16*(6):378–380, 1988.

De Montis, M. G., M. C. Olianas, B. Haber, and A. Tagliamonte. Increase in large neutral amino acid transport into brain by insulin. *Journal of Neurochemistry, 30:*121–124, 1978.

Evans, G.W. and L.K. Meyer. Life span is increased in rats supplemented with a chromium-pyridine 2 carbohydrate complex. *Advances in Scientific Research, 1:*19–23, 1994.

Evans, G.W., G. Swenson, and K. Walters. Chromium picolinate decreases calcium excretion and increases dehydroepiandrosterone acetate (DHEA) in postmenopausal women. Abstract presented at Annual Meeting of Federation of American Societies for Experimental Biology, 1995.

Lane, B. C. Calcium, chromium, protein, sugar and accommodation in myopia. *Documenta Ophthalmologica Proceedings Series, 28:*141–148, 1981.

Lane, B. C. Elevation of intraocular pressure with daily sustained closework stimulus to accommodation, lowered tissue chromium and dietary deficiency of ascorbic acid (vitamin C). *Documenta Ophthalmologica Proceedings Series, 28:*149–155, 1981.

McCarty, M. High-chromium yeast for acne? *Medical Hypotheses, 14:*307–310, 1984.

CHAPTER 6

Anderson, R. A., and N. Bryden. Concentration, insulin potentiation and absorption of chromium in beer. *Journal of Agricultural Food Chemistry, 31:*308–311, 1983.

Anderson, R. A., N. A. Bryden, M. M. Polansky, and P. A. Deuster. Exercise effects on chromium excretion of trained and untrained men consuming a constant diet. *Journal of Applied Physiology, 64*(1):249–252, 1988.

Anderson, R. A., and A. S. Kozlovsky. Chromium intake, absorption and excretion of subjects consuming self-selected diets. *American Journal of Clinical Nutrition, 41:*-1177–1183, 1985.

Anderson, R. A., M. M. Polansky, and N. A. Bryden. Acute effects on chromium, copper, zinc and selected clinical variables in urine and serum of male runners. *Biological Trace Element Research, 6:*327–336, 1984.

Anderson, R. A., M. M. Polansky, N. A. Bryden, and H. N. Guttman. Strenuous exercise may increase dietary needs for chromium and zinc. In F. I. Katch, ed., *The 1984 Olympic Scientific Congress Proceedings: Sport, Health and Nutrition, 2:*83–88, 1986.

Anderson, R. A., M. M. Polansky, N. A. Bryden, E. E. Roginski, K. Y. Patterson, and others. Effect of exercise (running) on serum glucose, insulin, glucagon and chromium excretion. *Diabetes, 31:*212–216, 1982.

Borel, J. S., T. C. Majerus, M. M. Polansky, P. B. Moser, and

R. A. Anderson. Chromium intake and urinary chromium excretion of trauma patients. *Biological Trace Element Research, 6:*317–326, 1984.

Bunker, V. W., M. S. Lawson, H. T. Delves, and B. E. Clayton. The uptake and excretion of chromium by the elderly. *American Journal of Clinical Nutrition, 39:*797–802, 1984.

Campbell, W. W., M. M. Polansky, N. A. Bryden, J. H. Soares, Jr., and R. A. Anderson. Exercise training and dietary chromium effects on glycogen, glycogen synthetase, phosphorylase and total protein in rats. *Journal of Nutrition, 119:*653–660, 1989.

Kozlovsky, A. S., P. B. Moser, S. Reiser, and R. A. Anderson. Effects of diets high in simple sugars on urinary chromium losses. *Metabolism, 35*(6):515–518, 1986.

Kumpulainen, J. T., W. R. Wolf, C. Veillon, and W. Mertz. Determination of chromium in selected United States diets. *Journal of Agricultural Food Chemistry, 27*(3):490–493, 1979.

Martinez, O. B., A. C. MacDonald, R. S. Gibson, and D. Bourn. Dietary chromium and effect of chromium supplementation on glucose tolerance of elderly Canadian women. *Nutrition Research, 5:*609–620, 1985.

Pekarek, R. S., E. C. Hauer, E. J. Rayfield, R. W. Wannemacher, and W. R. Beisel. Relationship between serum chromium concentration and glucose utilization in normal and infected subjects. *Diabetes, 24:*350–353, 1975.

Tipton, I. H., H. A. Schroeder, H. M. Perry, Jr., and M. J. Cook. Trace elements in human tissue. III. Subjects from Africa, the Near and Far East and Europe. *Health and Physiology, 11:*403–451, 1965.

CHAPTER 7

Bounous, G., P. A. L. Kongshavn, and P. Gold. The immunoenhancing property of dietary whey protein concentrate. *Clinical and Investigative Medicine, 11*(4): 271–278, 1988.

Bounous, G., R. Papenburg, P. A. L. Kongshavn, P. Gold, and D. Fleiszer. Dietary whey protein inhibits the development of dimethylhydrazine induced malignancy. *Clinical and Investigative Medicine, 11*(3):213–217, 1988.

Friedman, J. E., and P. W. R. Lemon. Effect of chronic endurance exercise on retention of dietary protein. *International Journal of Sports Medicine, 10*(2):118–223, 1989.

Lemon, P. W. R. Influence of dietary protein and total energy intake on strength development. *Sports Nutrition,* 2(14):1–5, 1989.

Lemon, P. W. R. Protein and exercise: Update 1987. *Medicine and Science in Sports and Exercise, 19* (5-supplement): s179–s190, 1987.

Lemon, P. W. R., K. E. Yarasheski, and D. G. Dolny. The importance of protein for athletes. *Sports Medicine, 1:*474–484, 1984.

Owen, O. E. Resting metabolic requirements of men and women. *Mayo Clinic Proceedings, 63:*503–510, 1988.

INDEX